CARING FOR THE OLDER ADULT WITH CANCER IN THE AMBULATORY SETTING

EDITORS

Lorraine K. McEvoy, DNP, MSN, RN, OCN®
Diane G. Cope, PhD, ARNP-BC, AOCNP®

Oncology Nursing Society
Pittsburgh, Pennsylvania

ONS Publications Department

Executive Director, Professional Practice and Programs:
Elizabeth M. Wertz Evans, RN, MPM, CPHQ, CPHIMS, FACMPE
Publisher and Director of Publications: Barbara Sigler, RN, MNEd
Managing Editor: Lisa M. George, BA
Technical Content Editor: Angela D. Klimaszewski, RN, MSN
Staff Editor II: Amy Nicoletti, BA
Copy Editor: Laura Pinchot, BA
Graphic Designer: Dany Sjoen

Library of Congress Cataloging-in-Publication Data

Caring for the older adult with cancer in the ambulatory setting / edited by Lorraine K. McEvoy and Diane G. Cope.
    p. ; cm.
Includes bibliographical references and index.
ISBN 978-1-935864-14-1 (alk. paper)
I. McEvoy, Lorraine K. II. Cope, Diane G. III. Oncology Nursing Society.
[DNLM: 1. Neoplasms–nursing. 2. Aged, 80 and over. 3. Aged. 4. Ambulatory Care. 5. Geriatric Assessment. WY 156]

616.99'40231–dc23

2011034903

Publisher's Note

This book is published by the Oncology Nursing Society (ONS). ONS neither represents nor guarantees that the practices described herein will, if followed, ensure safe and effective patient care. The recommendations contained in this book reflect ONS's judgment regarding the state of general knowledge and practice in the field as of the date of publication. The recommendations may not be appropriate for use in all circumstances. Those who use this book should make their own determinations regarding specific safe and appropriate patient-care practices, taking into account the personnel, equipment, and practices available at the hospital or other facility at which they are located. The editors and publisher cannot be held responsible for any liability incurred as a consequence from the use or application of any of the contents of this book. Figures and tables are used as examples only. They are not meant to be all-inclusive, nor do they represent endorsement of any particular institution by ONS. Mention of specific products and opinions related to those products do not indicate or imply endorsement by ONS. Web sites mentioned are provided for information only; the hosts are responsible for their own content and availability. Unless otherwise indicated, dollar amounts reflect U.S. dollars.

ONS publications are originally published in English. Publishers wishing to translate ONS publications must contact ONS about licensing arrangements. ONS publications cannot be translated without obtaining written permission from ONS. (Individual tables and figures that are reprinted or adapted require additional permission from the original source.) Because translations from English may not always be accurate or precise, ONS disclaims any responsibility for inaccuracies in words or meaning that may occur as a result of the translation. Readers relying on precise information should check the original English version.

Printed in the United States of America

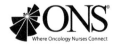

Oncology Nursing Society
Integrity • Innovation • Stewardship • Advocacy • Excellence • Inclusiveness

Contributors

EDITORS

Lorraine K. McEvoy, DNP, MSN, RN, OCN®
Nurse Leader, Ambulatory Services
Memorial Sloan-Kettering Cancer Center
New York, New York
Chapter 2. Physiology of Aging and Its Impact on the Older Adult; Chapter 4. Symptom Management

Diane G. Cope, PhD, ARNP-BC, AOCNP®
Oncology Nurse Practitioner
Florida Cancer Specialists
Fort Myers, Florida
Chapter 1. Cancer and the Aging Population

AUTHORS

Stewart M. Bond, PhD, RN, AOCN®
Research Assistant Professor
Vanderbilt University School of Nursing
Nashville, Tennessee
Chapter 2. Physiology of Aging and Its Impact on the Older Adult

Kimberly A. Christopher, PhD, RN, OCN®
Associate Professor and Chair
Department of Nursing
College of Health Professions
Towson University
Towson, Maryland
Chapter 6. Survivorship Issues

Nessa Coyle, PhD, ANP, ACHPN, FAAN
Nurse Practitioner, Pain and Palliative Care Service
Memorial Sloan-Kettering Cancer Center
New York, New York
Chapter 5. Hospice and Palliative Care

Mary Elizabeth Davis, RN, MSN, AOCNS®
Clinical Nurse Specialist, Ambulatory Care Services
Memorial Sloan-Kettering Cancer Center
New York, New York
Chapter 2. Physiology of Aging and Its Impact on the Older Adult; Chapter 4. Symptom Management

Dana Marcone DeDonato, MSW, LSW
Geriatric Oncology Social Work Specialist
Joan Karnell Cancer Center at Pennsylvania Hospital
Penn Medicine
Philadelphia, Pennsylvania
Chapter 7. Psychosocial Issues

Susan A. Derby, RN, MA, GNP-BC, ACHPN
Nurse Practitioner, Pain and Palliative Care Service
Memorial Sloan-Kettering Cancer Center
New York, New York
Chapter 4. Symptom Management

Sarah H. Kagan, PhD, RN
Lucy Walker Honorary Term Professor of
  Gerontological Nursing
Clinical Nurse Specialist
Abramson Cancer Center
University of Pennsylvania
Philadelphia, Pennsylvania
Chapter 8. Considering the Future of Nursing

Mary Pat Lynch, MSN, CRNP, AOCN®
Nurse Practitioner and Cancer Center
  Administrator
Joan Karnell Cancer Center at Pennsylvania
  Hospital
Penn Medicine
Philadelphia, Pennsylvania
Chapter 7. Psychosocial Issues

Janine A. Overcash, PhD, GNP-BC
Director of Nursing Research
James Cancer Hospital and Solove Research
  Institute
The Ohio State University
Columbus, Ohio
Chapter 3. Comprehensive Geriatric Assessment

Kathy Plakovic, FNP, ACHPN, AOCNP®
Nurse Practitioner, Pain and Palliative Care
  Service
Memorial Sloan-Kettering Cancer Center
New York, New York
Chapter 5. Hospice and Palliative Care

DISCLOSURE

Editors and authors of books and guidelines provided by the Oncology Nursing Society are expected to disclose to the readers any significant financial interest or other relationships with the manufacturer(s) of any commercial products.

A vested interest may be considered to exist if a contributor is affiliated with or has a financial interest in commercial organizations that may have a direct or indirect interest in the subject matter. A "financial interest" may include, but is not limited to, being a shareholder in the organization; being an employee of the commercial organization; serving on an organization's speakers bureau; or receiving research from the organization. An "affiliation" may be holding a position on an advisory board or some other role of benefit to the commercial organization. Vested interest statements appear in the front matter for each publication.

Contributors are expected to disclose any unlabeled or investigational use of products discussed in their content. This information is acknowledged solely for the information of the readers.

The contributors provided the following disclosure and vested interest information:

Nessa Coyle, PhD, ANP, ACHPN, FAAN: Visiting Nurse Service of New York Hospice and Palliative Care, board member

Mary Elizabeth Davis, RN, MSN, AOCNS®: Genentech, consultant

Contents

Preface... vii

Acknowledgments.. ix

Chapter 1. Cancer and the Aging Population..1
    Introduction...1
    Aging Population 1
    Cancer and Aging..2
    Ambulatory Oncology Care 4
    Role of the Ambulatory Care Oncology Nurse 4
    Conclusion...6
    References 6

Chapter 2. Physiology of Aging and Its Impact on the Older Adult................9
    Introduction...9
    Theories of Aging... 10
    Chronologic Age Versus Physiologic Age... 10
    Normal Aging.. 12
    Altered Response to Physiologic Stress... 13
    Physiologic Changes of Aging 14
    Pharmacokinetics 28
    Cytochrome P450 30
    Conclusion.. 30
    References 31

Chapter 3. Comprehensive Geriatric Assessment...................................... 37
    Introduction.. 37
    Definition and Development of a Comprehensive Geriatric Assessment 38
    Rapid Assessment Instruments to Include in a Comprehensive Geriatric
        Assessment 47
    Case Study Application of the Comprehensive Geriatric Assessment..................... 48
    Conclusion.. 50
    References 51

Chapter 4. Symptom Management 57
    Introduction.. 57
    Anorexia and Weight Loss 58
    Cognitive Impairment... 62
    Constipation 76

Dehydration 85
Dysphagia 89
Dyspnea 93
Fatigue 96
Pain 100
Sexuality 107
Conclusion 111
References 111

Chapter 5. Hospice and Palliative Care 125
Introduction 125
What Are Palliative Care and Hospice Care, and How Do They Differ? 126
Why Do Patients Need Access to Both Palliative and Hospice Care? 128
Transitions in Goals of Care and Communication 130
Ethical Issues 132
Symptom Assessment and Management 133
Examples of Palliative Care Symptom Management Procedures 133
Conclusion 138
References 138

Chapter 6. Survivorship Issues 143
Introduction 143
Demographics of the Older Adult Population 143
Transitioning to Survivorship Care 145
The Survivorship Care Plan: Facilitating Quality Care 146
Monitoring for Long-Term and Late Effects of Cancer and Cancer Therapy 147
Holistic Assessment: Integrating What We Know to Ensure Quality Care 150
Conclusion 153
References 153

Chapter 7. Psychosocial Issues 157
Introduction 157
Psychosocial Care 157
Psychosocial Assessment 158
Advance Care Planning 169
Conclusion 174
References 174

Chapter 8. Considering the Future of Nursing 177
Introduction 177
Ambulatory Oncology Care 178
Future Influences on Ambulatory Oncology Nursing Practice 178
Healthcare Reform and Effectiveness of Cancer Care 182
Leadership for the Future 183
Conclusion 185
References 185

Resources 191
Gerontology Centers 191
Associations and Societies 191
Statistics and Government Sites 192

Index 195

Preface

Aging will create the music of the coming century.

—Betty Friedan

The inspiration for this book came from the Oncology Nursing Society's (ONS's) forethought and recognition of the projected increase in the aging population and the need for specialization of geriatric oncology nursing in the future. In order to execute this vision, the ONS Gero-Oncology Think Tank Task Force met in December 2008, with the overall goal to create an organization-wide dedication to the special needs of older adults with cancer. Some of the task force's recommendations to support gero-oncology within ONS are as follows. The majority of these recommendations have been executed.

- Develop train-the-trainer gero-oncology regional workshops
- Develop a geriatric online course
- Ensure geriatric oncology content at future ONS conferences, including the ONS Advance Oncology Nursing Conference and ONS Annual Congress
- Dedicate the December 2009 *ONS Connect* issue to geriatrics
- Increase overall geriatric content on the ONS Web site
- Adapt oncology care competencies and the *Statement on the Scope and Standards of Oncology Practice* and the *Statement on the Scope and Standards of Advanced Practice Nursing in Oncology Nursing* to include geriatric-oncology perspectives
- Review ONS position statements for inclusion of gero-oncology perspectives
- Ensure that geriatric perspectives are included in existing and future educational materials and ONS Putting Evidence Into Practice resources
- Encourage geriatric-focused articles in the *Clinical Journal of Oncology Nursing* and *Oncology Nursing Forum*
- Support the development of an ONS Excellence in the Care of the Older Adult with Cancer Award in 2009.

Based on the work and recommendations of the Gero-Oncology Think Tank, the ONS Steering Committee continued discussions in an effort to identify additional areas for geriatric content and continue the development of ONS as a leader in geriatric oncology. From the work of both the Gero-Oncology Think Tank and the ONS Steering Committee, the development of evidence-based guidelines for ambulatory geriatric-oncology nursing was proposed.

This book opens with an introduction of the projected increase in our aging population and cancer incidence in the older adult over the next two decades, and the increasing trends of healthcare delivery and oncology care in the ambulatory setting. Subsequent chapters provide detailed geriatric content, including physiology of aging, assessment, management of common symptoms related to oncologic therapy, hospice and palliative care, survivorship issues, and psychosocial issues. The book concludes with a chapter focused on the future of oncology nursing as it relates to the care of the older adult with cancer.

In the future, oncology nurses will not only need to specialize in the field of oncology, but will also need to specialize in the field of gerontology. This book is envisioned as a textbook presenting geriatric content, a resource for the ambulatory oncology nurse to meet the special needs of the older adult with cancer, and an additional source of geriatric oncology educational material that supports the ONS's mission to bring the care of older adults to the forefront of oncology nursing practice. Oncology nurses are in the key position to become leaders in the novel field of gerontology/oncology, surrounded by the music of the future.

Diane G. Cope, PhD, ARNP-BC, AOCNP®

Acknowledgments

Today the experience of illness is not contained within hospital walls. Many people find that ambulatory care centers and their own homes have replaced the hospital setting at numerous points in their trajectory of illness. This is especially true when the illness is cancer. This book is the first large-scale effort to articulate clinical nursing practice and care management of older adults with cancer in the ambulatory setting. The project was truly a community effort. I am especially grateful to all of the authors who contributed their expertise to this work. I also wish to thank the friends and colleagues who reviewed drafts of the manuscript. They provided valuable ideas to improve the book.

Finally, I wish to thank my family, who were understanding and supportive and demonstrated great patience during this process. I hope that in some small way this endeavor will serve as an inspiration for them to pursue their creative interests.

Lorraine McEvoy, DNP, MSN, RN, OCN®

I would like to express my sincere gratitude to Barbara Sigler, Publisher and Director of Publications, for her vision of this textbook and for her ongoing support throughout the book process; to Judy Holmes, Laura Pinchot, and Lisa George with the ONS Publications Department for their expertise and assistance with this publication; to all of the expert authors who have made this book a reality; and to all my older adult patients with cancer who have shared and taught me about their life experience and the meaning of cancer and treatment at an advanced age. Finally, I would like to thank my husband, Steve, and son, Adam, for their constant love and support of all my oncology nursing endeavors.

Diane G. Cope, PhD, ARNP-BC, AOCNP®

CHAPTER 1

Cancer and the Aging Population

Diane G. Cope, PhD, ARNP-BC, AOCNP®

Introduction

The older adult population in the United States is expected to significantly increase over the next four decades. By 2050, the number of Americans age 65 years and older will comprise approximately 20% of the total population and is projected to reach 88.5 million, more than double the 40.2 million in 2010 (Vincent & Velkoff, 2010). Older adults are described as young-old (age 65–74), middle-old (age 75–84), and oldest-old (older than 85) and have a greater cancer incidence rate than younger people. The median age at diagnosis for cancer of all sites from 2003 to 2007 was 66 years of age with 46% of all cancers diagnosed in those younger than age 64 and 54% diagnosed in the 65-and-older age group (Altekruse et al., 2010). With the dramatic increase in the aging population and the increased incidence of cancer in older adults, healthcare providers need to be aware of the unique challenges in caring for the older adult with cancer. This chapter will discuss the aging population projections, cancer statistics, and trends in the older adult population, and the implications for oncology healthcare providers.

Aging Population

By 2030, the population of adults age 65 years and older is projected to increase by 40% and more than double by 2050 (Federal Interagency Forum on Aging-Related Statistics, 2011) (see Figure 1-1). The accelerated growth of older adults is due in part to the baby boomer generation born between 1946 and 1964, which totals approximately 75 million individuals (Vincent & Velkoff, 2010). Beginning January 1, 2011, approximately 8,000 baby boom-

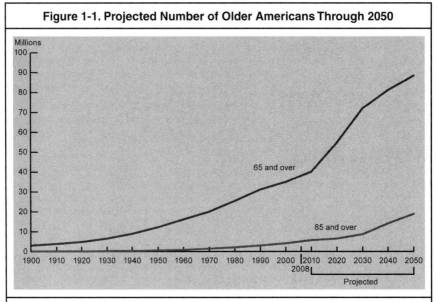

Figure 1-1. Projected Number of Older Americans Through 2050

Note. From *Older Americans 2010: Key Indicators of Well-Being* (p. 2), by the Federal Interagency Forum on Aging-Related Statistics, 2011. Retrieved from http://www.agingstats.gov/agingstatsdotnet/Main_Site/Data/2010_Documents/Docs/OA_2010.pdf.

ers will turn 65 each day for the next 18 years. Other factors contributing to the dramatic increase in the number of older adults are reduced death rates from chronic disease, improved public health measures, and increased life expectancy. The fastest growing segment of the population is the oldest old group of individuals (age 85 and older). Between 2008 and 2050, the 85-and-older population is expected to more than triple from 5.4 million to 19 million (Vincent & Velkoff, 2010).

Cancer and Aging

Incidence Rates

Cancer is a disease of the aging. In the United States, more than 65% of current cancer diagnoses occur among older adults, representing a 10-fold increased incidence rate for those older than 65 compared to incidence rates for individuals younger than 65 (Edwards et al., 2002; Institute of Medicine, 2008; Naeim & Keeler, 2005; Yancik, 2005).

Some major primary cancers that are common to men and women occur more frequently in individuals older than 65. These include cancers of the lung and bronchus, colon, rectum, stomach, urinary bladder, and pancreas

(Yancik, Ganz, Varricchio, & Conley, 2001). Approximately 75% of prostate cancer incidence in men and approximately 47% of breast cancer in women occur in patients older than 65 years of age (Smith, Smith, Hurria, Hortobagyi, & Buchholz, 2009).

Cancer incidence projections for 2000–2050 show a significant increase in the older adult age groups as a result of the aging baby boomers (see Figure 1-2). By 2010, when the baby boomers moved into the 45–64 age category, cancer incidence for males and females increased from 32% in 2000 to 37% (Hayat, Howlader, Reichman, & Edwards, 2007). This increase is evident for all of the top cancer sites. By 2030, baby boomers will reach the 65–84-year-old group, which represents the high-risk age group for cancer. From 2010 to 2030, the total projected cancer incidence will increase by approximately 45%, from 1.6 million to 2.3 million with the percentage of all cancers diagnosed in older adults increasing from 61% to 70% (Smith et al., 2009). A 67% increase in cancer incidence is expected in older adults age 65 or older, compared with an 11% increase for adults younger than 65 years of age

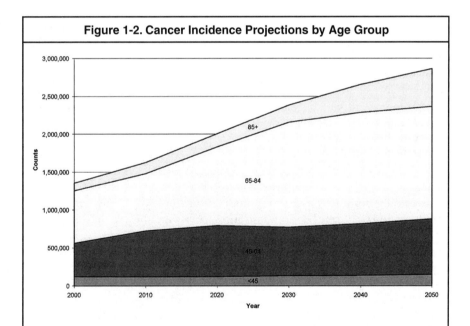

Figure 1-2. Cancer Incidence Projections by Age Group

Projected number of cancer cases for 2000–2050 by age group (< 45, 45–64, 65–84, 85+) based on projected census population estimates and delay-adjusted SEER-17 cancer incidence rates. Projections based on approximate single-year delay-adjusted SEER-17 incidence rates for 1998–2002 and population projections from the U.S. Census Bureau.

Note. From "Cancer Statistics, Trends, and Multiple Primary Cancer Analyses From the Surveillance, Epidemiology, and End Results (SEER) Program," by M.J. Hayat, N. Howlader, M.E. Reichman, and B.K. Edwards, 2007, *The Oncologist, 12*, p. 34. Copyright 2007 by AlphaMed Press, Inc. Reprinted with permission.

(Smith et al., 2009). The number of new patients with cancer is expected to more than double from 1.36 million in 2000 to almost 3 million in 2050 (Hayat et al., 2007). Certain primary cancers are expected to increase in incidence over the next 20 years. These include liver, stomach, pancreas, and lung (Smith et al., 2009).

Mortality Rates

Although cancer death rates overall have declined since 1990, cancer still accounts for more deaths than heart disease in people younger than 85, representing approximately 25% of total deaths in the United States (Siegel, Ward, Brawley, & Jemal, 2011). Approximately 50% of all cancer deaths are from lung, prostate, and colorectal cancer in men and lung, breast, and colorectal cancer in women (Siegel et al., 2011).

Ambulatory Oncology Care

The aging population and the projected increase in cancer incidence over the next 40 years will have a significant impact on healthcare systems, healthcare professionals, and the healthcare workforce. Recent trends in the provision of care suggest a significant shift from hospital-based care to a greater use of office-based services, specifically medical or surgical specialty care. The National Ambulatory Medical Care Survey and the U.S. Census Bureau reported that the percentage of physician office-based visits made by patients age 45 and older increased from 49% in 1998 to 57% in 2008 (Cherry, Lucas, & Decker, 2010). For patients age 65 and older, the percentage of visits to physicians with a medical or surgical specialty increased from 37% to 55% (Cherry et al., 2010) (see Figure 1-3).

Increasing multidrug cancer regimens and complexity in cancer therapies and increased treatment options and supportive therapies, as well as multidisciplinary involvement in the care of the older adult with cancer, have resulted in more physician and infusion room visits (Shulman et al., 2009). Data from 2001 to 2007 at an academic cancer center in New England found that the average number of physician visits per patient per year increased 25% for the first year of treatment (Shulman et al., 2009). Furthermore, during the first year of treatment, the number of infusion visits for a given patient increased by 111% (Shulman et al., 2009).

Role of the Ambulatory Care Oncology Nurse

Older adults with cancer presenting with comorbidities and normal aging decline will necessitate individualized, specialized nursing care in managing cancer and treatment side effects. Most oncologic care will take place in the

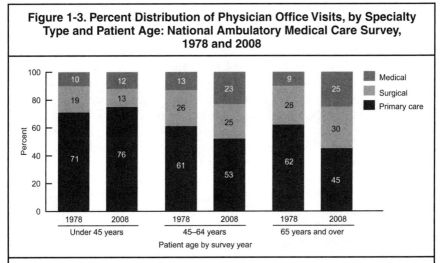

Figure 1-3. Percent Distribution of Physician Office Visits, by Specialty Type and Patient Age: National Ambulatory Medical Care Survey, 1978 and 2008

Note. From "Population Aging and the Use of Office-Based Physician Services," by D. Cherry, C. Lucas, and S.L. Decker, 2010, *NCHS Data Brief, 41.* Retrieved from http://www.cdc.gov/nchs/data/databriefs/db41.htm.

ambulatory setting, requiring a healthcare team that is able to anticipate and manage increased complexity of care. The older adult will require thorough, ongoing assessment, age-specific education regarding cancer and treatment, and prompt side effect management. Ambulatory care oncology nurses are in a key position to coordinate individualized care for the older adult with cancer.

Compounding factors for the older adult with cancer will require expert strategies and nursing interventions to ensure optimum patient outcomes. Factors that can affect treatment planning and care management may include limited income, minimal prescription coverage, lack of secondary insurance, lack of transportation, social isolation, lack of family or caregiver support, decreased sensory acuity, chronic diseases, and physical limitations or disabilities. Even fit older adults with minimal comorbidities will have normal aging decline that can place them at higher risk for complications when undergoing cancer treatment. In preparation for the complex needs of the older adult with cancer, ambulatory care oncology nurses will need educational preparation and resources specific to geriatric oncology. With the aging of the baby boomer generation and the associated projected increases in cancer incidence in the older adult population, awareness is heightened regarding the need for research and training specifically addressing the needs of older adults with cancer (Cohen, 2007; Nevidjon et al., 2010). Through these endeavors and resources such as this book, ambulatory care oncology nurses will be able to broaden their knowledge base and expand their clinical skills to provide optimum treatment and supportive care for this special population.

Conclusion

The U.S. 65-and-older population is expected to dramatically increase over the next four decades. Cancer is a disease of the aging, and therefore, the cancer incidence rate is projected to significantly increase in individuals older than 65 years. The ambulatory care oncology nurse is in a key position to educate patients and caregivers about cancer treatment and to anticipate, identify, and manage symptoms that may occur as a result of the disease, the cancer therapy, or a preexisting condition. Nurses will need to understand how the complexity of age-related physiologic changes, comorbid conditions, and the cancer diagnosis affect individual and family resources and dynamics. They must be able to coordinate the resources of a multidisciplinary team to meet patients' needs and to effectively manage the challenges associated with treatment and care.

References

Altekruse, S.F., Kosary, C.L., Krapcho, M., Neyman, N., Aminou, R., Waldron, W., ... Edwards, B.K. (Eds.). (2010). SEER cancer statistics review, 1975–2007. Retrieved from http://seer.cancer.gov/csr/1975_2007/

Cherry, D., Lucas, C., & Decker, S.L. (2010, August). Population aging and the use of office-based physician services. *NCHS Data Brief, 41*. Retrieved from http://www.cdc.gov/nchs/data/databriefs/db41.pdf

Cohen, H.J. (2007). The cancer aging interface: A research agenda. *Journal of Clinical Oncology, 25*, 1945–1948. doi:10.1200/JCO.2007.10.6807

Edwards, B.K., Howe, H.L., Ries, L.A., Thun, H.M., Rosenberg, R., Yancik, R., ... Feigal, E.G. (2002). Annual report to the nation on the status of cancer, 1973–1999, featuring implications of age and aging on U.S. cancer burden. *Cancer, 94*, 2766–2792. doi:10.1002/cncr.10593

Federal Interagency Forum on Aging-Related Statistics. (2011, January 14). *Older Americans 2010: Key indicators of well-being*. Retrieved from http://www.agingstats.gov/agingstatsdotnet/Main_Site/Data/2010_Documents/Docs/OA_2010.pdf

Hayat, M.J., Howlader, N., Reichman, M.E., & Edwards, B.K. (2007). Cancer statistics, trends, and multiple primary cancer analyses from the Surveillance, Epidemiology, and End Results (SEER) Program. *Oncologist, 12*, 20–37. doi:10.1634/theoncologist.12-1-20

Institute of Medicine. (2008). *Cancer care for the whole patient: Meeting psychosocial health needs*. Washington, DC: Author.

Naeim, A., & Keeler, E.B. (2005). Is adjuvant therapy for older patients with node (+) early breast cancer cost-effective? *Breast Cancer Research and Treatment, 94*, 95–103. doi:10.1007/s10549-004-8267-0

Nevidjon, B., Rieger, P., Murphy, C.M., Rosenzweig, M.Q., McCorkle, M.R., & Baileys, K. (2010). Filling the gap: Development of the oncology nurse practitioner workforce. *Journal of Oncology Practice, 6*, 2–6. doi:10.1200/JOP.091072

Shulman, L.N., Jacobs, L.A., Greenfield, S., Jones, B., McCabe, M.S., Syrjala, K., ... Ganz, P.A. (2009). Cancer care and cancer survivorship care in the United States: Will we be able to care for these patients in the future? *Journal of Oncology Practice, 5*, 119–123. doi:10.1200/JOP.0932001

Siegel, R., Ward, E., Brawley, O., & Jemal, A. (2011). Cancer statistics, 2011. *CA: A Cancer Journal for Clinicians, 61*, 212–236. doi:10.3322/caac.20121

Smith, B.D., Smith, G.L., Hurria, A., Hortobagyi, G.N., & Buchholz, T.A. (2009). Future of cancer incidence in the United States: Burdens upon an aging, changing nation. *Journal of Clinical Oncology, 27,* 2758–2765. doi:10.1200/JCO.2008.20.8983

Vincent, G.K., & Velkoff, V.A. (2010). *The next four decades: The older population in the United States: 2010 to 2050.* Retrieved from http://www.census.gov/prod/2010pubs/p25-1138

Yancik, R. (2005). Population aging and cancer: A cross-national concern. *Cancer Journal, 11,* 437–441. doi:10.1097/00130404-200511000-00002.pdf

Yancik, R., Ganz, P.A., Varricchio, C., & Conley, B. (2001). Perspectives on comorbidity and cancer in older patients: Approaches to expand the knowledge base. *Journal of Clinical Oncology, 19,* 1147–1151. Retrieved from http://jco.ascopubs.org/content/19/4/1147.full.pdf+html

CHAPTER 2

Physiology of Aging and Its Impact on the Older Adult

Stewart M. Bond, PhD, RN, AOCN®, Mary Elizabeth Davis, RN, MSN, AOCNS®, and Lorraine K. McEvoy, DNP, MSN, RN, OCN®

Introduction

Aging is a normal process that is inevitable and irreversible. An individual ages from conception to death. Although aging increases an individual's vulnerability to degenerative diseases, it is not directly responsible for disease and disability. A significant challenge to our understanding of aging and our ability to care for older adults is the unpredictability of the aging process. The process of aging varies both within and among individuals. Multiple lifestyle, genetic, and environmental factors contribute to the rate at which an individual ages. The exponential growth in the number of older adults and an increase in life expectancy make it even more imperative for nurses to understand the normal aging process.

Physical functioning or *functional status* refers to a person's ability to perform tasks necessary for normal living. These tasks are often referred to as activities of daily living. Instrumental activities of daily living include shopping, transportation, using a telephone, doing housework and yard work, taking medications, and handling finances. Physical activities of daily living include bathing, walking, eating, and using the bathroom. Changes associated with normal aging affect and limit physical function. The extent of functional defect is based on multiple factors, including cognitive function, physical disability, and comorbidity (Caserta et al., 2009).

This chapter provides an overview of normal biologic aging, or *senescence.* Common theories of aging will be presented. The relationship between chronologic age and physiologic age will be discussed. A distinction between the normal age-related changes and the onset of disease and disability is emphasized, and the concept of physiologic reserve capacity will be reviewed. The chapter concludes with a presentation of the age-related physiologic changes that occur in each organ system and a discussion of the relationship between normal aging and pharmacokinetics.

Theories of Aging

Aging is an intrinsically complex, multifactorial process. The progression of aging differs for each individual and is shaped by the interaction of genetic, lifestyle, and environmental factors. Ultimately, the interaction of these factors predisposes an individual to either having the increased likelihood of remaining in good health or developing age-related disease and disability (Kirkwood, 2003; Timiras, 2007c). Aging has been viewed as a genetically driven, programmed process to limit population and overcrowding. However, no single gene is responsible for aging (Kirkwood, 2002). Genes only contribute to 25% of individual variability in aging. Thus, 75% of aging is related to other lifestyle and environmental factors (Kirkwood, 2003). Lifestyle factors that affect aging include diet and nutrition, physical activity, tobacco use, and alcohol use. Environmental factors such as decreased social support, crime, and lower socioeconomic status affect aging by inhibiting positive lifestyle choices and increasing stress. These factors contribute to an acceleration of physical and psychological decline: disease, disability, and frailty (Adams & White, 2004; Kirkwood, 2005).

Numerous theories about aging have been proposed. These theories suggest that aging results from multiple detrimental mechanisms occurring at the molecular, cellular, and systemic levels. It is likely that the processes occurring at these different levels interact and overlap. A single theory does not exist that explains all the mechanics and causes underlying the biologic phenomenon of aging (Parker, 2009). Some of the more common theories of aging are presented in Table 2-1.

Chronologic Age Versus Physiologic Age

Aging is a highly individualized, multidimensional process reflected in chronologic as well as physiologic age. *Chronologic age* is simply one's age in years. It has been used to mark transitions from one stage of life to the next. As such, chronologic age has been used to define who is an "older adult." Until recently, 65 years old has been used as the benchmark to define who is an older adult. Unfortunately, this demarcation based solely on chronologic age has resulted in ageist views and false stereotypes. For example, the time from age 65 until death has been viewed "as a period of progressive decline in normal function and of inevitable increase in disease and disability" (Timiras, 2007c, p. 6). In addition, too often, treatment decisions for older adults have been based on chronologic age rather than physiologic age. Chronologic age alone cannot be used to predict comorbidity or the level of functional decline in an individual (Balducci & Beghe, 2000).

Table 2-1. Common Theories of Aging

Theory	Characteristics
Error	Progressive, random accumulation of errors can occur in the process of DNA transcription that eventually leads to aging or death of the cell (Parker, 2009).
Somatic mutation	The integrity of genetic material influences the process and rate of aging. Over a lifetime, molecular damage to DNA causing genetic mutation causes cells to deteriorate and malfunction over time (Carey & Zou, 2007).
Cross link	Advancing age causes proteins to become cross-linked or entwined and then impede metabolic processes. This suggests that as the immune system declines with age, the body's defenses cannot remove cross-linked agents and the accumulation of these agents can be the origin of disease in the elderly (Parker, 2009).
Telomere senescence	Telomeres are segments that protect the end of chromosomes; decline in cellular division is associated with telomere shortening. Telomeres act as an intrinsic counter of cell division, a protective mechanism against uncontrolled cell division, but aging is the price, and stress, particularly oxidative stress, increases telomere loss (Kirkwood, 2005).
Free radical	Environmental pollutants are believed to promote free radical activity. Free radicals are unpaired ions that are highly reactive. These unpaired ions can attach to other molecules, causing alterations in cellular structures (Parker, 2009).
Oxidative stress	Similar to free radical theory, byproducts (free radicals) from oxidative metabolism cause molecular damage; protective and repair mechanisms cannot keep up or prevent accumulation of damage with advancing calendar age (Auerhahn et al., 2007).
Mutation accumulation	Detrimental mutations that accumulate in the population are maintained and not selected during the reproductive years; after reproduction is complete, these mutations result in aging and pathology (Weinert & Timiras, 2003).
Disposable soma	Similar to mutation accumulation theory, repair and maintenance are focused on reproductive cells and tissues, and increased mutations and damage accumulates in nonreproductive tissues or soma (Weinert & Timiras, 2003).
Wear and programmed aging	Tissues have a preprogrammed amount of energy available to them. Over time, injury and insults of daily living accumulate cellular defects, which eventually wear out and result in dysfunction or disease (Hayflick, 2004).

(Continued on next page)

Table 2-1. Common Theories of Aging *(Continued)*	
Theory	**Characteristics**
Rate of living	Theory states that people (and other creatures) have a finite number of breaths, heartbeats, or other measures. The modern version of this theory recognizes that the number of heartbeats does not predict life span. Instead, researchers examine the speed at which an organism processes oxygen. When comparing species, some evidence shows that creatures with faster oxygen metabolisms die younger (Carey & Zou, 2007; Lints,1989).
Immunity	Immune function diminishes with age (Jin, 2010). These changes result in decreased resistance to tumor cells and increased incidence of cancer and autoimmune diseases (Hunt et al., 2010).
Neuroendocrine	Neuroendocrine control of homeostasis declines with age, which leads to age-related physiologic changes (Carey & Zou 2007).

Today, many individuals older than 65 are healthy with few functional limitations. Because aging among individuals is highly variable, some who are 75 years old may be as fit or more fit than many at age 60 (Aapro, 2005). Therefore, the physiology of aging or physiologic age rather than chronologic age should be used to define who is "old." Because chronologic age is a straightforward and practical way of defining a target population, 70 years old is most commonly used as the cutoff for defining "older adults" in geriatric oncology (Kristjansson & Wyller, 2010). However, in the healthcare setting, clinicians need to evaluate older adults individually, objectively, and independently from chronologic age (Bond, 2010).

Normal Aging

The observable or phenotypic changes in aging are distinct from diseases of aging; all older adults inevitably experience changes associated with aging, whereas diseases of aging affect only a subpopulation (Kim, 2003). Over the past several decades, our understanding of aging has shifted. Rather than focusing on aging as a process of declining function and health, the focus now is on the preservation of function and healthy living. A clear distinction is made between aging with disease and disability and successful aging (Rowe & Kahn, 1987).

Rowe and Kahn (1997), expounding on their theory of successful aging, suggested that three aging trajectories exist. The first involves the development of disease and disability with aging. The second, which encompasses the majority of older adults, is labeled as usual aging. With usual aging, overt pathology is absent, but some people decline in function and are at risk for developing chronic disease. The third trajectory is successful aging. Older adults who are aging successfully exhibit little or no physiologic or functional loss and are at low risk for developing disease (Rowe & Kahn, 1997). Additionally, in Rowe and Kahn's definition of successful aging, older adults who successfully age maintain high cognitive and physical functioning and active engagement with life. A criticism of Rowe and Kahn's definition of successful aging is that it does not allow for successful aging among individuals with any level of chronic disease or disability. Others have defined successful aging more broadly (Baltes & Carstensen, 1996; Pruchno, Wilson-Genderson, & Cartwright, 2010; Schmidt, 1994; Strawbridge, Wallhagen, & Cohen, 2002). Schmidt (1994) defined successful aging as having minimal interruption in one's usual function. Baltes and Carstensen's (1996) definition portrays successful aging as doing the best one can with what one has. Strawbridge and colleagues (2002) let individuals rate their own aging success. Pruchno and colleagues (2010) based their definition on two dimensions: objective success and subjective success. These definitions permit individuals to have chronic illnesses and disability and still age successfully.

Altered Response to Physiologic Stress

Normal aging in the absence of disease is associated with physiologic changes in all organ systems. Over time, these changes result in a reduction in the physiologic or functional reserve capacity of organ systems. *Physiologic reserve capacity* refers to the spare capacity that is not being used by organ systems to maintain homeostasis but is available if needed. The spare capacity enables organ systems to maintain function or increase function in response to homeostatic challenges or physiologic stressors. This decreased ability to respond to homeostatic challenges has been called *homeostenosis* (Taffet, 2003).

The decline in physiologic reserve capacity occurs over a number of years without altering the functional capacity of organ systems. In other words, aged organ systems generally remain efficient and effective. Declines in reserve capacity resulting from normal age-related changes may not be evident when an individual is in an unstressed or low stress state. However, when the individual is stressed beyond a certain threshold, functional limitations resulting from age-related changes may become readily apparent. This threshold is the point at which the physiologic reserve capacity of organ systems is depleted or so diminished that homeostasis cannot be maintained (Taffet, 2003; Timiras, 2007a).

Figure 2-1 presents this process. Although depicted as a linear process, the response to physiologic stress and maintenance of homeostasis are dynamic

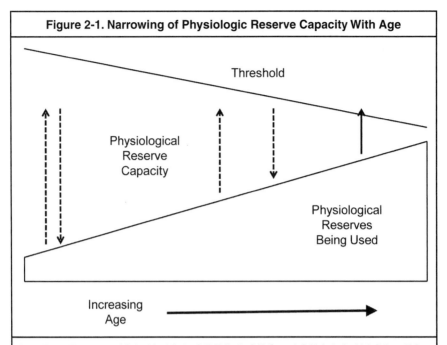

Figure 2-1. Narrowing of Physiologic Reserve Capacity With Age

Note. From "Physiology of Aging" (p. 31), by G.E. Taffet in C.K. Cassel, R.M. Leipzig, H.J. Cohen, E.B. Larson, and D.E. Meier (Eds.), *Geriatric Medicine: An Evidence-Based Approach* (4th ed.), 2003, New York, NY: Springer-Verlag. Copyright 2003 by Springer. Adapted with kind permission of Springer Science+Business Media and the author.

processes that are constantly changing (Taffet, 2003). An organ system's ability to adequately respond to physiologic stressors depends upon the type, level, and duration of the stressor, the level of physiologic reserves already in use, and the system's reserve capacity. Aged organ systems use more physiologic reserves to compensate for normal age-related changes. When demands on organ systems are high or when increased physiologic reserves are being used to compensate for normal changes, the available reserve capacity may be too limited to respond to demands of additional stressors, and the threshold is crossed. When organ systems reach or exceed their threshold, organ dysfunction and systems failure occur. For example, delirium, a common neuropsychiatric syndrome in older adults, occurs when the reserve capacity of the neurophysiologic system is depleted and the system is no longer able to respond adaptively to stressors.

Physiologic Changes of Aging

Physiologic changes associated with aging involve every organ system. It is suggested that many organ systems accrue impairments at a rate of about

5%–10% every decade after an individual reaches 30 years old (Mobbs, 2003). This section presents the common age-related physiologic changes that occur in the major organ systems.

Neurologic

Brain weight decreases with age, especially within the white matter. Between the ages of 20 and 90, the brain loses 5%–10% of its weight (Mobbs, 2006). Ventricular size increases with loss of brain volume, with normal-pressure hydrocephalus commonly associated with increasing age (American Association of Neuroscience Nurses [AANN], 2007).

Older adults develop decreased cerebral blood flow (CBF) with increased cerebrovascular resistance. By age 80, a 20%–25% reduction in CBF can be measured primarily due to the loss of elasticity and lumen diameter in aged blood vessels (Knight & Nigam, 2008c; Sehl, Sawhney, & Naeim, 2005). Decreased ability of the cerebral blood vessels to regulate pressures by vasodilation and constriction affects older adults' adaptation to postural changes (Narayanan, Collins, Hamner, Mukai, & Lipsitz, 2001). Lower CBF along with lower cerebral oxygen consumption reduces older adults' responsiveness to hypercapnia, and as a result, confusion, syncope, and falls can occur. Atherosclerotic changes, commonly seen in the blood vessels of the brain and spinal cord, can increase risk for transient ischemic attacks and vascular dementia in older adults with underlying vascular disease and comorbid conditions such as diabetes (Knight & Nigam, 2008c).

Nearly 40% reduction in the amount of hair in the semicircular canals of the vestibular apparatus located in the inner ear can occur after the age of 70 (Rauch, Velazquez-Villasenor, Dimitri, & Merchant, 2001). Loss of these labyrinth hair cells, nerve fibers, and vestibular ganglion cells (Scarpa's ganglion) has been shown to affect the vestibulo-ocular reflex in older individuals (Ishiyama, 2009). Such changes affect balance and may cause dizziness and falls.

Reaction time is the time it takes to initiate a motor response following a stimulus. Reaction times have generally been found to slow with increasing age, and the extent of this slowing increases as the movement increases in complexity (Kolev, Falkenstein, & Yordanova, 2006). The slowing of response rates and reaction times seen with aging is associated with changes in the number and density of peripheral nerve fibers and the loss of synapses between neurons (AANN, 2007). Changes in the synthesis of many neurotransmitters and their receptors, including the catecholamines (adrenaline and noradrenalin), dopamine, and serotonin, may slow reactions and impair the processing of information. Despite reduced speed, most older adults are able to maintain accuracy of movement. The extent that slowed reaction time interferes with activities of daily living varies greatly among individuals.

At approximately age 70, amyloid deposits or plaques can increase in the small and midsized vessels of the cerebral cortex and leptomeninges (AANN, 2007). Although these protein deposits have been recognized as one of the morphologic hallmarks of Alzheimer disease, they have also been found in the brains of older adults who are neurologically healthy. These plaques may increase risk of dementia, intracranial hemorrhage, or transient neurologic events (Menon, Merino, & Hachinski, 2010).

Cognitive functioning refers to the way in which individuals perceive and react to the world around them. Changes associated with aging are not uniform among individuals and are influenced by many factors, including genetics, lifestyle, education, and past experiences. Intellectual performance in the absence of disease changes little during adult life. Some functions, including vocabulary and practical judgment, have been found to improve between the third and seventh or eighth decade of life, whereas other tasks, such as processing large amounts of new information, may deteriorate with age. With accumulation of experience and maturity, older adults can handle abstract material efficiently but at the cost of slowing down tasks typically measured in reaction time experiments (Knight, 2004). Memory is known to decrease with age, although the specific age when this occurs has been debated. Some studies suggest that declines in memory begin as early as the third or fourth decade of life, whereas other studies suggest that the decline may be much less precipitous and is gradual, at least until the seventh decade of life (Caserta et al., 2009).

Sensory

Vision: Usually by the fourth decade, adults begin to experience presbyopia, the inability to focus or properly accommodate. Stiffening and reduced elasticity of the lens, decreases in the size of the resting pupil (senile miosis), and changes in eye muscles (sphincter pupillae) cause slower reflex reaction to light and accommodation (Meisami, Brown, & Emerle, 2007; Nigam & Knight, 2008b). Increased opacities of the lens and cataract development impair visual acuity and can alter depth perception and contrast sensitivity (Larner, 2006). Difficulty adapting to a change in illumination and night vision is related to degeneration of photoreceptors in the retina (Nigam & Knight, 2008b). Drusen are tiny yellow-white accumulations of extracellular material that build up in Bruch membrane of the eye. The presence of a few small drusen is normal with advancing age; however, the presence of larger and more numerous drusen in the macula is a common early sign of age-related macular degeneration (National Eye Institute, 2010a). Yellowing of the lens contributes to changes in color perception and a decreasing ability to discriminate between colors, especially in differentiating between the green-blue-violet regions of the light spectrum. Losses in peripheral vision also occur with aging. Peripheral vision may be reduced to two-thirds by age 75 and to half by age 90; these age-related changes in vision increase vulnerability to hazards while driving or walking (Schiffman, 2007).

With age, the vitreous humor, a gel-like substance between the lens and the retina composed of a network of thin collagen fibrils, shrinks. As the vitreous shrinks, the fibrils pull on the retinal surface, causing decreased adhesion and liquidation of the gel. Strands from the fibrils cast tiny shadows on the retina and can appear as "floaters." Vitreous detachment itself does not affect vision, but it plays a pivotal role in a number of common eye diseases associated with blindness, including rhegmatogenous retinal detachment, proliferative diabetic retinopathy, and macular hole formation (Bishop, Holmes, Kadler, McLeod, & Bos, 2004). Vitreous detachment is a common condition that usually affects people older than age 50 and is very common after age 80 (National Eye Institute, 2010b). Lacrimal secretions also decrease with advancing age, causing dry eye, increased sensitivity to irritation, and inflammation. As a result, increased tearing may occur to compensate (AANN, 2007).

Hearing: Age-related hearing loss is commonly called *presbycusis* and represents contributions of aging and noise damage, plus genetic susceptibility, comorbid conditions, and exposures to ototoxic agents (Gates & Mills, 2005). Presbycusis is characterized by reduced hearing sensitivity and speech understanding in noisy environments, slowed central processing of acoustic information, and impaired localization of sound sources (Huang & Tang, 2010). It can begin in young adulthood, but is initially evident at 60 years. Decreased blood supply, loss of hair cells in the basal end of the cochlea, and degeneration of the stria vascularis (the spiral ligament of the cochlea duct) contribute to presbycusis and associated high-frequency loss (Huang & Tang, 2010). Over time, the threshold elevation progresses to lower and lower frequency areas (Gates & Mills, 2005).

With aging, the number and density of neurons and synapses in the cochlea nuclei and auditory centers of the brain decrease. This, combined with a reduction in the size and changes in the neurochemical makeup of cells, contributes to a decline of the central auditory system. Slower processing caused by degeneration of the spiral ganglion (cell bodies of the auditory nerve fibers) or loss of neuronal fibers plays a role in abnormal auditory perception and processing seen in older individuals (Rawool, 2007). Changes typically affect speed of processing and result in poorer speech understanding with noise or rapid or degraded speech (Gates & Mills, 2005).

Accumulation of cerumen (ear wax) in the middle ear also can affect hearing. With aging, the concentration of keratin in cerumen increases and cerumen becomes drier, causing accumulation and obstruction of the ear canal. Impaction is a common cause of hearing impairment in older patients (McCartner, Courtney, & Pollart, 2007).

Smell: Smell identification deteriorates progressively with age. The best odor performance occurs between ages 20 and 40 (Kovacs, 2004) with more than half of individuals 65–80 years old showing major olfactory decline (Wrobel & Leopold, 2004). These changes are thought to be related to degeneration of the number of fibers in the olfactory bulb as well as continuous damage to the nasal epithelium, which lead to a loss of olfactory receptors (Bhutto & Morley, 2008; Boyce & Shone, 2006). A common misperception is that the loss of smell decreases the ability to taste or perceive sweet, sour, bitter, and salty sensations via cranial nerves VII, IX, and X. However, smell loss has no meaningful influence on taste function, and when clinical associations between smell and taste dysfunction are observed, they likely reflect comorbid influences such as smoking, medications, and poor dentition (Stinton, Atif, Barkat, & Doty, 2010). However, altered smell function can adversely influence food preferences, food intake, and appetite and can have significant quality-of-life, nutritional, and safety consequences (Doty & Mishra, 2001).

Taste: True loss of taste is extremely rare; in most cases, the sense of taste is not totally absent (ageusia) in older adults but rather is reduced (hypogeusia) or distorted (dysgeusia). Most patients who complain of a loss of taste actually suffer from olfactory dysfunction with inability to perceive the flavors of food (Wrobel & Leopold, 2004). The aging process adversely affects the sense of taste but to a lesser degree than the sense of smell. Atrophy of the tongue and the progressive loss of the number of taste buds/papillae are an explanation for the alterations in taste perception among older people. Small studies have suggested that taste buds in specific anatomic areas such as the epiglottis may decline with age (Kano, Shimizu, Okayama, & Kikuchi, 2007), but the large variation in taste bud density among individuals makes it difficult to draw absolute conclusions (Bhutto & Morley, 2008). Altered taste perception might reflect altered functioning of ion channels in the taste cell membrane rather than an actual loss of taste cells or taste receptors (Bhutto & Morley, 2008; Schiffman & Graham, 2000). In the older adult, medications are the most significant yet underappreciated contributors to taste changes (Schiffman, 2009). Alterations in saliva, mouth hygiene, zinc deficiency, and smoking also may play a greater role in altered taste perception than aging (Bhutto & Morley, 2008).

Sleep

Aging is accompanied by an increased susceptibility to sleep disturbances. This lack of sleep can cause decreased physical function and energy and can affect quality of life. Older adults take longer to fall asleep and, once asleep, spend less time in deep sleep with more periods of light sleep, causing frequent awakenings. Older adult men have more difficulty staying asleep, lighter sleep periods, and more incidence of sleep pathology (e.g., sleep apnea) than women (Floyd, 2002). Although they spend a longer amount of time in bed, older adults experience less overall sleep time (Loiselle, Means, & Edinger, 2005). Older adults also experience changes in their circadian rhythms, causing a shift associated with earlier bedtimes and rising times. Women tend to have greater shifts in circadian rhythms and are prone to sleep disturbances during menopause (Bliwise, 2011).

Cardiovascular

Normal age-related physiologic changes occur in the cardiovascular system and are primarily associated with alterations in blood pressure, myocardial function, and a reduction in baroreceptor sensitivity. The size of the heart increases modestly with age, primarily because of increases in the thickness of the left ventricular wall from hypertrophy of cardiac muscle cells (Karavidas, Lazaros, Tsiachris, & Pyrgakis, 2010). Changes in the elastin and collagen within these muscles cause decreased elasticity and increased stiffness in a similar process as with other age-related muscle changes.

Systolic blood pressure (BP) rises linearly with advancing age in contrast to diastolic BP, which usually peaks around ages 45–55 then decreases after age 60; this results in a widening of pulse pressure with age (Karavidas et al., 2010). Although peripheral vascular resistance primarily dictates BP in younger adults, central arterial stiffness is the main determinant of BP in older adults (Aalami, Fang, Song, & Nacamuli, 2003). Atherosclerotic and arteriosclerotic changes causing decreases in lumen size and decreased compliance in blood vessels play a role. For example, the compliance of the common carotid artery decreases by approximately 40%–50% from age 25 to 75 (Karavidas et al., 2010). Baroreceptors are stretch receptors that serve to minimize fluctuations in BP that result from abrupt changes in peripheral resistance, heart rate, or blood volume. Baroreceptor sensitivity declines with age and is thought to be mediated by reduced adrenergic sensitivity at receptors as well as changes in myocyte signal transduction (Karavidas et al., 2010). Changes in baroreceptor sensitivity put older adults at increased risk for orthostatic hypotension and resultant falls. Cardiac rhythm at rest may be stable or only slightly decreased in older adults; however, the maximal heart rate in response to stress or exercise is lower, reflecting decreased reserves of cardiac output and decreased stimulation of the sympathetic nervous system. This, along with changes in the pacemaker cells within the sinoatrial node, increases the potential for cardiac arrhythmias in older adults (Karavidas et al., 2010; Knight & Nigam, 2008a).

Pulmonary

Lung maturity occurs between 12 and 20–25 years of age when the maximal respiratory functioning is reached; after this age, the lungs begin to lose some of their tissue and structural integrity and progressively decrease in performance (Timiras & De Martinis, 2007). Normal structural and physiologic age-related changes alone are not usually responsible for impaired gas exchange. The contributions of other factors must not be overlooked. These include exposure to tobacco smoke, respiratory infections, air pollutants (dust and fumes), comorbid conditions (chronic obstructive pulmonary disease and coronary artery disease), sedentary lifestyle, and nutritional status (Timiras & De Martinis, 2007). The interaction of these factors with normal aging affects the reserve capacity of the respiratory system. The older adult can become more symptomatic with minimal stress and is less able to adapt to a changing respiratory environment.

Structurally, the number of alveoli decreases, and a corresponding decrease in lung capillaries occurs. The alveoli flatten and collapse sooner with expiration, trapping air within the alveolar duct rather than in the alveoli where oxygen exchange is most efficient. This hyperinflation is termed *senile emphysema*, and the net effect is decreased alveolar surface area. Surface area at age 30 is approximately $75/m^2$ and decreases by 4% per decade thereafter (Timiras & De Martinis, 2007). This affects the diffusion of oxygen from the alveolar air into the blood. In healthy older adults, this decrease has little effect on the amount of oxygen carried into tissues, and blood gas exchange is maintained within normal limits even during periods of heavy exercise (Taylor & Johnson, 2010). Changes in respiratory drive also occur with age. Older adults have a decreased sensation of dyspnea and a diminished response to hypoxia and hypercapnia; these changes make them more vulnerable during high demand states (e.g., heart failure, surgery, pneumonia) and contribute to poor outcomes (Sharma & Goodwin, 2006). The chest wall becomes more rigid with advancing age because of calcifications in rib cartilage. The shape of the thorax may change as a result of osteoporosis, kyphosis, or scoliosis. These changes affect chest wall compliance and may modify the curvature and strength of the diaphragm muscle. Lung elasticity is reduced and, combined with decreased muscle strength (sarcopenia), results in increased air trapping, increased residual volumes, and decreased expiratory flow rates and vital capacity (the amount of air that can be expired after full inspiration). These changes highlight the greater difficulty of the older lung to empty adequately with each expiration (Timiras & De Martinis, 2007). Total lung capacity, the volume of air within the lungs following full inspiration, does not change significantly with age. It is hypothesized that the reduction in lung elasticity is counterbalanced by the increased rigidity of the chest wall (Knight & Nigam, 2008b). Tidal volume, the amount of air exchanged during normal breathing, also does not significantly change with age. Table 2-2 displays the changes in pulmonary function tests usually seen with normal aging. The decline in pulmonary function tests depends on peak lung function achieved during adulthood, the duration of the plateau phase, and the rate of lung function decline (Sharma & Goodwin, 2006).

The cilia in the lungs are responsible for trapping inhaled dust and bacteria within the mucus and clearing mucus from the lungs. The movement of mucus from the lungs to the pharynx, where it is swallowed and passed through the stomach, is accomplished via a mechanism called the mucociliary escalator. With age, evidence supports a slowing of this escalator (Knight & Nigam, 2008b). Along with a gradual decrease in the number of cilia and reduced sensitivity of the cough reflex, older adults are vulnerable to respiratory infections. Despite these age-related changes in the respiratory system, no evidence supports that the changes have an impact on older adults' day-to-day function. They may, however, become evident if physiologic demands stress the limits of supply (Zeleznik, 2003).

Gastrointestinal

Aging of the gastrointestinal tract can be subtle, as many of the changes are of small magnitude and may go unnoticed unless excessive stress takes

Table 2-2. Age-Related Changes in Pulmonary Function Tests	
Parameter	Change With Aging
Vital capacity	↓
Expiratory flow rate	↓
Residual volume	↑
Tidal volume	Stable
Total lung capacity	Stable
Note. Based on information from Knight & Nigam, 2008b; Timiras & De Martinis, 2007.	

place (Morley, 2007). The number of acinar (saliva-producing) cells on the tongue decreases, although salivary production is usually stable. The loss of acinar cells causes a lack of secretory reserve. Salivary gland dysfunction in older adults is more likely due to medications or medical comorbidities such as Sjögren syndrome and other rheumatologic disorders, diabetes, and liver disease (Turner & Ship, 2007; von Bültzingslöwen et al., 2007). With physiologic stressors (e.g., surgery, disease) or prescribed medications that impair salivation (e.g., anticholinergics), the salivary reserve cannot meet increased demands; hence, older adults may experience xerostomia (dry mouth). Additionally, the oral microflora within saliva changes with age, particularly after age 70. Percival, Challacombe, and Marsh (1991) investigated the microflora and immunoglobulin levels within saliva of healthy older adults; results revealed increased counts of lactobacilli and potential opportunistic pathogens such as yeast and staphylococci that were unrelated to denture wearing. Subsequent studies revealed declines in the secretion rates and concentrations of salivary immunoglobulins (Challacombe, Percival, & Marsh, 1995; Percival, Marsh, & Challacombe, 1997). The combination of altered microflora, decreased saliva, and changes in salivary antibodies creates opportunity for infection in the oral mucosa. Changes in dentition and chewing difficulties can occur from a combination of factors, including osteoporotic changes, decreasing levels of calcium in bone, and shrinkage of mandibular and maxillary bones, causing slow erosion of the tooth sockets and eventual tooth loss (Nigam & Knight, 2008a).

Swallowing is a timed sequence of contraction and relaxation of muscles and sphincters. Age-related atrophy and weakness of skeletal muscles can cause changes in the propulsion of food and desynchronization of swallowing. Pharyngeal peristalsis increases in amplitude and duration with age (Sawheny, Sehl, & Naeim, 2005). Decreases in esophageal peristalsis and reduced compliance of the upper esophageal sphincter interfere with the passage of food from the throat into the esophagus. In addition, approximately one-third of older adults develop narrowing in the opening of the upper esophageal sphincter (Leonard, Kendall, & McKenzie, 2004). Decreased pressure in the lower esophageal sphincter contributes to heartburn and gastrointestinal reflux and can increase the risk of aspiration pneumonia in older adults. Controversy exists as to whether gastric acid secretion is affected by age, but evidence has shown that acid secretion is decreased in the presence of *Helicobacter pylori* infection (Morley, 2007; Nigam & Knight, 2008a).

Changes in gastrointestinal motility and delayed gastric emptying contribute to early satiety, which is often seen in older adults. Early satiety plays a role in the concept of "anorexia of aging." This term is used to define an age-associated physiologic reduction in appetite and food intake, leading to unintentional weight loss and undernutrition (Chapman, 2007). Anorexia associated with aging, which is more marked in men than women (Morley, 2007), makes older adults highly vulnerable to developing cachexia (Morley, Thomas, & Wilson, 2006).

In the small bowel, a reduction in the height of intestinal villi decreases surface area and can lead to absorption disorders, specifically of calcium and carbohydrates, although this may be inconsistent and may not be clinically significant (Aalami et al., 2003). References to malabsorption of nutrients, such as vitamin D, vitamin B_{12}, iron, and folate, may relate more broadly to nutrient bioavailability rather than to a specific reduced enzymatic capacity for nutrient absorption or to changes to absorptive surfaces (Jensen, McGee, & Binkley, 2001). There is no doubt, however, that nutrient deficiencies contribute to anemia, malnutrition, and osteoporosis (Doerflinger, 2009).

Age-related changes in the large intestines include an increased prevalence of diverticula and thickening of the colonic muscle layers. Thickening of the muscular layers occurs due to elastin buildup between the myocytes. After age 60, the rate of thickening increases. The tinea coli (longitudinal muscles of the colon) are affected more than the circular muscles around the colon. This thickening affects muscle contraction, slows colonic transit time, and contributes to hard stool, constipation, and fecal impaction (Aalami et al., 2003). Diverticula occur as a result of weakening of the muscularis propria. These pocket-like mucosal herniations occur at locations where arteries and veins cross the bowel wall. The incidence of diverticulosis increases with age, from less than 5% before age 40 to greater than 65% by age 85 (Nguyen, Chudasama, Dea, & Cooperman, 2009). Complications of diverticula include diverticulitis (inflammation of one or more diverticula), abscess formation, intestinal rupture, peritonitis, and fistula formation.

Hepatic

The liver plays an important role in metabolizing the body's waste products and medications. Hepatic mass declines approximately 40% by age 80, with a proportionate decline in hepatic and visceral blood flow (Sawheny et al., 2005). The quantitative loss of hepatic mass and blood flow accounts for most of the decline in functional reserve of the liver. Interestingly, liver function test results generally remain stable. Age-related changes in hepatocytes are associated with impairment in many hepatic metabolic and detoxification activities, with implications for systemic aging and age-related disease (Everitt, Le Couteur, & Lebel, 2009). For example, the age-related impairment of the hepatic metabolism of lipoproteins predisposes individuals to cardiovascular disease, and age-related declines in the hepatic clearance of most medications cause an increased risk of adverse drug reactions. The production and flow of bile decreases with aging and bile becomes thicker with higher cholesterol content, increasing the likelihood of gallstones (Nigan & Knight, 2008a).

Genitourinary

Similar to the liver, aging of the kidney is marked by a decrease in renal mass and weight due to cortical tissue loss. The average kidney increases in weight from birth to approximately age 50 and then gradually decreases by 20%–30% (Pannarale et al., 2010). Arteriosclerosis causes narrowing of the vascular lumen and thickened arterial walls with subsequent reduction in renal blood flow. In young adults, blood flow is estimated at 600 ml/minute, although this can be reduced by half in older adults (Cukuranovic & Vlajkovic, 2005). Reduced flow with reduced oxygenation can lead to ischemia, particularly in the renal cortex (Andrade & Knight, 2008). Dysregulation of the renin-angiotensin system with impaired responsiveness to antidiuretic hormone (ADH) alters the ability to concentrate or dilute urine and excrete water and electrolytes; this can increase the vulnerability of older adults to volume depletion and pre-renal azotemia (Sawheny et al., 2005). Thirst can also be impaired. Creatinine clearance and glomerular filtration rate decrease with age; however, the clinical significance of this is usually negligible until an acute or chronic illness further impairs the kidney's reserve capacity (Colloca, Santoro, & Gambassi, 2010). Despite these reductions in renal function, because of reduced creatinine production and decreased lean body mass in older adults, serum creatinine concentration remains within normal limits (Luckey & Parsa, 2003).

Epidemiologic data suggest a high prevalence of reduced renal function in older patients, but recognition of this condition is limited by the measurement of serum creatinine, which is an insensitive surrogate marker for glomerular filtration rate (Coresh et al., 2003). Renal function is only one factor that contributes to serum creatinine concentrations. Other factors include creatinine production in muscles and secretion by renal tubules.

Numerous studies have detailed age-related changes in the structure and function of the bladder that may contribute to the high prevalence of disrupted bladder control in the older population, but the relationship of these changes to symptoms remains unclear (Goepel, Hoffmann, Piro, Rubben, & Michel, 2002).

Disrupted bladder function manifested as urinary incontinence is increased with age in both men and women. Health issues such as obesity, frequent constipation, and chronic cough may contribute to incontinence, as does menopause for women and an enlarged prostate for men (Goepel et al., 2002). Urinary incontinence is classified into two categories: transient and established incontinence. Transient incontinence occurs unexpectedly during an acute illness or exacerbation of a chronic medical problem or condition. When the causes of transient incontinence are treated, continence is restored. Established incontinence is due to a functional alteration of the lower urinary tract and requires further evaluation for treatment or management (Lekan-Rutledge, 2004). Structural changes leading to established incontinence include overactive bladder, benign prostatic hypertrophy, bladder prolapse, and urethral prolapse.

Overactive bladder is a symptomatic condition characterized by urinary frequency and urgency with or without incontinence and is highly prevalent in the geriatric population, affecting up to 46% of older adults in the United States (Sexton et al., 2011). Overactive bladder is associated with relaxation of the urethral sphincter, resulting in diminished control of voiding. The etiology is thought to be related to changes within the transmission of synapses in the central nervous system through multiple comorbid conditions such as peripheral vascular disease, stroke, benign prostatic hypertrophy, diabetic neuropathy. Urethral strictures contribute to symptoms and cause reduced blood flow, bladder ischemia, and obstruction (Chu & Dmochowski, 2006).

Benign prostatic hypertrophy is a bladder outlet obstruction associated with detrusor overactivity. However, symptoms may remain in up to 33% of patients after surgical removal of the obstruction, suggesting that central nervous system alterations may contribute to the urinary dysfunction (Andersson, 2003).

Two common age-related structural alterations in women are bladder prolapse (cystocele) and urethral prolapse (urethrocele). A cystocele occurs when the wall of the bladder presses against and moves the wall of the vagina. A urethrocele occurs when the tissues surrounding the urethra sag downward into the vagina. The front wall of the vagina supports the bladder, and this wall can weaken or loosen with age. These changes are commonly associated with menopause. Prior to menopause, women produce estrogen, which maintains muscle strength in and around the vagina. After menopause, the reduction in estrogen results in weakened vaginal muscles (Lentz, 2007). Lower urinary tract symptoms can be caused by numerous, often overlapping mechanisms, which may contribute to variations in symptoms and response to treatment (Andersson, 2003).

Integumentary

Intrinsic aging, also known as the natural aging process, is noted as functional alterations in the skin of older adults, which include a decreased growth rate of the epidermis, hair, and nails; delayed wound healing; reduced dermal clearance of fluids and foreign materials; and compromised vascular responsiveness. Hormones and chemical signals that are important in skin growth and repair are reduced, and the receptors that detect them (e.g., vitamin D receptors) decline (Nigam & Knight, 2008c).

With aging, a drastic reduction in dermal blood vessels and a shortening of capillary loops in the dermal papillae are noted. The dermal papillae are the boundary between the dermis and epidermis where fingerlike formations (or interdigitation) serve to strengthen the epidermal/dermal junction. The effects of aging can lead to the two layers of tissues becoming separated from each other. This separation contributes to the pallor, decreased temperature, and impaired thermoregulation often found in the skin of older adults. Thermoregulatory mechanisms such as vasoconstriction and shivering are less effective and less responsive with age, thus predisposing older adults to hypothermia in cold environments (Aalami et al., 2003). Also, a loss of sensory nerve endings in the epidermis and dermis causes older adults to be less able to detect changes in environmental stimuli, causing increased risk for traumatic injury or less awareness of physiologic alterations, such as vascular insufficiency or infection (Farage, Miller, & Maibach, 2010).

An extrinsic factor known as photoaging occurs as a result of cumulative damage from the ultraviolet radiation of sun exposure. Photoaging superimposes changes to the skin caused by chronologic aging, affecting the epidermis and causing irreparable damage to cellular DNA and disruption of collagen synthesis, leading to acute collagen loss in the skin (Moyal & Fourtanier, 2004). With advancing age, the biochemical composition of tissues change, physiologic capacity is progressively reduced, and the ability to respond to environmental stimuli is decreased.

Musculoskeletal

Age-associated loss of skeletal muscle mass is related to a reduction in the number and size of muscle fibers, as well as denervation (loss of nerve supply) and reduced stimulation of muscle groups (Knight & Nigam, 2008d). Electrophysiologic studies have found declining nerve conduction velocity related to decreased myelin size, thickness, and loss of fibers. The aging nerve fibers have diminished ability to regenerate and reinnervate (Visovsky, 2006). Muscle contraction time is increased, reaction times are prolonged, and deep tendon reflexes may be slowed (Doerflinger, 2009). Peak muscle strength occurs between the ages of 20 and 30 and declines continuously thereafter, although the rate depends on the muscle group and physical activity (Timiras & Navazio, 2007). The muscles become smaller in size (atrophy), and the resulting reduction in muscle mass and muscle strength is referred to as sarcopenia. The prevalence of sarcopenia has been reported to be 12% in individuals older than 60 and 30% among adults older than 80 (Fielding et al., 2011).

With regard to skeletal integrity, peak bone mass is reached during adolescence, and with increasing age, bone mass decreases and bones become weaker (Freemont & Hoyland, 2007). The onset and magnitude of this loss depends on age, type of bone, and gender. Among women, vertebral bone loss may begin as early as the third decade, whereas appendicular bone loss begins after age 50. This loss especially accelerates after menopause, contributing to the high prevalence of osteoporosis in older women. In men, bone loss begins at a much later age. Menopause triggers a rapid phase of bone loss in women that can be prevented by estrogen replacement. Bone resorption (breakdown), as assessed by biochemical markers, increases by 90% at menopause, whereas bone formation markers increase by only 45%. This imbalance between bone resorption and bone formation leads to accelerated bone loss (Khosla & Riggs, 2005). An increasing body of evidence supports that bone-resorbing cytokines, such as interleukin-1, interleukin-6, tumor necrosis factor-alpha, macrophage colony-stimulating factor, and prostaglandins, may be potential candidates for mediating bone loss following estrogen deficiency (Freemont & Hoyland, 2007; Khosla & Riggs, 2005). Declining bioavailable estrogen levels may play a significant role in mediating age-related bone loss in men. Because testosterone has some antiresorptive effects and is important for maintaining bone formation, declining bioavailable testosterone levels may also contribute (Khosla & Riggs, 2005). Also threatening skeletal integrity in older adults is a decrease in cutaneous production of vitamin D_3, diminished 1-hydroxylation of 25-hydroxyvitamin D by the kidney, decreased intestinal calcium absorption, and increased parathyroid hormone levels (Knight & Nigam, 2008d; Timiras & Navazio, 2007).

Within the joints, cartilage generally becomes thicker with increasing age, with the exception of the patella, which becomes thinner, especially in women (Timiras & Navazio, 2007). Decreased activity of the chondrocytes (cartilage-forming cells) leads to a reduction in the amount of cartilage present (Freemont & Hoyland, 2007). Aging cartilage loses elasticity and becomes stretched, resulting in reduced joint mobility. Hormone-mediated regulatory mechanisms play a role in aging bone and cartilage as seen with estrogen level reductions in postmenopausal women and testosterone levels in aging men (Freemont & Hoyland, 2007; Hanna et al., 2005).

Hematopoiesis and Immune Function

Normal hematopoiesis is the process of producing diverse, differentiated blood cell types in a manner responsive to physiologic requirements. Aging of the hematopoietic stem cell compartment is believed to contribute to the onset of a variety of age-dependent blood cell pathologies. Drivers of hematopoietic stem cell aging include a reduction in the capacity of aged hematopoietic stem cells to regenerate, resulting in reduced bone marrow reserves (Sehl et al., 2005). This reduced capacity is known as *immunosenescence*. Immunosenescence is a multifactorial condition in which the immune system of older adults is perceived as declining in reliability and efficiency with age, resulting in an increased susceptibility to infectious diseases and inflammatory conditions. The individual contributing factors to immunosenescence are many and varied because of the multifactorial complexity of the immune system (Licastro et al., 2005). An example of this complexity is lymphocytes, wherein the interaction between B cells and T cells is crucial for effective responses (Bruunsgaard, 2006). In older adults, therefore, immunosenescence increases susceptibility to infectious diseases as well as being at the root of the biologic mechanisms responsible for inflammatory age-related diseases (Hunt, Walsh, Voegeli, & Roberts, 2010).

According to Rothstein (2003), as people age, modulation of hematopoiesis becomes disordered, impairing the ability of older people to respond appropriately to the physiologic demand for hematopoietic cell replacement triggered by stimuli such as infection, blood loss, or cytoreductive chemotherapy. In older adults, normal hematopoiesis is disrupted, and the hematopoietic system becomes populated with cells that are quantitatively and functionally deficient (Beerman et al., 2010). These defects in the production and maturation of the various differentiated blood cells are so tightly associated with aging that they are considered to be geriatric conditions that can lead to anemia, neutropenia, thrombocytopenia, and acute hematopoietic disorders (Rothstein, 2003). The decline of hematopoietic function and immune responsiveness is a clinically significant consequence of aging (Rossi et al., 2005).

Committed bone marrow red blood cell precursor concentrations are reduced in healthy older adults, suggesting that the marrow proliferative capacity becomes attenuated. Although the hematopoietic system is affected by age as the continuous decrease in bone marrow hematopoietic elements indicates, normal aging does not cause significant decreases in blood cell count parameters (Berkahn & Keating, 2004). Anemia slightly increases in prevalence with aging, but this is thought to be related to chronic diseases, bleeding, or vitamin and mineral deficiencies (Navazio & Testa, 2007). Anemia may reduce the ability to carry oxygen to the muscles and other organs and can be a special concern in patients with cancer in whom both the disease and the treatment may contribute to its manifestation and severity (Balducci & Hardy, 2004).

Endocrine

Age-related endocrine changes include alterations in the secretion, circulating levels, metabolism, and biologic activity of hormones. There is significant individual heterogeneity in the ability to maintain homeostasis in response to age-related changes in physiology, metabolism, and function (Timiras, 2007b). The clinical significance of these age-related alterations is variable and includes (Chahal & Drake, 2007)

- Reduced protein synthesis
- Decreased lean body mass
- Decreased bone mass
- Increased fat mass
- Increased insulin resistance

- Systemic vascular insufficiency with increasing disease risk of multiple organ systems
- Increased vasomotor symptoms, fatigue, depression, anemia, poor libido, erectile deficiency, and a decline in immune function.

Although most glands decrease their levels of secretion, normal aging usually does not lead to a deficiency state. For example, while the adrenal cortex decreases its secretion of cortisol, negative feedback mechanisms maintain normal plasma levels. Blood and tissue concentrations of many other hormones (thyroid-stimulating hormone, thyroid hormones, ADH, parathyroid hormone, prolactin, and glucocorticoids) remain unchanged. Yet, despite unchanging hormone levels, some endocrine tissues become less responsive to stimulation. For example, less growth hormone and insulin are secreted after a carbohydrate-rich meal or during a glucose tolerance test in older adults than in younger people. In addition, peripheral tissues become less responsive to some hormones, particularly glucocorticoids and ADH, as people reach older adulthood. The failure to produce enough glucocorticoids can affect metabolism and the ability to deal with stress. A decline in production will reduce anti-inflammatory and immunosuppressive qualities. Subsequently, older adults are more prone to experience pain and infections (Walston et al., 2006).

Because endocrinology and metabolism are broad and complex subjects that incorporate many bodily functions, the interplay between the extrinsic corrections of one hormonal imbalance can affect numerous other metabolic processes and organ systems. The role of the endocrine system is coordinating, integrating, regulating, stimulating, suppressing, and modulating to maintain optimum health. Age-related alterations within the endocrine system can impair the highly regulated coordination of continuously changing metabolic processes and affect an individual's ability to efficiently respond to external stressors (Becker, Nylen, & Snider, 2001).

Pharmacokinetics

Pharmacokinetics is the way that the body absorbs, distributes, metabolizes, and excretes medication. The previously described age-related physiologic changes that affect multiple body systems alter the pharmacokinetics of many medications. Table 2-3 outlines common pharmacokinetic changes that occur in conjunction with the physiologic changes of aging.

The use of pharmacologic agents in older patients is one of the most challenging aspects of patient care. An understanding of the common physiologic changes expected with aging is helpful to anticipate changes expected in pharmacokinetic parameters. Distribution, metabolism, and excretion are significantly altered for many drugs.

The liver is the major organ of drug metabolism in the body. With aging comes a decrease in blood flow and liver size. However, in the absence of

Table 2-3. Common Pharmacokinetic Changes Caused by Physiologic Changes of Aging

Mechanism	Physiologic Change	Effect on Pharmacokinetics
Absorption	Decreased intestinal motility Diminished blood flow to gut	Delayed peak effect Delayed signs and symptoms of toxicity
Distribution	Decreased fluid volume Increased body fat percentage Decreased plasma proteins Decreased lean body mass	Increased concentration of water-soluble drugs Increased half-life of fat-soluble drugs Increased amount of active drug Increased drug concentration
Metabolism	Decreased blood flow to liver Decreased liver function	Decreased rate of clearance by liver Increased accumulation of some drugs
Excretion	Decreased kidney function Decreased creatinine clearance	Increased accumulation of drugs that are normally excreted by the kidneys

Note. Based on information from Hutchison & O'Brien, 2007.

disease, function is maintained. Decreased size and hepatic blood flow may slow the clearance of certain drugs, and reduced dosages may be required.

Diminished clearance via renal structure and physiology is frequently responsible for altered drug levels. Even in healthy adults, renal function declines steadily with age as a result of decreased renal blood flow, loss of cortical mass, a resultant progressive reduction of glomerular filtration rate, and reduced tubular secretion. In older adults, serum creatinine levels may appear normal or low due to an age-related decline in creatinine production and loss of lean body mass. Thus, serum creatinine should not be used as a measure of renal function. Creatinine clearance estimates can be determined using various equations, which are convenient but less accurate in older adults (Wasil & Lichtman, 2005). Body mass changes may lead to changes in total body content of drugs in older patients. With aging, body fat increases by up to 50%, and body water percentage decreases 10%–15% (Elmadfa & Meyer, 2008). A water-soluble drug (low volume of distribution [Vd]) is absorbed more readily by lean tissue or muscle and attains higher serum concentrations in patients with less body water or lean tissue. Conversely, a lipid-soluble (high Vd) drug is retained in body fat, resulting in a higher Vd for some drugs (Hutchison & O'Brien, 2007).

It is important for clinicians to be aware that pharmaceutical manipulations may inadvertently cause devastating consequences to older adults. Homeostatic changes encountered during normal aging may alter sensitivity to a given medication, resulting in pharmacokinetic effects. Responses may differ markedly from reactions seen in younger patients. Multiple drugs, drug side effects, drug interactions, and drug-disease interactions contribute to the risks assumed when treating older adult patients (Lynch & Price, 2007).

Cytochrome P450

Cytochrome P450 proteins in humans are drug-metabolizing enzymes and enzymes that are used to make cholesterol, steroids, and other important lipids (Byrd & Luther, 2010). Many drug interactions are a result of inhibition or induction of cytochrome P450 enzymes (CYP450). The CYP450 superfamily is a large and diverse group of enzymes. The function of most CYP enzymes is to catalyze the oxidation of organic substances. CYP450 tests may be used to help determine which medications may be effective for specific individuals. Medications affect each individual differently because of inherited genetic traits. By examining DNA for certain gene variations, CYP450 tests can offer information related to an individual's ability to respond to a particular drug. For example, CYP450 tests are being used to determine whether certain cancer medications are likely to be effective. CYP450 tests and other genotyping tests can provide the ability to predict the therapeutic effects of drug treatments and identify individuals at risk for drug interactions and adverse events (Johansson & Ingelman-Sundberg, 2011).

Conclusion

Changes associated with normal aging affect older adults' functional status and ability to carry out activities of daily living. However, the severity of limitations is determined by many factors. Awareness of normal age-related changes will allow nurses to identify and differentiate normal changes of aging and disease. In caring for older adults, it is important to accurately interpret signs and symptoms and the results of diagnostic tests to avoid medicalizing normal aging phenomena (Zeleznik, 2003).

Although wrinkles develop, hair turns gray, and arteries stiffen, the normal changes of aging are unlikely to be a cause of death. Rather, the normal changes of aging reduce reserve capacity. Individuals die from disease, some of which might not have caused problems in younger years. Therefore, injuries or infections can cause a cascade of health problems that can lead to rapid decline in health and function. Aging results in a diminished ability to maintain homeostasis and regulate body systems. Everyone ages differently, and the rate of change in the function of organ systems can vary markedly. It is important to know that the rate of physiologic decline can be modified.

A tremendous diversity exists among individuals of similar chronologic age. A physically fit older adult can have the functional capacity of someone much younger, while an individual who smokes and is sedentary may be physiologically and functionally similar to someone several decades older. Healthy aging is an issue of increasing importance as the size of the older population continues to grow. Poor health in later life is not inevitable. Modifying lifestyle factors to include a healthy diet, physical activity, social connections, and management of health issues can reduce the incidence of illness and disability associated with aging.

References

Aalami, O.O., Fang, T.D., Song, H.M., & Nacamuli, R.P. (2003). Physiologic features of aging persons. *Archives of Surgery, 138,* 1068–1076. doi:10.1001/archsurg.138.10.1068

Aapro, M.S. (2005). The frail are not always elderly. *Journal of Clinical Oncology, 23,* 2121–2122. doi:10.1200/JCO.2005.10.976

Adams, J.M., & White, M. (2004). Biological ageing: A fundamental, biological link between socioeconomic status and health? *European Journal of Public Health, 14,* 331–334. doi:10.1093/eurpub/14.3.331

American Association of Neuroscience Nurses. (2007). *Neurologic assessment of the older adult: A guide for nurses. AANN Clinical Practice Guideline Series.* Glenview, IL: Author.

Andersson, K.E. (2003). Storage and voiding symptoms: Pathophysiologic aspects. *Urology, 62*(Suppl. 2), 3–10. doi:10.1016/j.urology.2003.09.030

Andrade, M., & Knight, J. (2008). Exploring the anatomy and physiology of ageing. Part 4—The renal system. *Nursing Times, 104*(34), 22–23.

Auerhahn, C., Capezuti, E., Flaherty, E., & Resnick, B. (Eds.). (2007). *Geriatric nursing review syllabus: A core curriculum in advanced practice geriatric nursing* (2nd ed.). New York, NY: American Geriatrics Society.

Balducci, L., & Beghe, C. (2000). The application of the principles of geriatrics to the management of the older person with cancer. *Critical Reviews in Oncology/Hematology, 35,* 147–154. doi:10.1016/S1040-8428(00)00089-5

Balducci, L., & Hardy, C.L. (2004). Anemia and aging: Relevance to the management of cancer. In L. Balducci, G.H. Lyman, W.B. Ershler, & M. Extermann (Eds.), *Comprehensive geriatric oncology* (2nd ed., pp. 444–450). Boca Raton, FL: Taylor & Francis.

Baltes, M.M., & Carstensen, L.L. (1996). The process of successful aging. *Ageing and Society, 16,* 397–422. doi:10.1017/S0144686X00003603

Becker, K.L., Nylen, E.S., & Snider, R.H. (2001). Endocrinology and the endocrine patient. In K.L. Becker, J.P. Bilerikian, W.J. Bremner, W. Hung, C.R. Kahn, D.L. Loriaux, … L. Wartofsky (Eds.), *Principles and practice of endocrinology and metabolism* (3rd ed., pp. 2–7). Philadelphia, PA: Lippincott Williams & Wilkins.

Beerman, I., Bhattacharya, D., Zandi, S., Sigvardsson, M., Weissman, I.L., Bryder, D., & Rossi, D.J. (2010). Functionally distinct hematopoietic stem cells modulate hematopoietic lineage potential during aging by a mechanism of clonal expansion. *Proceedings of the National Academy of Sciences, 107,* 5465–5470. doi:10.1073/pnas.1000834107

Berkahn, L., & Keating, A. (2004). Hematopoiesis in the elderly. *Hematology, 9,* 159–163. doi:10.1080/10245330410001701468

Bhutto, A., & Morley, J.E. (2008). The clinical significance of gastrointestinal changes with aging. *Current Opinion in Clinical Nutrition and Metabolic Care, 11,* 651–660. doi:10.1097/MCO.0b013e32830b5d37

Bishop, P.N., Holmes, D.F., Kadler, K.E., McLeod, D., & Bos, K.J. (2004). Age-related changes on the surface of vitreous collagen fibrils. *Investigative Ophthalmology and Visual Science, 45,* 1041–1046. doi:10.1167/iovs.03-1017

Bliwise, D.L. (2011). Normal aging. In M. Kryger, T. Roth, & W. Dement (Eds.), *Principles and practice of sleep medicine* (5th ed., pp. 27–41). St. Louis, MO: Elsevier Saunders.

Bond, S.M. (2010). Physiologic aging in older adults with cancer: Implications for treatment decision making and toxicity management. *Journal of Gerontological Nursing, 36,* 26–37. doi:10.3928/00989134-20091103-98

Boyce, J.M., & Shone, G.R. (2006). Effects of ageing on smell. *Postgraduate Medical Journal, 82,* 239–241. doi:10.1136/pgmj.2005.039453

Bruunsgaard, H. (2006). The clinical impact of systemic low-level inflammation in elderly populations. With special reference to cardiovascular disease, dementia and mortality. *Danish Medical Bulletin, 53,* 285–309.

Byrd, L., & Luther, C. (2010). Cytochrome P450: Drug metabolism—Why it's so important to understand. *Geriatric Nursing, 31,* 385–387.

Carey, J.R., & Zou, S. (2007). Theories of lifespan and aging. In P.S. Timiras (Ed.), *Physiologic basis of aging and geriatrics* (4th ed., pp. 55–68). New York, NY: Informa Healthcare.

Caserta, M.T., Bannon, Y., Fernandez, F., Giunta, B., Schoenberg, M.R., & Tan, J. (2009). Normal brain aging: Clinical, immunological, neuropsychological, and neuroimaging features. *International Review of Neurobiology, 84,* 1–19. doi:10.1016/S0074-7742(09)00401-2

Chahal, H., & Drake, W. (2007). The endocrine system and ageing. *Journal of Pathology, 211,* 173–180. doi:10.1002/path.2110

Challacombe, S.J., Percival, R.S., & Marsh, P.D. (1995). Age-related changes in immunoglobulin isotypes in whole and parotid saliva and serum in healthy individuals. *Oral Microbiology and Immunology, 10,* 202–207. doi:10.1111/j.1399-302X.1995.tb00143.x

Chapman, I.M. (2007). The anorexia of aging. *Clinics in Geriatric Medicine, 23,* 735–756. doi:10.1016/j.cger.2007.06.001

Chu, F.F., & Dmochowski, R. (2006). Pathophysiology of overactive bladder. *American Journal of Medicine, 119*(Suppl. 3), 3–8. doi:10.1016/j.amjmed.2005.12.010

Colloca, G., Santoro, M., & Gambassi, G. (2010). Age-related physiologic changes and perioperative management of elderly patients. *Surgical Oncology, 19,* 124–130. doi:10.1016/j.suronc.2009.11.011

Coresh, J., Selvin, E., Stevens, L.A., Manzi, J., Kusek, J.W., Eggers, P., … Levey, A.S. (2003). Prevalence of chronic kidney disease and decreased kidney function in the adult U.S. population: Third National Health and Nutrition Examination Survey. *American Journal of Kidney Diseases, 41,* 1–12. doi:10.1053/ajkd.2003.50007

Cukuranovic, R.C., & Vlajkovic, S. (2005). Age-related anatomical and functional characteristics of the human kidney. *Medicine and Biology, 12,* 61–69.

Doerflinger, D.M. (2009). Normal changes of aging and their impact on care of the older surgical patient. *Thoracic Surgery Clinics, 19,* 289–299.

Doty, R.L., & Mishra, A. (2001). Olfaction and its alternation by nasal obstruction, rhinitis, and rhinosinusitis. *Laryngoscope, 111,* 409–423. doi:10.1097/00005537-200103000-00008

Elmadfa, I., & Meyer, A.L. (2008). Body composition, changing physiological functions and nutrient requirements of the elderly. *Annals of Nutrition and Metabolism, 52*(Suppl. 1), 2–5. doi:10.1159/000115339

Everitt, A., Le Couteur, D.G., & Lebel, M. (2009, July 1). The aging liver. Retrieved from http://www.healthplexus.net/article/aging-liver

Farage, M.A., Miller, K.W., & Maibach, H.L. (2010). Degenerative changes in aging skin. In M.A. Farage, K.W. Miller, & H.I. Maibach (Eds.), *Textbook of aging skin* (pp. 25–36). Berlin, Germany: Springer-Verlag.

Fielding, R.A., Vellas, B., Evans, W.J., Bhasin, S., Morley, J.E., Newman, A.B., … Zamboni, M. (2011). Sarcopenia: An undiagnosed condition in older adults. Current consensus definition: Prevalence, etiology, and consequences. *Journal of the American Medical Directors Association, 12,* 249–256. doi:10.1016/j.jamda.2011.01.003

Floyd, J. (2002). Sleep and aging. *Nursing Clinics of North America, 37,* 719–731. doi:10.1016/S0029-6465(02)00034-8

Freemont, A.J., & Hoyland, J.A. (2007). Morphology, mechanisms and pathology of musculoskeletal ageing. *Journal of Pathology, 211,* 252–259. doi:10.1002/path.2097

Gates, G.A., & Mills, J.H. (2005). Presbycusis. *Lancet, 366,* 1111–1120. doi:10.1016/S0140 -6736(05)67423-5

Goepel, M., Hoffmann, J.A., Piro, M., Rubben, H., & Michel, M.C. (2002). Prevalence and physician awareness of symptoms of urinary bladder dysfunction. *European Urology, 41,* 234–239.

Hanna, F., Ebeling, P.R., Wang, Y., O'Sullivan, R., Davis, S., Wluka, A.E., & Cicuttini, F.M. (2005). Factors influencing longitudinal change in knee cartilage volume measured from magnetic resonance imaging in healthy men. *Annals of the Rheumatic Diseases, 64,* 1038–1042. doi:10.1136/ard.2004.029355

Hayflick, L. (2004). "Anti-aging" is an oxymoron. *Journals of Gerontology Series A: Biological Sciences and Medical Sciences, 59,* B573–B578.

Huang, Q., & Tang, J. (2010). Age-related hearing loss or presbycusis. *European Archives of Otorhinolaryngology, 267,* 1179–1191. doi:10.1007/s00405-010-1270-7

Hunt, K.J., Walsh, B.M., Voegeli, D., & Roberts, H.C. (2010). Inflammation in aging—Part 1: Physiology and immunological mechanisms. *Biological Research for Nursing, 11,* 245–252. doi:10.1177/1099800409352237

Hutchison, L.C., & O'Brien, C.E. (2007). Changes in pharmacokinetics and pharmacodynamics in the elderly patient. *Journal of Pharmacology Practice, 20,* 4–12. doi:10.1177/0897190007304657

Ishiyama, G. (2009). Imbalance and vertigo: The aging human vestibular periphery. *Seminars in Oncology, 29,* 491–499. doi:10.1055/s-0029-1241039

Jensen, G.L., McGee, M., & Binkley, J. (2001). Nutrition in the elderly. *Gastroenterology Clinics of North America, 30,* 313–334. doi:10.1016/S0889-8553(05)70184-9

Jin, K. (2010). Modern biological theories of aging. *Aging and Disease, 1,* 72–74.

Johansson, I., & Ingelman-Sundberg, M. (2011). Genetic polymorphism and toxicology—With emphasis on cytochrome P450. *Toxicological Sciences, 120,* 1–13. doi:10.1093/toxsci/kfq374

Kano, M., Shimizu, Y., Okayama, K., & Kikuchi, M. (2007). Quantitative study of ageing epiglottal taste buds in humans. *Gerodontology, 24,* 169–172. doi:10.1111/j.1741 -2358.2007.00165.x

Karavidas, A., Lazaros, G., Tsiachris, D., & Pyrgakis, V. (2010). Aging and the cardiovascular system. *Hellenic Journal of Cardiology, 51,* 421–427. Retrieved from http://www.hellenicjcardiol .org/archive/full_text/2010/5/2010_5_421.pdf

Khosla, S., & Riggs, B.L. (2005). Pathophysiology of age-related bone loss and osteoporosis. *Endocrinology Metabolism Clinics of North America, 34,* 1015–1030. doi:10.1016/j .ecl.2005.07.009

Kim, S. (2003). Molecular biology of aging. *Archives of Surgery, 138,* 1051–1054. doi:10.1001/ archsurg.138.10.1051

Kirkwood, T.B.L. (2002). Evolution of aging. *Mechanisms of Aging and Development, 123,* 737–745. doi:10.1016/S0047-6374(01)00419-5

Kirkwood, T.B.L. (2003). The most pressing problem of our age. *BMJ, 326,* 1297–1299. doi:10.1136/bmj.326.7402.1297

Kirkwood, T.B.L. (2005). Understanding the odd science of aging. *Cell, 120,* 437–447. doi:10.1016/j.cell.2005.01.027

Knight, B.G. (2004). *Psychotherapy with older adults* (3rd ed.). Thousand Oaks, CA: Sage.

Knight, J., & Nigam, Y. (2008a). Exploring the anatomy and physiology of ageing: Part 1— The cardiovascular system. *Nursing Times, 104*(31), 26–27.

Knight, J., & Nigam, Y. (2008b). Exploring the anatomy and physiology of ageing: Part 2— The respiratory system. *Nursing Times, 104*(32), 24–25.

Knight, J., & Nigam, Y. (2008c). Exploring the anatomy and physiology of ageing: Part 5— The nervous system. *Nursing Times, 104*(35), 18–19.

Knight, J., & Nigam, Y. (2008d). Exploring the anatomy and physiology of ageing: Part 10—Muscles and bone. *Nursing Times, 104*(48), 22–23.

Kolev, V., Falkenstein, M., & Yordanova, J. (2006). Motor-response generation as a source of aging-related behavioral slowing in choice-reaction tasks. *Neurobiology of Aging, 27,* 1719–1730. doi:10.1016/j.neurobiolaging.2005.09.027

Kovacs, T. (2004). Mechanisms of olfactory dysfunction in aging and neurodegenerative disorders. *Ageing Research Reviews, 3,* 215–232. doi:10.1016/j.arr.2003.10.003

Kristjansson, S.R., & Wyller, T.B. (2010). Introduction. In D. Schrijvers, M. Aapro, B. Zakotnik, R. Audisio, H. van Halteren, & A. Hurria (Eds.), *European Society for Medical Oncology handbook of cancer in the senior patient* (pp. 1–7). New York, NY: Informa Healthcare.

Larner, A.J. (2006). Neurological signs of aging. In M.S.J. Pathy, A.J. Sinclair, & J.E. Morley (Eds.), *Principles and practice of geriatric medicine* (4th ed., pp. 743–750). Hoboken, NJ: Wiley.

Lekan-Rutledge, D. (2004). Urinary incontinence strategies for frail elderly women. Retrieved from http://www.medscape.com/viewarticle/488559

Lentz, G.M. (2007). Anatomic defects of the abdominal wall and pelvic floor. In V.L. Katz, R.A. Lobo, G. Lentz, & D. Gershenson (Eds.), *Comprehensive gynecology* (5th ed., pp. 501–536). Philadelphia, PA: Elsevier Mosby.

Leonard, R., Kendall, K., & McKenzie, S. (2004). UES opening and cricopharyngeal bar in nondysphagic elderly and nonelderly adults. *Dysphagia, 19,* 182–191. doi:10.1007/s00455-004-0005-6

Licastro, F., Candore, G., Lio, D., Porcellini, E., Colonna-Romano, G., & Franceschi, C. (2005). Innate immunity and inflammation in ageing: A key for understanding age-related diseases. *Immunity and Ageing, 2,* 8. doi:10.1186/1742-4933-2-8

Lints, F.A. (1989). The rate of living theory revisited. *Gerontology, 35,* 36–57. doi:10.1159/000212998

Loiselle, R.C.M., Means, M.K., & Edinger, J.D. (2005). Sleep disturbances in aging. *Advances in Cell Aging and Gerontology, 17,* 33–59. doi:10.1016/S1566-3124(04)17002-8

Luckey, A.E., & Parsa, C.J. (2003). Fluid and electrolytes in the aged. *Archives of Surgery, 138,* 1055–1060. doi:10.1001/archsurg.138.10.1055

Lynch, T., & Price, A. (2007). The effect of cytochrome P450 metabolism on drug response, interactions, and adverse effects. *American Academy of Family Physicians, 76,* 391–396.

McCartner, D.F., Courtney, U., & Pollart, S.M. (2007). Cerumen impaction. *American Family Physician, 75,* 1523–1528. Retrieved from http://www.aafp.org/afp/2007/0515/p1523.html

Meisami, E., Brown, C.M., & Emerle, H.F. (2007). Sensory systems: Normal aging, disorders and treatment of vision and hearing in humans. In P.S. Timiras (Ed.), *Physiologic basis of aging and geriatrics* (4th ed., pp. 109–136). New York, NY: Informa Healthcare.

Menon, R.S., Merino, J.G., & Hachinski, V.C. (2010). Cerebral amyloid angiopathy. Retrieved from http://emedicine.medscape.com/article/1162720-overview

Mobbs, C. (2003). Molecular and biological factors in aging. In C.K. Cassel, R.M. Leipzig, H.J. Cohen, E.B. Larson, & D.E. Meier (Eds.), *Geriatric medicine: An evidence-based approach* (4th ed., pp. 15–26). New York, NY: Springer-Verlag.

Mobbs, C. (2006). Aging of the brain. In M.S.J. Pathy, A.J. Sinclair, & J.E. Morley (Eds.), *Principles and practice of geriatric medicine* (4th ed., pp. 59–67). Hoboken, NJ: Wiley.

Morley, J.E. (2007). The aging gut: Physiology. *Clinics in Geriatric Medicine, 23,* 757–767. doi:10.1016/j.cger.2007.06.002

Morley, J.E., Thomas, D.R., & Wilson, M.M. (2006). Cachexia: Pathophysiology and clinical relevance. *American Journal of Clinical Nutrition, 83,* 735–743.

Moyal, D., & Fourtanier, A. (2004). Acute and chronic affects of UV on skin. In S. Rigel, R.A. Weiss, H.W. Lim, & J.S. Dover (Eds.), *Photoaging* (pp. 15–26). New York, NY: Marcel Dekker.

Narayanan, K., Collins, J.J., Hamner, J., Mukai, S., & Lipsitz, L.A. (2001). Predicting cerebral blood flow response to orthostatic stress from resting dynamics: Effects of healthy aging. *American Journal of Physiology—Regulatory, Integrative and Comparative Physiology, 281,* R716–R722. Retrieved from http://ajpregu.physiology.org/content/281/3/R716.full.pdf+html

National Eye Institute. (2010a, August). Facts about age-related macular degeneration. Retrieved from http://www.nei.nih.gov/health/maculardegen/armd_facts.asp

National Eye Institute. (2010b, February). Facts about vitreous detachment. Retrieved from http://www.nei.nih.gov/health/vitreous/vitreous.asp#1

Navazio, F.M., & Testa, M. (2007). Benefits of physical exercise. In P.S. Timiras (Ed.), *Physiological basis of aging and geriatrics* (4th ed., pp. 382–391). New York, NY: Informa Healthcare.

Nguyen, M.C.T., Chudasama, Y.N., Dea, S.K., & Cooperman, A. (2009). Diverticulitis. Retrieved from http://emedicine.medscape.com/article/173388-overview

Nigam, Y., & Knight, J. (2008a). Exploring the anatomy and physiology of ageing: Part 3— The digestive system. *Nursing Times, 104*(33), 22–23.

Nigam, Y., & Knight, J. (2008b). Exploring the anatomy and physiology of ageing: Part 6— The eye and ear. *Nursing Times, 104*(36), 22–23.

Nigam, Y., & Knight, J. (2008c). Exploring the anatomy and physiology of ageing: Part 11—The skin. *Nursing Times, 104*(49), 24–25.

Pannarale, G., Carbone, R., Del Mastro, G., Gallo, C., Gattullo, V., Natalicchio, L., ... Tedesco, A. (2010). The aging kidney: Structural changes. *Journal of Nephrology, 23*(Suppl. 15), S37–S40.

Parker, P. (2009). Theories of aging. In P. Gillman, P. Parker, & P. Tabloski (Eds.), *Gerontological nursing: ANCC review and resource manual* (pp. 43–54). Silver Spring, MD: American Nurses Credentialing Center.

Percival, R.S., Challacombe, S.J., & Marsh, P.D. (1991). Age-related microbiological changes in the salivary and plaque microflora of healthy adults. *Journal of Medical Microbiology, 35,* 5–11. doi:10.1099/00222615-35-1-5

Percival, R.S., Marsh, P.D., & Challacombe, S.J. (1997). Age-related changes in salivary antibodies to commensal oral and gut biota. *Oral Microbiology and Immunology, 12,* 57–63. doi:10.1111/j.1399-302X.1997.tb00367.x

Pruchno, R.A., Wilson-Genderson, M., & Cartwright, F. (2010). A two-factor model of successful aging. *Journals of Gerontology Series B: Psychological Sciences and Social Sciences, 65,* 671–679. doi:10.1093/geronb/gbq051

Rauch, S.D., Velazquez-Villasenor, L., Dimitri, P., & Merchant, S.N. (2001). Decreasing hair cell counts in aging humans. *Annals of the New York Academy of Sciences, 942,* 220–227.

Rawool, V.W. (2007, August). The aging auditory system, part 2: Slower processing and speech recognition. *Hearing Review.* Retrieved from http://www.hearingreview.com/issues/articles/2007-08_04.asp

Rossi, D.J., Bryder, D., Zahn, J.M., Ahlenius, H., Sonu, R., Wagers, A.J., & Weissman, I.L. (2005). Cell intrinsic alterations underlie hematopoietic stem cell aging. *Proceedings of the National Academy of Sciences, 102,* 9194–9199. doi:10.1073/pnas.0503280102

Rothstein, G. (2003). Disordered hematopoiesis and myelodysplasia in the elderly. *Journal of the American Geriatrics Society, 51*(Suppl. 3), 22–26. doi:10.1046/j.1532-5415.51.3s.3.x

Rowe, J.W., & Kahn, R.L. (1987). Human aging: Usual and successful. *Science, 237,* 143–149.

Rowe, J.W., & Kahn, R.L. (1997). Successful aging. *Gerontologist, 37,* 433–440.

Sawhney, R., Sehl, M., & Naeim, A. (2005). Physiologic aspects of aging: Impact on cancer management and decision making, part I. *Cancer Journal, 11,* 449–460. doi:10.1097/00130404-200511000-00004

Schiffman, S.S. (2007). Critical illness and changes in sensory perception. *Proceedings of the Nutrition Society, 66,* 331–345. doi:10.1017/S0029665107005599

Schiffman, S.S. (2009). Effects of aging on the human taste system. *International Symposium on Olfaction and Taste: Annals of the New York Academy of Sciences, 1170,* 725–729. doi:10.1111/j.1749-6632.2009.03924.x

Schiffman, S.S., & Graham, B.G. (2000). Taste and smell perception affect appetite and immunity in the elderly. *European Journal of Clinical Nutrition, 54*(Suppl.), 54–63.

Schmidt, R.M. (1994). Healthy aging into the 21st century. *Contemporary Gerontology, 1,* 3–6.

Sehl, M., Sawhney, R., & Naeim, A. (2005). Physiologic aspects of aging: Impact on cancer management and decision making, part II. *Cancer Journal, 11,* 461–473. doi:10.1097/00130404-200511000-00005

Sexton, C.C., Coyne, K.S., Thompson, C., Bavendam, T., Chen, C., & Markland, A. (2011). Prevalence and effect on health-related quality of life of overactive bladder in older Americans: Results from the epidemiology of lower urinary tract symptoms study. *Jour-*

nal of the American Geriatrics Society. Advance online publication. doi:10.1111/j.1532 -5415.2011.03492.x

Sharma, G., & Goodwin, J. (2006). Effect of aging on respiratory system physiology and immunology. *Clinical Interventions in Aging, 1,* 253–260. doi:10.2147/ciia.2006.1.3.253

Stinton, N., Atif, M.A., Barkat, N., & Doty, R.L. (2010). Influence of smell loss on taste function. *Behavioral Neuroscience, 4,* 256–264.

Strawbridge, W.J., Wallhagen, M.I., & Cohen, R.D. (2002). Successful aging and well-being: Self-rated compared with Rowe and Kahn. *Gerontologist, 42,* 727–733. doi:10.1093/geront/42.6.727

Taffet, G.E. (2003). Physiology of aging. In C.K. Cassel, R.M. Leipzig, H.J. Cohen, E.B. Larson, & D.E. Meier (Eds.), *Geriatric medicine: An evidence-based approach* (4th ed., pp. 27–36). New York, NY: Springer-Verlag.

Taylor, B.J., & Johnson, B.D. (2010). The pulmonary circulation and exercise response in the elderly. *Seminars in Respiratory and Critical Care Medicine, 31,* 528–538. doi:10.1055/s-0030-1265894

Timiras, P.S. (2007a). Comparative aging, geriatric functional assessment, aging, and disease. In P.S. Timiras (Ed.), *Physiological basis of aging and geriatrics* (4th ed., pp. 23–40). New York, NY: Informa Healthcare.

Timiras, P.S. (2007b). The endocrine pancreas, obesity and diffuse endocrine and chemical mediators. In P.S. Timiras (Ed.), *Physiological basis of aging and geriatrics* (4th ed., pp. 220–230). New York, NY: Informa Healthcare.

Timiras, P.S. (2007c). Old age as a stage of life: Common terms related to aging and methods used to study aging. In P.S. Timiras (Ed.), *Physiological basis of aging and geriatrics* (4th ed., pp. 3–10). New York, NY: Informa Healthcare.

Timiras, P.S., & De Martinis, M. (2007). The pulmonary respiration, hematopoiesis, and erythrocytes. In P.S. Timiras (Ed.), *Physiological basis of aging and geriatrics* (4th ed., pp. 277–296). New York, NY: Informa Healthcare.

Timiras, P.S., & Navazio, F.M. (2007). The skeleton, joints, and skeletal and cardiac muscles. In P.S. Timiras (Ed.), *Physiological basis of aging and geriatrics* (4th ed., pp. 329–344). New York, NY: Informa Healthcare.

Turner, M.D., & Ship, J.A. (2007). Dry mouth and its effects on the oral health of elderly people. *Journal of the American Dental Association, 138*(Suppl. 1), 15S–20S. Retrieved from http://jada.ada.org/content/138/suppl_1/15S.long

Visovsky, C. (2006). The effects of neuromuscular alterations in elders with cancer. *Seminars in Oncology Nursing, 22,* 36–42. doi:10.1016/j.soncn.2005.10.010

von Bültzingslöwen, I., Sollecito, T.P., Fox, P.C., Daniels., T., Jonsson, R., Lockhart, P.B., ... Schiødt, M. (2007). Salivary dysfunction associated with systemic diseases: Systematic review and clinical management recommendations. *Oral Surgery, Oral Medicine, Oral Pathology, Oral Radiology, and Endodontology, 103*(Suppl. 1), S57.e1–S57.e15. doi:10.1016/j.tripleo.2006.11.010

Walston, J., Hadley, E.C., Ferrucci, L., Guralnik, J.M., Newman, A.B., Studenski, S.A., ... Fried, L.P. (2006). Research agenda for frailty in older adults: Toward a better understanding of physiology and etiology: Summary from the American Geriatrics Society/National Institute on Aging Research Conference on Frailty in Older Adults. *Journal of the American Geriatrics Society, 54,* 991–1001. doi:10.1111/j.1532-5415.2006.00745.x

Wasil, T., & Lichtman, S.M. (2005). Clinical pharmacology issues relevant to the dosing and toxicity of chemotherapy drugs in the elderly. *Oncologist, 10,* 602–612. doi:10.1634/theoncologist.10-8-602

Weinert, B.T., & Timiras, P.S. (2003). Invited review: Theories of aging. *Journal of Applied Physiology, 95,* 1706–1716. doi:10.1152/japplphysiol.00288.2003

Wrobel, B.B., & Leopold, D.A. (2004). Clinical assessment of patients with smell and taste disorders. *Otolaryngologic Clinics of North America, 37,* 1127–1142. doi:10.1016/j.otc.2004.06.010

Zeleznik, J. (2003). Normative aging of the respiratory system. *Clinics in Geriatric Medicine, 19,* 1–18. doi:10.1016/S0749-0690(02)00063-0

CHAPTER 3

Comprehensive Geriatric Assessment

Janine A. Overcash, PhD, GNP-BC

Introduction

The older adult with cancer often has complex cancer care needs interwoven with comorbid conditions and associated symptoms. Recognizing risks and health problems before functional limitations or threats to independence occur can be critical to the quality of life (QOL) and well-being of the older person with cancer. One method of identifying potentially health-limiting issues is to conduct a comprehensive geriatric assessment (CGA). The CGA is a global assessment that delves beyond the boundaries of a traditional history and physical examination into issues affecting health and QOL of an older adult (Overcash, 2008; Overcash, Beckstead, Extermann, & Cobb, 2005). CGA is a battery of instruments that can be individualized by choosing specific assessment tools to address needs and limitations for all types of patients with cancer (e.g., inpatient, outpatient, all tumor sites).

CGA has been found to be effective in predicting patients who are able to tolerate chemotherapy (Aaldriks et al., 2011; Hurria et al., 2007), predicting frailty (Kristjansson et al., 2010), and identifying people who are at risk for falls (Overcash & Beckstead, 2008). Another benefit of administering a CGA to patients with cancer is to identify older adults who are more likely to benefit from aggressive chemotherapy (Tucci et al., 2009) and various surgical oncology procedures (Audisio et al., 2008). This chapter will discuss components of a CGA that relate to nonmalignant and cancer-related problems that can arise for the older adult while undergoing treatment for a malignancy, such as cognitive function impairment, depression, falls, fatigue, pain, sexual problems, and sleep disturbances. A case study illustrating use of the CGA in clinical practice will be presented to assist the ambulatory care oncology nurse when caring for the older adult with cancer.

Definition and Development of a Comprehensive Geriatric Assessment

The premise of using a CGA for patients diagnosed with cancer is to identify concerns in the health and general functioning that can be proactively addressed so that cancer therapy can be tolerated and beneficial (Balducci, Colloca, Cesari, & Gambassi, 2010; Hurria, Lachs, Cohen, Muss, & Kornblith, 2006). The National Comprehensive Cancer Network (NCCN) recommends using CGA as a tool to determine cancer treatment strategies and to identify which patients should receive palliative care versus curative care (NCCN, 2011b). The full version of the NCCN Comprehensive Geriatric Assessment tool is presented in Figure 3-1 (NCCN, 2011b). It is important to remember that assessment tools are only used to screen and not to diagnose. Depending on the issue, more in-depth diagnostic procedures should be performed by specialists.

A broad range of factors, such as nutrition, pain, comorbid conditions, cancer-associated signs and symptoms, independent functioning, transportation, or lack of an available caregiver, must be considered when evaluating health and social issues. Although it is not possible to explore every assessment question, it is important to consider what items should be included in a CGA that will be useful for ambulatory oncology care. CGA items differ among healthcare settings, tumor types, age, and sex of the patient. Most CGAs are developed to assess issues that are very common for older adults, such as depression (Filipović, Filipović, Kerkez, Milinić, & Ranđelović, 2007), functional limitations (Luciani et al., 2008), transportation (Goodwin, Hunt, & Samet, 1993), dementia (Gorin, Heck, Albert, & Hershman, 2005; Louwman et al., 2005), and a history of falls with or without injury (Overcash, 2007). However, other types of instruments can be included to facilitate the completion of a thorough, oncology-oriented assessment. When developing a CGA for ambulatory oncology care, the following questions should be addressed.

- What types of problems that can act as barriers to cancer treatment are generally present in a particular patient group?
- What limitations can be feasibly addressed in the ambulatory oncology setting?

Prior to conducting a CGA, it is important to consider how management of identified limitations would be addressed. Managing other comorbid conditions can be difficult in the ambulatory oncology setting. Therefore, it is important to proactively plan to work with the patient's primary care provider to discuss and manage findings from the CGA.

Components of a Comprehensive Geriatric Assessment Specific to Oncology

Both cancer-related and comorbid problems have been found to influence QOL in patients receiving chemotherapy (Cheng & Lee, 2011; So et al.,

Figure 3-1. National Comprehensive Cancer Network Guidelines: Comprehensive Geriatric Assessment

National Comprehensive Cancer Network®

NCCN Guidelines™ Version 1.2011
Senior Adult Oncology

NCCN Guidelines Index
Senior Adult Oncology TOC
Discussion

COMPREHENSIVE GERIATRIC ASSESSMENT (1 of 2)

Comorbidity
- May affect treatment decisions in 4 ways:
  ‣ Cancer treatment may interact with comorbidity to impact functional status or worsen the comorbidity (i.e renal insufficiency). This includes any drug-drug interactions.
  ‣ Cancer treatment may be too risky because of the type and severity of comorbidity (i.e. cardiomyopathy). These may include cardiovascular problems, congestive heart failure, mild dementia, depressions, anemia, and osteoporosis.
  ‣ Cancer treatment may not impact future life expectancy due to risk of morbidity[1] associated with comorbid condition. The effect of comorbidity on life expectancy should be evaluated before patient receives treatment. Renal insufficiency, diabetes, lung disease, tobacco use and heart failure all decrease life expectancy.
  ‣ Comorbidity may affect treatment outcome
- Seriousness of comorbid conditions (comorbidity index)
- The following should be specifically considered as part of the comorbidity evaluation:
  ‣ GI problems
  ‣ Renal Insufficiency
  ‣ Cardiomyopathy (cardiovascular problems)
  ‣ Diabetes
  ‣ Neuropathy
  ‣ Anemia
  ‣ Dementia
  ‣ Depression
  ‣ Osteoporosis
  ‣ Lung Disease
  ‣ Tobacco or Alcohol Use

Function
- Activities of daily living (ADL) - Eating, dressing, continence, grooming, transferring, using the bathroom
- Instrumental activities of daily living (IADL) - Using transportation, managing money, taking medications, shopping, preparing meals, doing laundry, doing housework, using telephone
- Performance status

Socioeconomic issues
- Living conditions
- Presence and adequacy of care giver
- Income
- Access to transportation
- Financial counsel to discuss cost, coverage options etc.

Common geriatric syndromes
- Dementia
- Depression
- Delirium
- Falls
- Osteoporosis (spontaneous fractures)
- Neglect and abuse
- Failure to thrive
- Persistent dizziness
- Nutritional deficiency

[1]Mortality can be predicted using weight, body mass index, nutrition, fatigue and existing medical conditions.

Note: All recommendations are category 2A unless otherwise indicated.
Clinical Trials: NCCN believes that the best management of any cancer patient is in a clinical trial. Participation in clinical trials is especially encouraged.

SAO-D
1 of 2

(Continued on next page)

Figure 3-1. National Comprehensive Cancer Network Guidelines: Comprehensive Geriatric Assessment (Continued)

NCCN National Comprehensive Cancer Network®

NCCN Guidelines™ Version 1.2011
Senior Adult Oncology

NCCN Guidelines Index
Senior Adult Oncology TOC
Discussion

COMPREHENSIVE GERIATRIC ASSESSMENT (2 of 2)

Polypharmacy
• Drug-drug interactions[2]
• Number of medications
• Avoid inappropriate drugs
  ‣ Medication Appropriateness Index[3]
  ‣ Beers Criteria[4]
• Use caution when using medications that can contribute to delirium[5,6]
  ‣ Benzodiazepines
  ‣ Anticholinergics
  ‣ Antipsychotics
  ‣ Opioids
  ‣ Corticosteroids

Screening Tools for Common Geriatric Syndromes
• Dementia - Mini Mental State Examination (MMSE)[7,8]
• Depression - Geriatric Depression Scale (GDS)[9,10]
• Delirium - NCCN Distress Management Guidelines
• Osteoporosis - DEXA scan, NCCN Bone Health Task Force
• Fatigue - NCCN Fatigue Guidelines
• Nutrition deficiency- Mini-Nutritional Assessment (MNA)[11,12]

[2]Riechelmann RP, Saad ED. A systemic review on drug interactions in oncology. Cancer Investigation. 2006; 24: 704-712.
[3]Samsa GP, Hanlon JT, Schmader KE, Weinberger M, Clipp EC, Uttech KM, Lewis IK, Landsman, Cohen HJ. A summated score for the medication appropriateness index: development and assessment of clinimetric properties including content validity. J Clin Epidemiology. 1994; 47(8): 891-6
[4]Fick DM, Cooper JW, Wade WE, Waller JL, Maclean JR, Beers MH. Updating the Beers criteria for potentially inappropriate medications use in older adults: results of a US consensus panel of experts. Archives of Internal Medicine. 2003; 163(22): 2716-24.
[5]Hilmer SN, Mager DE, Simonsick EM, Cao Y, Ling SM, Windham, G, Harris TB, Hanlon JT, Rubin SM, Shorr RI, Bauer DC, Abernathy DR. A drug burden index to define the functional burden of medications in older people. Archives of Internal Medicine. 2007; 167: 781-787.
[6]Chew, ML, Mulsant BH, Pollock BG, Lehman ME, Greenspan A, Mahmoud RA, Kirshner MA, Sorisio DA, Bies RR, Gharabawi G. Anticholinergic activity of the 107 medications commonly used by older adults. Journal of the American Geriatrics Society. 2008 May 26 (e-pub, in press).
[7]Tombaugh TN, McIntyre NJ. The mini-mental state examination: a comprehensive review. J Am Geriatr Soc.1992;40(9):922-935.
[8]Crum RM, Anthony JC, Bassett SS, Folstein MF. Population-based norms for the Mini-Mental State Examination by age and educational level. JAMA. 1993;269(18):2386-2391.
[9]Yesavage JA, Brink TL, Rose TL, et al. Development and validation of a geriatric depression screening scale: a preliminary report. J Psychiatr Res. 1982;17(1):37-49).
[10]Yath P, Katona C, Mullan E, Evans S, Katona C. Screening, Detection and Management of Depression in Elderly Primary Care Attenders: The Acceptability and Performance of the 15 Item Geriatric Depression Scale (GDS15) and the Development of Short Versions. Fam. Pract. 1994;11(3):260-266.
[11]Vellas B, Guigoz Y, Garry PJ, et al. The Mini Nutritional Assessment (MNA) and its use in grading the nutritional state of elderly patients. Nutrition. 1999;15(2):116-122.
[12]Rubenstein LZ, Harker JO, Salva A, Guigoz Y, Vellas B. Screening for Undernutrition in Geriatric Practice: Developing the Short-Form Mini-Nutritional Assessment (MNA-SF). J Gerontol A Biol Sci Med Sci. 2001;56(6):M366-372.

Note: All recommendations are category 2A unless otherwise indicated.
Clinical Trials: NCCN believes that the best management of any cancer patient is in a clinical trial. Participation in clinical trials is especially encouraged.

Version 1.2011, 01/11/11 © National Comprehensive Cancer Network, Inc. 2011. All rights reserved. The NCCN Guidelines™ and this illustration may not be reproduced in any form without the express written permission of NCCN®.

SAO-D
2 of 2

2009). Common problems may include fatigue, pain, insomnia, sexual concerns, caregiver issues, anxiety, and depression. Various instruments have been developed to address oncology-related problems. By identifying and monitoring distressing problems, patients may be able to maintain independence while undergoing cancer treatment.

Comorbid Conditions

A diagnosis of cancer may be only one of several comorbidities. In a classic study at Johns Hopkins University, people who were 70 years old and older were found to have a mean of 5.6 diagnoses (Fried et al., 2001). Health limitations may be the result of the culmination of several comorbidities interacting with the cancer diagnosis and treatment (Reiner & Lacasse, 2006). Older patients with cancer and multiple comorbidities who are hospitalized more than 120 days are likely to die in the hospital (Koroukian, 2009; Kozyrskyi, Black, Chateau, & Steinbach, 2005). People who present to emergency departments often have a diagnosis of cancer, are age 85 and older, and have three or more comorbidities (Sikka & Ornato, in press). The more severe the comorbidity, the greater the threat to survival at one year and five years following a diagnosis of cancer (Iversen, Nørgaard, Jacobsen, Laurberg, & Sørensen, 2009). Seniors diagnosed with a moderate to severe comorbid condition between 6 and 18 months prior to a diagnosis of cancer have been associated with lower survival (Shack, Rachet, Williams, Northover, & Coleman, 2010). Patients who are diagnosed with the comorbid condition of diabetes have a twofold risk of recurrence or development of a new breast cancer as compared to people who do not have diabetes (Patterson et al., 2010). Conversely, people who have three or more stable comorbid conditions generally use mammography services and are diagnosed at earlier stages of breast cancer (Yasmeen, Xing, Morris, Chlebowski, & Romano, 2011). Assessing for the presence, extent, and management of comorbid conditions can help provide the ambulatory care oncology nurse with critical information for the care and management of the older adult with cancer.

Fatigue

Older adults who are diagnosed with cancer tend to experience more symptoms associated with fatigue as compared to younger individuals (Butt et al., 2010). Fatigue is defined as an exhaustion or general weakness unrelieved by rest (National Cancer Institute, 2011). Fatigue is a syndrome of symptoms that are multicausal and can be difficult to address. Problems with chemotherapy tolerance, anemia, and insomnia can also be associated with fatigue (Yellen, Cella, Webster, Blendowski, & Kaplan, 1997). One assessment instrument to consider is a visual analog scale, which is a simple clinical assessment procedure, designed to understand the intensity of fatigue (Van Belle et al., 2005) (see Figure 3-2). Also, simply asking the patient to rate the severity of fatigue

---

Figure 3-2. Assessment Instrument References for Cancer-Related Concerns

Fatigue
- Visual analog scale (Van Belle et al., 2005)

Pain
- Faces Pain Scale (Kim & Buschmann, 2006)
- Brief Pain Inventory (Cleeland, 1991)
- Numeric pain rating (De Conno et al., 1994)

Sexual Function
- Brief Male Sexual Function Inventory (Mykletun et al., 2006)
- Female Sexual Functional Index (Rosen et al., 2000)

Sleep
- Pittsburgh Sleep Quality Index (Buysse et al., 1989)
- Iowa Sleep Disturbance Scale (Koffel & Watson, 2010)
- Caregiver Concerns
- Modified Caregiver Strain Index (Thornton & Travis, 2003)

---

from 0 (no fatigue) to 10 (the worse fatigue) is a reasonable method of evaluating fatigue (NCCN, 2011a).

Fatigue should be monitored at each ambulatory visit. Depending on the time interval from the last cancer treatment, fatigue can be more or less pronounced. Assessing trends in a patient's fatigue intensity levels while receiving cancer treatment can help predict and anticipate days that may yield lower energy levels. Planning can occur for tasks such as household chores and family and employment responsibilities.

Pain

Pain assessment is a cardinal aspect of an oncology nursing assessment. Questions assessing pain and the effectiveness of pain medication with a numeric pain rating scale are reasonable components of a CGA in the older adult with cancer. The numeric pain rating scale has been shown to be an effective and easily administered pain measure in patients with cancer (De Conno et al., 1994), and the pain visual analog scale (Price, McGrath, Rafii, & Buckingham, 1983) is also a reasonable clinical pain assessment tool. For pain intensity assessment, the Faces Pain Scale has been shown to be valid and reliable specific to older adults (Kim & Buschmann, 2006). Other pain instruments, such as the Brief Pain Inventory (Cleeland, 1991), exist but are frequently used in research as opposed to clinical needs, and a fee is associated with using these tools.

For patients with pain control issues, a referral to a supportive cancer care team or pain specialist can be very helpful in specifying the type of pain and related pain management strategies (Yennurajalingam et al., 2010). Pain assessment and management are vital components during an ambulatory oncology care visit and should be included in the CGA.

Insomnia

Approximately 45% of patients with cancer report sleep problems (National Cancer Institute, 2010). Insomnia has been found to affect physical and mental function and performance of activities of daily living in older adults (Grov, Fosså, & Dahl, 2010). Insomnia is often accompanied by pain and fatigue and can directly affect QOL (Eyigor, Eyigor, & Uslu, 2009).

As women age and reach menopause, sleep impairments often escalate (Tom, Kuh, Guralnik, & Mishra, 2010). Additionally, women 50 years old and older who are receiving chemotherapy or hormonal therapy may experience increased problems with insomnia (Enderlin et al., 2010). Lack of sleep is not only a problem with the patient, but it can also include the caregiver. One method used to clinically assess insomnia is the Pittsburgh Sleep Quality Index (PSQI) (Buysse, Reynolds, Monk, Berman, & Kupfer, 1989), a 19-item instrument that generally requires about 10 minutes to administer. The PSQI can be used for research or clinical assessments. The PSQI is recommended by the Hartford Institute for Geriatric Nursing for use in older patients. The Iowa Sleep Disturbance scale was developed more recently, but it is mainly used for research purposes and not clinical care (Koffel & Watson, 2010). The Insomnia Severity Index is also often used in clinical settings (Morin, Belleville, Bélanger, & Ivers, 2011).

Sexual Dysfunction

Problems with sexual function are often reported by patients with cancer (Shell, Carolan, Zhang, & Meneses, 2008). The incidence of patients who experience sexual dysfunction after chemotherapy has been reported as high as 100% (Derogatis & Kourlesis, 1981). Issues associated with sexual dysfunction include relationship quality, depression, and anxiety (Nelson, Choi, Mulhall, & Roth, 2007). Various cancer treatments can cause problems with sexual function and interest and concerns associated with body image. Few sexual function assessment tools exist. The Brief Male Sexual Function Inventory is both a research and clinical assessment tool that can be included in a CGA (Mykletun, Dahl, O'Leary, & Fosså, 2006). The Female Sexual Function Index (Rosen et al., 2000) includes domains of desire, subjective arousal, lubrication, orgasm, satisfaction, and pain and can be used as a clinical instrument.

Creating a nonthreatening environment in which to assess issues of sexuality can help promote productive discussion. Consulting a social worker or psychologist who is experienced in the science of sexual dysfunction is another option for patient evaluation and assistance.

Caregiver Considerations

Having a caregiver can be critical for the older adult with cancer receiving oncologic treatment. A classic study found that lack of transportation is a chief reason many people do not receive cancer treatment (Goodwin, Hunt, & Samet, 1991). Conversely, many older patients with cancer are caregivers to other people. Asking questions about the availability of a caregiver who is able to be present in the home is important to the plan of care. For some patients who are starting treatment, a caregiver is neither needed nor present in the home. Proactively identifying potential caregivers who could spend reasonable time providing transportation and performing essential tasks such as housekeeping and cooking can be an important element to the plan of care.

The strain and stress of daily medical treatments and the effects of chemotherapy can be overwhelming for some caregivers. The Modified Caregiver Strain Index (CSI) is a reasonable assessment instrument to include in the CGA (Thornton & Travis, 2003) (see Figure 3-2). It is composed of 13 items, with a score of 0 meaning no strain and 26 meaning high strain. The CSI is recommended for use in older adults by the Hartford Geriatric Nursing Initiative as a clinical instrument for patient/caregiver assessment. The presence of caregiver strain can be challenging to address. It is important to work with patients and caregivers to anticipate problems that can lead to stressful situations and to develop strategies for resolutions that can affect QOL and effective cancer treatment.

Functional Status

Functional status refers to the ability to conduct everyday activities that maintain some degree of independence. Functional status is a key oncologic component of the CGA. It has been shown to be predictive of cancer treatment tolerance and is an important element when considering cancer treatment options and selection of participants for clinical trials (Garman & Cohen, 2002; Leonard & Malinovszky, 2005; Townsley, Selby, & Siu, 2005). Self-report methods of assessing functional status are the Activities of Daily Living scale (Katz, Downs, Cash, & Grotz, 1970) or the Independent Activities of Daily Living Scale (Lawton & Brody, 1969) (see Figure 3-3). The scales prompt the clinician to ask about concerns such as bathing, dressing, walking, and housework and require about five minutes to conduct. Changes in chemotherapy dosages or cycle timing can be augmented to accommodate failing functional status resulting from chemotherapy toxicity (Chen et al., 2003).

Proactive interventions in high-risk patients can help avoid further functional decline and chemotherapy dosage reductions or treatment delays. Decisions to maintain independence are best made at the beginning of functional decline and often require joint patient-healthcare team input in order to develop a realistic plan. Functional decline may first be noted when patients begin having problems performing activities of independence such as dress-

---

Figure 3-3. Assessment Instruments for Nonmalignant Concerns for Older Adults

Functional Status
- Activities of Daily Living (Katz et al., 1970)
- Instrumental Activities of Daily Living (Lawton & Brody, 1969)

Depression
- 5-Item Geriatric Depression Scale (Hoyl, Alessi, et al., 1999; Hoyl, Valenzuela, et al., 1999)

Cognitive Function
- Mini-Cog (Borson et al., 2000)

Falls
- *Clinical Practice Guideline: Prevention of Falls in Older Persons* (American Geriatrics Society and British Geriatrics Society Panel on the Clinical Practice Guideline on the Prevention of Falls in Older Persons, 2010)

---

ing, cooking, and walking. Once decisions are made and the care plan is formulated, ongoing assessments and subsequent treatment plan changes must be made to accommodate fluctuation in functional status.

Depression

More than 6.5 million Americans who are 65 years old or older are diagnosed with depression (National Alliance on Mental Illness, 2009). Depression can be very common in newly diagnosed patients with cancer (Filipović et al., 2007). Prevalence of a depressive disorder in patients with cancer is approximately 24% (Mitchell et al., 2011). The emotional state of the older adult with cancer is a critical element in the comprehensive assessment (Mitchell et al., 2011; Patrick et al., 2004). In patients with metastatic breast cancer, depression has been found to be associated with alterations in autonomic regulation such as respiratory sinus arrhythmia (Giese-Davis et al., 2006), alterations in breast cancer surgery recovery (Caban et al., 2006), and lower patient satisfaction regarding quality of medical care (Bui, Ostir, Kuo, Freeman, & Goodwin, 2005).

Identifying depression and associated risk factors is within the scope of practice for the nurse taking care of the older adult (Pasquini et al., 2006), and early intervention can be vital to the patient's QOL (Akechi et al., 2006). Risk factors for depression include age, poor general health, decreased feeling of well-being, social isolation, and neuroticism (de Jonge et al., 2006). Other risk factors include lower socioeconomic level, a change in marital status, inability to work, and pain (McCorkle, Tang, Greenwald, Holcombe, & Lavery, 2006).

The Geriatric Depression Scale (GDS) is a 15-item "yes" and "no" scale that helps clinicians screen for depression. More than five items scored as indicating depression are considered a positive screen, and the patient should be referred for additional diagnostic assessment (Yesavage et al., 1982–1983). A five-item short form, developed from the GDS, is also available and is very quick to administer (Hoyl, Alessi, et al., 1999).

Cognitive Function

Dementia screening is important to the care of the older adult with cancer. Determining if the dementia is a result of a metastatic process, previous treatment with chemotherapy or radiation therapy, or a comorbid condition is important when planning oncologic treatment. Dementia has been found to be a predictor of postoperative complications (Fukuse, Satoda, Hijiya, & Fujinaga, 2005), a barrier to curative cancer treatment (Gorin et al., 2005; Louwman et al., 2005), and a predictor of one-year mortality in patients who are in a nursing home (van Dijk et al., 2005).

The CGA can help the nurse and healthcare team determine the cognitive limitations associated with dementia and the extent to which the patient can participate in cancer treatment decisions. Dementia may be accompanied by delirium that can magnify cognitive dependency. The Mini-Cog is an assessment instrument that combines the clock-drawing test with a three-item recall. The three-item recall is an assessment of short-term memory and is used as part of the Mini-Mental State Exam (Folstein, Folstein, & McHugh, 1975). It is a valid and reliable clinical instrument that can help to detect dementia and is recommended by the Hartford Geriatric Nursing Initiative for clinical assessment and patient care.

Interventions to measure dementia are generally specific to the type of dementia. For some patients, cancer therapies or disease processes can cause dementia, and by treating the cause, the cognitive changes may improve.

Falls

The general definition of a fall considers the experience of unintentionally dropping to the ground for reasons other than trauma or loss of consciousness (Kellogg International Work Group, 1987). In 2003, falls accounted for approximately 13,000 deaths in the United States for people age 65 years and older, and from 2001 to 2005, the data for fall-related mortality were unchanged (Centers for Disease Control and Prevention, 2006). A 21% mortality rate exists for older patients who undergo internal reduction of a hip resulting from trauma associated with a fall (Vidal, Coeli, Pinheiro, & Camargo, 2006).

For patients with a diagnosis of cancer, falls can be related to fatigue and anemia, which are often associated with cancer treatment (Holley, 2002). Issues such as bone metastasis, neuropathy, dementia, and general weakness can also contribute to a fall (Bylow et al., 2008; Tofthagen, Overcash, & Kip, 2011). Injury from a fall can further complicate treatment and QOL of the older adult with cancer. Falls can be reflective of frailty and other comorbidities such as depression (Tinetti & Williams, 1998; Turcu et al., 2004).

The occurrence of prior falls can be assessed by asking whether a fall has occurred within the last year (American Geriatrics Society and British Geriatrics Society Panel on the Clinical Practice Guideline for the Prevention of Falls in Older Persons, 2010). Often, healthcare decisions concerning the patient who has a history of falls and is at risk for future falls focus on safety in the home and community. Including an assessment for falls as a component in the CGA can provide an important panorama to clinicians developing the plan of care.

Geriatric Syndromes

Geriatric syndromes are health concerns that are multifactorial and rather complex. Issues such as skin breakdown, functional impairment, incontinence, and many other challenging problems are examples of geriatric syndromes. Generally, the three most common geriatric syndromes in outpatient care are dementia, depression, and gait problems (Boongird, Thamakaison, & Krairit, 2010). Older patients with cancer who have been diagnosed with geriatric syndromes are unlikely to undergo surgical intervention, and the presence of two or more geriatric syndromes is associated with poor survival outcomes (Koroukian, 2009; Koroukian et al., 2010). The probability of acquiring geriatric syndromes is associated with age, with people who are older than 85 being at greatest risk (Koroukian, Murray, & Madigan, 2006).

Rapid Assessment Instruments to Include in a Comprehensive Geriatric Assessment

Conducting a CGA can often require more time in comparison to the traditional assessments performed in the ambulatory oncology setting. Medicare does not reimburse at a higher rate for the additional time spent on conducting a CGA. One timesaving option is to use instruments in the CGA that are brief and require only a few minutes to administer. *Rapid assessment technique* refers to options that shorten or accelerate the evaluation process. Clinical instruments such as the Timed Up and Go (Podsiadlo & Richardson, 1991), grip strength measurement with dynamometer (Rantanen et al., 2003), Five-Item Geriatric Depression Scale (Hoyl, Valenzuela, & Marin, 1999), and Clock Drawing Test (Cohen et al., 1993) are all examples of practical instruments that can be included in the CGA and require minimal time to complete. When constructing a CGA for ambulatory cancer care, it is important to consider respondent burden and the feasibility of completing all of the assessment instruments at one visit.

Another option to expedite the CGA process is to send the instrument to the patient via post or e-mail prior to the initial clinic visit. Self-administered assessment instruments can be reliable and returned with the patient at the clinical visit (Ingram et al., 2002; Stuck et al., 2002). Phone administration is an option for several of the commonly used CGA instruments. The Activities of Daily Living Scale (Katz et al., 1970) and the GDS have both been shown to be valid and reliable when administered to patients via the telephone (Burke, Roccaforte, Wnegel, Conley, & Potter, 1995; Ciesla, Stoskopf, & Samuels, 1993). Another prescreening measure is the Abbreviated Comprehensive Geriatric Assessment (aCGA) (Overcash et al., 2005). The aCGA considers three domains: (a) depression as measured by the GDS, (b) cognition as measured by the MMSE, and (c) functional status as measured by Activities of Daily Living Scale and the Instrumental Activities of Daily Living (Lawton & Brody, 1969). Prescreening measures such as the aCGA can help to identify patients who may benefit from more extensive screening with the CGA and patients who are fit and most likely will not benefit from a CGA.

Case Study Application of the Comprehensive Geriatric Assessment

Presentation

Mrs. S presents to the ambulatory care clinic at the regional cancer center. At 70 years old, Mrs. S was diagnosed with breast cancer, underwent lumpectomy, and is maintained on antihormonal therapy. In addition to breast cancer, Mrs. S has osteoporosis, hypertension, and hyperlipidemia. Mrs. S reported some complaints, including the inability to maintain sleep throughout the night, occasional urinary frequency at night, and several near falls. Mrs. S recently became widowed when her husband of many years passed away. Mrs. S is active, playing golf three times per week, playing occasional tennis, and walking each morning with friends in her retirement community. Over the past three weeks, Mrs. S has become less active and is grieving the loss of her husband. Mrs. S told the oncology ambulatory nurse that there is little reason for her to continue her antihormonal therapy. Mrs. S states she feels lonely and nervous since the death of her husband.

Assessment

Overt problems detected in this case study are potential depression, potential for falls, urinary urgency and potential incontinence, and sleep disorder, in addition to osteoporosis, hypertension, and hyperlipidemia. Detection of such health problems necessitates screening with valid and reliable instruments. When the screening tools are positive for problems, further diagnostics must be arranged.

The ambulatory care oncology nurse, along with the other members of the healthcare team, can select instruments to incorporate in the CGA. Mrs. S said that she intends to discontinue her antihormonal therapy and states, "I have nothing to live for." Mrs. S has been grieving her husband and has detached from her usual activities. Sleep difficulties are another limitation requiring further assessment. The GDS is useful to screen for depression.

Deciding when to readminister the CGA is important. As in this situation, assessment should occur at various intervals of cancer treatment. Often the intervals of assessment are at the initiation of cancer treatment, at some time midpoint, and after treatment is complete (Extermann, 2003a, 2003b; Extermann et al., 2004; Repetto et al., 2002). When using many instruments, it may be prudent to assess the patient with some of the questionnaires on one clinic visit and save the remaining for the following visit or provide the instruments prior to the clinical visit. Overburdening the patient with multiple questions should be avoided.

In reviewing the tools included in the CGA, the GDS was positive for depression, and the PSQI found that Mrs. S was falling asleep in 30 minutes or less but not remaining asleep. Frequent urination during the night was a problem in her sleep routine. The PSQI suggested that sleepiness would occur when lying and resting in the afternoon, and napping accentuated the sleep problem at night. The Urinary Incontinence Assessment in Older Adults revealed no incontinence, but clinical assessment revealed a urinary tract infection. The Fall Risk Assessment suggested that depressive symptoms were the most likely risk for falls.

Implementation of a Treatment Plan

After discussion at the team conference, Mrs. S was sent to psychosocial oncology for further diagnostics and treatment of depression. Urinalysis, culture, and sensitivity were obtained and found to be positive for more than 100,000 white blood cells. Mrs. S was prescribed sulfamethoxazole, two tablets orally twice daily for seven days. Because frequent urination and depression may be the culprits for the sleep problems, no other medicine was prescribed at this time. Sleep will continue to be monitored. The patient was encouraged to verbalize feelings of grief concerning the loss of her husband. Education was provided to the patient regarding breast cancer treatment and her probability of cancer recurrence with and without hormonal therapy.

The primary care nurse in the ambulatory oncology clinic communicated with the primary care provider (PCP). The PCP will follow the patient for fall risk, urinary tract infection, and any further signs and symptoms of depression in addition to the comorbid conditions. The oncology team recommended that the patient continue her antihormonal therapy to reduce the probability of cancer recurrence. The patient was asked to return to the oncology clinic in three months for evaluation of her cancer and nonmalignant problems.

Decisions made as a result of the CGA were to

- Diagnose and treat depression, which can potentially interfere with cancer treatment
- Treat a urinary tract infection, which could increase the occurrence of falls and urinary incontinence
- Not prescribe any additional sleep medications but to treat the underlying causes
- Communicate with the PCP
- Have fall risk monitored by the PCP.

The healthcare team's treatment decisions to manage the nonmalignant conditions were essential to the cancer treatment plan. Mrs. S was considering discontinuing antihormonal therapy because she was grieving the loss of her husband and because of lack of knowledge about her cancer diagnosis. Providing information and allowing grieving helped the patient make reasonable decisions about cancer treatment.

Follow-Up and Outcomes

Another important element of using the CGA in making cancer treatment decisions is the establishment of follow-up care (Cefalu, Kaslow, Mims, & Simpson, 1995). Interventions as a result of an outpatient CGA can be difficult to evaluate (Stuck et al., 2002). Healthcare treatment decisions are often based on the notion that patients will adhere to the interventions established in the treatment plan. Patients are less likely to comply with the treatment plan if a high number of recommendations are presented and if they have inadequate caregiver support (Bogardus et al., 2004; Esmail, Brazil, & Lam, 2000). Ambulatory care oncology nurses can develop a specific patient follow-up schedule to facilitate patient adherence with treatment plans.

For Mrs. S, the patient follow-up schedule consisted of the ambulatory care oncology nurse making monthly calls to assess for medication adherence and side effects. Mrs. S reported that she was taking her medication daily and expressed gratitude to the nurse and her healthcare team for their thorough evaluation and care that has improved her QOL.

Conclusion

The CGA is a versatile and practical instrument that is a beneficial addition to an ambulatory oncology care practice. Understanding the extent of health and psychosocial limitations is vital so that they can be addressed. Enhancing the opportunity to undergo and complete more aggressive cancer therapy is a function of the CGA. Taking the time to make the CGA part of the ambulatory oncology nursing care process will culminate in better care and improved patient outcomes for older adults with cancer and their caregivers.

References

Aaldriks, A.A., Maartense, E., le Cessie, S., Giltay, J., Verlaan, H.A., van der Geest, L.G., ... Nortier, J.W. (2011). Predictive value of geriatric assessment for patients older than 70 years, treated with chemotherapy. *Critical Reviews in Oncology/Hematology, 79,* 205–212. doi:10.1016/j.critrevonc.2010.05.009

American Geriatrics Society and British Geriatrics Society Panel on the Clinical Practice Guideline for the Prevention of Falls in Older Persons. (2010). *Clinical practice guideline: Prevention of falls in older persons.* Retrieved from http://www.americangeriatrics.org/files/documents/health_care_pros/Falls.Summary.Guide.pdf

Akechi, T., Akizuki, N., Okamura, M., Shimizu, K., Oba, A., Ito, T., ... Uchitomi, Y. (2006). Psychological distress experienced by families of cancer patients: Preliminary findings from psychiatric consultation of a cancer center hospital. *Japanese Journal of Clinical Oncology, 36,* 329–332. doi:10.1093/jjco/hyl029

Audisio, R.A., Pope, D., Ramesh, H.S., Gennari, R., van Leeuwen, B.L., West, C., ... Marshall, E. (2008). Shall we operate? Preoperative assessment in elderly cancer patients (PACE) can help. A SIOG surgical task force prospective study. *Critical Reviews in Oncology/Hematology, 65,* 156–163. doi:10.1016/j.critrevonc.2007.11.001

Balducci, L., Colloca, G., Cesari, M., & Gambassi, G. (2010). Assessment and treatment of elderly patients with cancer. *Surgical Oncology, 19,* 117–123. doi:10.1016/j.suronc.2009.11.008

Bogardus, S.T., Jr., Bradley, E.H., Williams, C.S., Maciejewski, P.K., Gallo, W.T., & Inouye, S.K. (2004). Achieving goals in geriatric assessment: Role of caregiver agreement and adherence to recommendations. *Journal of the American Geriatrics Society, 52,* 99–105. doi:10.1111/j.1532-5415.2004.52017.x

Boongird, C., Thamakaison, S., & Krairit, O. (2010). Impact of a geriatric assessment clinic on organizational interventions in primary health-care facilities at a university hospital. *Geriatrics and Gerontology International, 10,* 204–210. doi:10.1111/j.1447-0594.2010.00671.x

Borson, S., Scanlon, J., Brush, M., Vitallano, P., & Dolmak, A. (2000). The Mini-Cog: A cognitive "vital signs" measure for dementia screening in multi-lingual elderly. *International Journal of Geriatric Psychiatry, 15,* 1021–1027. doi:10.1002/1099-1166(200011)15:11<1021::AID-GPS234>3.0.CO;2-6

Bui, Q.U., Ostir, G.V., Kuo, Y.F., Freeman, J., & Goodwin, J.S. (2005). Relationship of depression to patient satisfaction: Findings from the barriers to breast cancer study. *Breast Cancer Research and Treatment, 89,* 23–28. doi:10.1007/s10549-004-1005-9

Burke, W.J., Roccaforte, W.H., Wnegel, S.P., Conley, D.M., & Potter, J.F. (1995). The reliability and validity of the Geriatric Depression Rating Scale administered by telephone. *Journal of the American Geriatrics Society, 43,* 674–679.

Butt, Z., Rao, A.V., Lai, J.S., Abernethy, A.P., Rosenbloom, S.K., & Cella, D. (2010). Age-associated differences in fatigue among patients with cancer. *Journal of Pain and Symptom Management, 40,* 217–223. doi:10.1016/j.jpainsymman.2009.12.016

Buysse, D.J., Reynolds, C.F., III, Monk, T.H., Berman, S.R., & Kupfer, D.J. (1989). The Pittsburgh Sleep Quality Index: A new instrument for psychiatric practice and research. *Psychiatry Research, 28,* 193–213. doi:10.1016/0165-1781(89)90047-4

Bylow, K., Dale, W., Mustian, K., Stadler, W.M., Rodin, M., Hall, W., ... Mohile, S.G. (2008). Falls and physical performance deficits in older patients with prostate cancer undergoing androgen deprivation therapy. *Urology, 72,* 422–427. doi:10.1016/j.urology.2008.03.032

Caban, M.E., Freeman, J.L., Zhang, D.D., Jansen, C., Ostir, G., Hatch, S.S., & Goodwin, J.S. (2006). The relationship between depressive symptoms and shoulder mobility among older women: Assessment at one year after breast cancer diagnosis. *Clinical Rehabilitation, 20,* 513–522. doi:10.1191/0269215506cr966oa

Centers for Disease Control and Prevention. (2006, November 15). Fatalities and injuries from falls among older adults—United States, 1993–2003 and 2001–2005. *MMWR: Morbidity and Mortality Weekly Report, 55,* 1221–1224. Retrieved from http://www.cdc.gov/mmwr/preview/mmwrhtml/mm5545a1.htm

Cefalu, C.A., Kaslow, L.D., Mims, B., & Simpson, S. (1995). Follow-up of comprehensive geriatric assessment in a family medicine residency clinic. *Journal of the American Board of Family Practice, 8,* 337–340.

Chen, H., Cantor, A., Meyer, J., Corcoran, M.B., Grendys, E., Cavanaugh, D., ... Extermann, M. (2003). Can older cancer patients tolerate chemotherapy? A prospective pilot study. *Cancer, 97,* 1107–1114. doi:10.1002/cncr.11110

Cheng, K.K.F., & Lee, D.T.F. (2011). Effects of pain, fatigue, insomnia, and mood disturbance on functional status and quality of life of elderly patients with cancer. *Critical Reviews in Oncology/Hematology, 78,* 127–137. doi:10.1016/j.critrevonc.2010.03.002

Ciesla, J.R., Stoskopf, C.H., & Samuels, M.E. (1993). Reliability of Katz's Activities of Daily Living Scale when used in telephone interviews. *Evaluation and the Health Professions, 16,* 190–203.

Cleeland, C. (1991). Research in cancer pain. What we know and what we need to know. *Cancer, 67*(3 Suppl.), 823–827. doi:10.1002/1097-0142(19910201)67:3+<823::AID-CNCR2820671412>3.0.CO;2-S

Cohen, C.A., Gold, D.P., Shulman, K.I., Wortley, J.T., McDonald, G., & Wargon, M. (1993). Factors determining the decision to institutionalize dementing individuals: A prospective study. *Gerontologist, 33,* 714–720.

De Conno, F., Caraceni, A., Gamba, A., Mariani, L., Abbattista, A., Brunelli, C., ... Ventifridda, V. (1994). Pain measurement in cancer patients: A comparison of six methods. *Pain, 57,* 161–166. doi:10.1016/0304-3959(94)90219-4

de Jonge, P., Kempen, G.I., Sanderman, R., Ranchor, A.V., van Jaarsveld, C.H., van Sonderen, E., ... Ormel, J. (2006). Depressive symptoms in elderly patients after a somatic illness event: Prevalence, persistence, and risk factors. *Psychosomatics, 47,* 33–42. doi:10.1176/appi.psy.47.1.33

Derogatis, L.R., & Kourlesis, S.M. (1981). An approach to evaluation of sexual problems in the cancer patient. *CA: A Cancer Journal for Clinicians, 31,* 46–50. doi:10.3322/canjclin.31.1.46

Enderlin, C.A., Coleman, E.A., Cole, C., Richards, K.C., Hutchins, L.F., & Sherman, A.C. (2010). Sleep across chemotherapy treatment: A growing concern for women older than 50 with breast cancer. *Oncology Nursing Forum, 37,* 461–468. doi:10.1188/10.ONF.461-468

Esmail, R., Brazil, K., & Lam, M. (2000). Short report: Compliance with recommendations in a geriatric outreach assessment service. *Age and Ageing, 29,* 353–356. doi:10.1093/ageing/29.4.353

Extermann, M. (2003a). Comprehensive geriatric assessment basics for the cancer professional. *Journal of Oncology Management, 12*(2), 13–17.

Extermann, M. (2003b). Studies of comprehensive geriatric assessment in patients with cancer. *Cancer Control, 10,* 463–468.

Extermann, M., Meyer, J., McGinnis, M., Crocker, T.T., Corcoran, M., Yoder, J., ... Balducci, L. (2004). A comprehensive geriatric intervention detects multiple problems in older breast cancer patients. *Critical Reviews in Oncology/Hematology, 49,* 69–75. doi:10.1016/S1040-8428(03)00099-4

Eyigor, S., Eyigor, C., & Uslu, R. (2009). Assessment of pain, fatigue, sleep and quality of life (QoL) in elderly hospitalized cancer patients. *Archives of Gerontology and Geriatrics, 51,* 57–61. doi:10.1016/j.archger.2009.11.018

Filipović, B.R., Filipović, B.F., Kerkez, M., Milinić, N., & Ranđelović, T. (2007). Depression and anxiety levels in therapy-naive patients with inflammatory bowel disease and cancer of the colon. *World Journal of Gastroenterology, 13,* 438–443. Retrieved from http://www.wjgnet.com/1007-9327/full/v13/i3/438.htm

Folstein, M., Folstein, S.E., & McHugh, P.R. (1975). "Mini-mental state": A practical method for grading the cognitive state of patients for the clinician. *Journal of Psychiatric Research, 12,* 189–198. doi:10.1016/0022-3956(75)90026-6

Fried, L.P., Tangen, C.M., Walston, J., Newman, A.B., Hirsch, C., Gottdiener, J., ... McBurnie, M.A. (2001). Frailty in older adults: Evidence for a phenotype. *Journals of Gerontology: Series A, Biological Sciences and Medical Sciences, 56*(3), M146–M156.

Fukuse, T., Satoda, N., Hijiya, K., & Fujinaga, T. (2005). Importance of a comprehensive geriatric assessment in prediction of complications following thoracic surgery in elderly patients. *Chest, 127,* 886–891. doi:10.1378/chest.127.3.886

Garman, K.S., & Cohen, H.J. (2002). Functional status and the elderly cancer patient. *Critical Reviews in Oncology/Hematology, 43,* 191–208. doi:10.1016/S1040-8428(02)00062-8

Giese-Davis, J., Wilhelm, F.H., Conrad, A., Abercrombie, H.C., Sephton, S., Yutsis, M., ... Spiegel, D. (2006). Depression and stress reactivity in metastatic breast cancer. *Psychosomatic Medicine, 68,* 675–683. doi:10.1097/01.psy.0000238216.88515.e5

Goodwin, J.S., Hunt, W.C., & Samet, J.M. (1991). A population-based study of functional status and social support networks of elderly patients newly diagnosed with cancer. *Archives of Internal Medicine, 151,* 366–370. doi:10.1001/archinte.151.2.366

Goodwin, J.S., Hunt, W.C., & Samet, J.M. (1993). Determinants of cancer therapy in elderly patients. *Cancer, 72,* 594–601. doi:10.1002/1097-0142(19930715)72:2<594::AID-CNCR2820720243>3.0.CO;2-#

Gorin, S.S., Heck, J.E., Albert, S., & Hershman, D. (2005). Treatment for breast cancer in patients with Alzheimer's disease. *Journal of the American Geriatrics Society, 53,* 1897–1904. doi:10.1111/j.1532-5415.2005.00467.x

Grov, E.K., Fosså, S.D., & Dahl, A.A. (2010). Insomnia in elderly cancer survivors—A population-based controlled study of associations with lifestyle, morbidity, and psychosocial factors. Results from the Health Survey of North Trondelag County (HUNT-2): Insomnia in elderly cancer survivors [Online version]. *Supportive Care in Cancer.* Retrieved from http://www.springerlink.com/content/g572q27035887m63/fulltext.pdf

Holley, S. (2002). A look at the problem of falls among people with cancer. *Clinical Journal of Oncology Nursing, 6,* 193–197. doi:10.1188/02.CJON.193-197

Hoyl, M.T., Alessi, C.A., Harker, J.O., Josephson, K.R., Pietruszka, F.M., Koelfgen, M., ... Rubenstein, L.Z. (1999). Development and testing of a five-item version of the Geriatric Depression Scale. *Journal of the American Geriatrics Society, 47,* 873-878.

Hoyl, T., Valenzuela, E., & Marin, P.P. (1999). [Depression in the aged: Preliminary evaluation of the effectiveness, as a screening instrument, of the 5-item version of the Geriatric Depression Scale]. *Reviews in Medicine Chilean, 128,* 1199–1204.

Hurria, A., Lachs, M.S., Cohen, H.J., Muss, H.B., & Kornblith, A.B. (2006). Geriatric assessment for oncologists: Rationale and future directions. *Critical Reviews in Oncology/Hematology, 59,* 211–217. doi:10.1016/j.critrevonc.2006.03.007

Hurria, A., Lichtman, S.M., Gardes, J., Li, D., Limaye, S., Patil, S., ... Kelly, E. (2007). Identifying vulnerable older adults with cancer: integrating geriatric assessment into oncology practice. *Journal of the American Geriatrics Society, 55,* 1604–1608. doi:10.1111/j.1532-5415.2007.01367.x

Ingram, S.S., Seo, P.H., Martell, R.E., Clipp, E.C., Doyle, M.E., Montana, G.S., & Cohen, H.J. (2002). Comprehensive assessment of the elderly cancer patient: The feasibility of self-report methodology. *Journal of Clinical Oncology, 20,* 770–775. doi:10.1200/JCO.20.3.770

Iversen, L.H., Nørgaard, M., Jacobsen, J., Laurberg, S., & Sørensen, H.T. (2009). The impact of comorbidity on survival of Danish colorectal cancer patients from 1995 to 2006—A population-based cohort study. *Diseases of the Colon and Rectum, 52,* 71–78. doi:10.1007/DCR.0b013e3181974384

Katz, S., Downs, T.D., Cash, H.R., & Grotz, R.C. (1970). Progress in the development of the index of ADL. *Gerontologist, 10,* 20–30.

Kellogg International Work Group. (1987). The prevention of falls in later life: A report of the Kellogg International Work Group on the Prevention of Falls by the Elderly. *Danish Medical Bulletin, 34*(Suppl. 4), 1–24.

Kim, E.J., & Buschmann, M.T. (2006). Reliability and validity of the Faces Pain Scale with older adults. *International Journal of Nursing Studies, 43,* 447–456. doi:10.1016/j.ijnurstu.2006.01.001

Koffel, E., & Watson, D. (2010). Development and initial validation of the Iowa Sleep Disturbances Inventory. *Assessment, 17,* 423–439. doi:10.1177/1073191110362864

Koroukian, S.M. (2009). Assessment and interpretation of comorbidity burden in older adults with cancer. *Journal of the American Geriatrics Society, 57*(Suppl. 2), S275–S278. doi:10.1111/j.1532-5415.2009.02511.x

Koroukian, S.M., Murray, P., & Madigan, E. (2006). Comorbidity, disability, and geriatric syndromes in elderly cancer patients receiving home health care. *Journal of Clinical Oncology, 24*, 2304–2310. doi:10.1200/JCO.2005.03.1567

Koroukian, S.M., Xu, F., Bakaki, P.M., Diaz-Insua, M., Towe, T.P., & Owusu, C. (2010). Comorbidities, functional limitations, and geriatric syndromes in relation to treatment and survival patterns among elders with colorectal cancer. *Journals of Gerontology: Series A, Biological Sciences and Medical Sciences, 65*, 322–329. doi:10.1093/gerona/glp180

Kozyrskyi, A.L., Black, C., Chateau, D., & Steinbach, C. (2005). Discharge outcomes in seniors hospitalized for more than 30 days. *Canadian Journal on Aging, 24*(Suppl. 1), 107–119. doi:10.1353/cja.2005.0048

Kristjansson, S.R., Nesbakken, A., Jordhoy, M.S., Skovlund, E., Audisio, R.A., Johannessen, H.O., … Wyller, T.B. (2010). Comprehensive geriatric assessment can predict complications in elderly patients after elective surgery for colorectal cancer: A prospective observational cohort study. *Critical Reviews in Oncology/Hematology, 76*, 208–217. doi:10.1016/j.critrevonc.2009.11.002

Lawton, M.P., & Brody, E.M. (1969). Assessment of older people: Self-maintaining and instrumental activities of daily living. *Gerontologist, 9*, 179–186.

Leonard, R.C., & Malinovszky, K.M. (2005). Chemotherapy for older women with early breast cancer. *Clinical Oncology, 17*, 244–248. doi:10.1016/j.clon.2005.02.002

Louwman, W.J., Janssen-Heijnen, M.L., Houterman, S., Voogd, A.C., van der Sangen, M.J., Nieuwenhuijzen, G.A., & Coebergh, J.W. (2005). Less extensive treatment and inferior prognosis for breast cancer patient with comorbidity: A population-based study. *European Journal of Cancer, 41*, 779–785. doi:10.1016/j.ejca.2004.12.025

Luciani, A., Jacobsen, P.B., Extermann, M., Foa, P., Marussi, D., Overcash, J.A., & Balducci, L. (2008). Fatigue and functional dependence in older cancer patients. *American Journal of Clinical Oncology, 31*, 424–430. doi:10.1097/COC.0b013e31816d915f

McCorkle, R., Tang, S.T., Greenwald, H., Holcombe, G., & Lavery, M. (2006). Factors related to depressive symptoms among long-term survivors of cervical cancer. *Health Care for Women International, 27*, 45–58. doi:10.1080/07399330500377507

Mitchell, A.J., Chan, M., Bhatti, H., Halton, M., Grassi, L., Johansen, C., & Meader, M. (2011). Prevalence of depression, anxiety and adjustment disorder in oncological, haematological, and palliative-care settings: A meta-analysis of 94 interview-based studies. *Lancet Oncology, 12*, 160–174. doi:10.1016/S1470-2045(11)70002-X

Morin, C.M., Belleville, G., Bélanger, L., & Ivers, H. (2011). The Insomnia Severity Index: Psychometric indicators to detect insomnia cases and evaluate treatment response. *Sleep, 34*, 601–608.

Mykletun, A., Dahl, A.A., O'Leary, M.P., & Fosså, S.D. (2006). Assessment of male sexual function by the Brief Sexual Function Inventory. *BJU International, 97*, 316–323. doi:10.1111/j.1464-410X.2005.05904.x

National Alliance on Mental Illness. (2009, October). Depression in older persons fact sheet. Retrieved from http://www.nami.org/Template.cfm?Section=Depression&Template=/ContentManagement/ContentDisplay.cfm&ContentID=88876

National Cancer Institute. (2010, January 8). Sleep disorders (PDQ®) [Patient version]. Retrieved from http://www.cancer.gov/cancertopics/pdq/supportivecare/sleepdisorders

National Cancer Institute. (2011, June 16). Fatigue PDQ® [Health professional version]. Retrieved from http://www.cancer.gov/cancertopics/pdq/supportivecare/fatigue/HealthProfessional/page1

National Comprehensive Cancer Network. (2011a). *NCCN Clinical Practice Guidelines in Oncology: Cancer-related fatigue* [v.1.2011]. Retrieved from http://www.nccn.org/professionals/physician_gls/pdf/fatigue.pdf

National Comprehensive Cancer Network. (2011b). *NCCN Clinical Practice Guidelines in Oncology: Senior adult oncology* [v.2.2011]. Retrieved from http://www.nccn.org/professionals/physician_gls/pdf/senior.pdf

Nelson, C.J., Choi, J.M., Mulhall, J.P., & Roth, A.J. (2007). Determinants of sexual satisfaction in men with prostate cancer. *Journal of Sexual Medicine, 4,* 1422–1427. doi:10.1111/j.1743-6109.2007.00547.x

Overcash, J. (2007). Prediction of falls in older adults with cancer: A preliminary study. *Oncology Nursing Forum, 34,* 341–346. doi:10.1188/07.ONF.341-346

Overcash, J.A. (2008). Health needs of the older cancer patient: Constructing a comprehensive geriatric assessment. *Advance for Nurse Practitioner, 16,* 53–54, 56–58.

Overcash, J.A., & Beckstead, J. (2008). Predicting falls in older patients using components of a comprehensive geriatric assessment. *Clinical Journal of Oncology Nursing, 12,* 941–949. doi:10.1188/08.CJON.941-949

Overcash, J.A., Beckstead, J., Extermann, M., & Cobb, S. (2005). The abbreviated comprehensive geriatric assessment (aCGA): A retrospective analysis. *Critical Reviews in Oncology/Hematology, 54,* 129–136. doi:10.1016/j.critrevonc.2004.12.002

Pasquini, M., Biondi, M., Costantini, A., Cairoli, F., Ferrarese, G., Picardi, A., & Sternberg, C. (2006). Detection and treatment of depressive and anxiety disorders among cancer patients: Feasibility and preliminary findings from a liaison service in an oncology division. *Depression and Anxiety, 23,* 441–448. doi:10.1002/da.20198

Patrick, D.L., Ferketich, S.L., Frame, P.S., Harris, J.J., Hendricks, C.B., Levin, B., ... Vernon, S.W. (2004). National Institutes of Health State-of-the-Science Conference Statement: Symptom management in cancer: Pain, depression, and fatigue, July 15–17, 2002. *Journal of the National Cancer Institute Monographs, 2004*(32), 9–16. doi:10.1093/jnci monographs/djg014

Patterson, R.E., Flatt, S.W., Saquib, N., Rock, C.L., Caan, B.J., Parker, B.A., ... Pierce, J.P. (2010). Medical comorbidities predict mortality in women with a history of early stage breast cancer. *Breast Cancer Research and Treatment, 122,* 859–865. doi:10.1007/s10549-010-0732-3

Podsiadlo, D., & Richardson, S. (1991). The timed "Up & Go": A test of basic functional mobility for frail elderly persons. *Journal of the American Geriatrics Society, 39,* 142–148.

Price, D.D., McGrath, P.A., Rafti, A., & Buckingham, B. (1983). The validation of visual analogue scales as ratio scale measures for chronic and experimental pain. *Pain, 17,* 45–56. doi:10.1016/0304-3959(83)90126-4

Rantanen, T., Volpato, S., Ferrucci, L., Heikkinen, E., Fried, L.P., & Guralnik, J.M. (2003). Handgrip strength and cause-specific and total mortality in older disabled women: Exploring the mechanism. *Journal of the American Geriatrics Society, 51,* 636–641. doi:10.1034/j.1600-0579.2003.00207.x

Reiner, A., & Lacasse, C. (2006). Symptom correlates in the gero-oncology population. *Seminars in Oncology Nursing, 22,* 20–30. doi:10.1016/j.soncn.2005.10.004

Repetto, L., Fratino, L., Audisio, R.A., Venturino, A., Gianni, W., Vercelli, M., ... Zagonel, V. (2002). Comprehensive geriatric assessment adds information to Eastern Cooperative Oncology Group performance status in elderly cancer patients: An Italian Group for Geriatric Oncology Study. *Journal of Clinical Oncology, 20,* 494–502. doi:10.1200/JCO.20.2.494

Rosen, R., Brown, C., Heiman, J., Leiblum, S., Meston, C., Shabsigh, R., ... D'Agostino, R., Jr. (2000). The Female Sexual Function Index (FSFI): A multidimensional self-report instrument for the assessment of female sexual function. *Journal of Sex and Marital Therapy, 26,* 191–208.

Shack, L.G., Rachet, B., Williams, E.M., Northover, J.M., & Coleman, M.P. (2010). Does the timing of comorbidity affect colorectal cancer survival? A population-based study. *Postgraduate Medical Journal, 86*(1012), 73–78. doi:10.1136/pgmj.2009.084566

Shell, J.A., Carolan, M., Zhang, Y., & Meneses, K.D. (2008). The longitudinal effects of cancer treatment on sexuality in individuals with lung cancer. *Oncology Nursing Forum, 35,* 73–79. doi:10.1188/08.ONF.73-79

Sikka, V., & Ornato, J.P. (in press). Cancer diagnosis and outcomes in Michigan EDs vs other settings. *American Journal of Emergency Medicine.* doi:10.1016/j.ajem.2010.11.029

So, W.K., Marsh, G., Ling, W.M., Leung, F.Y., Lo, J.C., Yeung, M., & Li, G.K. (2009). The symptom cluster of fatigue, pain, anxiety, and depression and the effect on the quality of life of women receiving treatment for breast cancer: A multicenter study [Online exclusive]. *Oncology Nursing Forum, 36,* E205–E214. doi:10.1188/09.ONF.E205-E214

Stuck, A.E., Elkuch, P., Dapp, U., Anders, J., Iiffe, S., & Swift, C.G. (2002). Feasibility and yield of a self-administered questionnaire for health risk appraisal in older people in three European countries. *Age and Ageing, 31,* 463–467. doi:10.1093/ageing/31.6.463

Thornton, M., & Travis, S.S. (2003). Analysis of the reliability of the modified caregiver strain index. *Journals of Gerontology: Series B. Psychological Sciences and Social Sciences, 58,* S127–S132.

Tinetti, M.E., & Williams, C.S. (1998). The effect of falls and fall injuries on functioning in community-dwelling older persons. *Journals of Gerontology: Series A. Biological Sciences and Medical Sciences, 53,* M112–M119.

Tofthagen, C., Overcash, J., & Kip, K. (2011). Falls in persons with chemotherapy-induced peripheral neuropathy. *Supportive Care in Cancer.* Advance online publication. doi:10.1007/s00520-011-1127-7

Tom, S.E., Kuh, D., Guralnik, J.M., & Mishra, G.D. (2010). Self-reported sleep difficulty during the menopausal transition: Results from a prospective cohort study. *Menopause, 17,* 1128–1135. doi:10.1097/gme.0b013e3181dd55b0

Townsley, C.A., Selby, R., & Siu, L.L. (2005). Systematic review of barriers to the recruitment of older patients with cancer onto clinical trials. *Journal of Clinical Oncology, 23,* 3112–3124. doi:10.1200/JCO.2005.00.141

Tucci, A., Ferrari, S., Bottelli, C., Borlenghi, E., Drera, M., & Rossi, G. (2009). A comprehensive geriatric assessment is more effective than clinical judgment to identify elderly diffuse large cell lymphoma patients who benefit from aggressive therapy. *Cancer, 115,* 4547–4553. doi:10.1002/cncr.24490

Turcu, A., Toubin, S., Mourey, F., D'Athis, P., Manckoundia, P., & Pfitzenmeyer, P. (2004). Falls and depression in older people. *Gerontology, 50,* 303–308. doi:10.1159/000079128

Van Belle, S., Paridaens, R., Evers, G., Kerger, J., Bron, D., Foubert, J., … Rosillon, D. (2005). Comparison of proposed diagnostic criteria with FACT-F and VAS for cancer-related fatigue: Proposal for use as a screening tool. *Supportive Care in Cancer, 13,* 246–254.

van Dijk, P.T., Mehr, D.R., Ooms, M.E., Madsen, R., Petroski, G., Frijters, D.H., … Ribbe, M.W. (2005). Comorbidity and 1-year mortality risks in nursing home residents. *Journal of the American Geriatrics Society, 53,* 660–665. doi:10.1111/j.1532-5415.2005.53216.x

Vidal, E.I., Coeli, C.M., Pinheiro, R.S., & Camargo, K.R., Jr. (2006). Mortality within 1 year after hip fracture surgical repair in the elderly according to postoperative period: A probabilistic record linkage study in Brazil. *Osteoporosis International, 17,* 1569–1576. doi:10.1007/s00198-006-0173-3

Yasmeen, S., Xing, G., Morris, C., Chlebowski, R.T., & Romano, P.S. (2011). Comorbidities and mammography use interact to explain racial/ethnic disparities in breast cancer stage at diagnosis. *Cancer.* Advance online publication. doi:10.1002/cncr.25857

Yellen, S.B., Cella, D.F., Webster, K., Blendowski, C., & Kaplan, E. (1997). Measuring fatigue and other anemia-related symptoms with the Functional Assessment of Cancer Therapy (FACT) measurement system. *Journal of Pain and Symptom Management, 13,* 63–74. doi:10.1016/S0885-3924(96)00274-6

Yennurajalingam, S., Urbauer, D.L., Casper, K.L., Reyes-Gibby, C.C., Chacko, R., Poulter, V., … Bruera, E. (2010). Impact of a palliative care consultation team on cancer-related symptoms in advanced cancer patients referred to an outpatient supportive care clinic. *Journal of Pain and Symptom Management, 41,* 49–56. doi:10.1016/j.jpainsymman.2010.03.017

Yesavage, J., Brink, T.L., Rose, T.L., Lum, O., Huang, V., Adey, M., & Leirer, V.O. (1982–1983). Development and validation of a geriatric depression scale: A preliminary report. *Journal of Psychiatric Research, 17,* 37–49.

CHAPTER 4

Symptom Management

Mary Elizabeth Davis, RN, MSN, AOCNS®, Susan A. Derby, RN, MA, GNP-BC, ACHPN, and Lorraine K. McEvoy, DNP, MSN, RN, OCN®

Introduction

The treatment of cancer in the older adult is made more complex by issues of diminished functional status, comorbid conditions, and altered physical, physiologic, and psychosocial capacity. For the older adult, activities of daily living (ADLs) can influence decision making related to cancer treatment. With a greater emphasis on ambulatory treatment and care, patients and their caregivers are participating as active members of the care team, and treatment decisions are made collaboratively. Inherent in these discussions are the extent of disease, treatment options, risks and benefits, and the goals and expectations of treatment. This is paralleled by an increased interest in choosing care that matches the patient's values and optimizes quality of life (QOL). The patient's chronologic age should not be the only determinant of cancer treatment.

Managing chronic conditions when cancer is not the only health concern becomes significant as cancer treatment planning is undertaken. As cancer treatment is planned, the patient care team should understand that symptoms may be a result of disease, cancer therapy, or a complex interaction with a preexisting condition. Understanding the interplay of aging, comorbidities, and cancer allows ambulatory care oncology nurses to anticipate patients' needs and effectively manage the competing demands for treatment and care. Interaction among symptoms may exist, or symptoms may present simultaneously. Treatment side effects may be more severe and debilitating in older adults, resulting in compromised function, delayed recovery, more frequent hospital admissions, increased length of stay, and loss of independent living (Berg, 2006).

When care is delivered in an ambulatory setting, significant demands will be placed on patients and caregivers. Nurses should include patients and caregivers in the care plan development and provide education to make self-care possible. All efforts should be directed at preventing, promptly recognizing, and intervening with and controlling problems as they arise. The collaborative multidisciplinary team's goals are to maintain patients' functional status and independence consistent with their usual pattern of living, minimize disruptions to the treatment protocol, and facilitate care delivery.

This chapter will provide oncology nurses in the ambulatory care setting a framework for addressing symptom management in the older adult with cancer. The principles for symptom management are similar to those in other care settings; however, the ambulatory care setting presents unique challenges. Patient visits are time limited, and patients are often anxious and stressed. Time dedicated to teaching is often less than optimal, and the complexity of older adults' care needs can be overwhelming. In the outpatient setting, assessments are often conducted over the telephone with only verbal reports from the patient or caregiver to guide the nurse's appraisal of the situation and intervention. Knowledge of common and significant symptoms associated with the treatment of cancer in older adults and their interrelatedness to aging is necessary to develop interventions to minimize severity, reduce distress, maintain level of function, and improve QOL. This chapter will discuss anorexia and weight loss, cognitive impairment, constipation, dehydration, dysphagia, dyspnea, fatigue, pain, and sexuality.

Anorexia and Weight Loss

Overview

Maintaining weight and adequate nutrition is integral to supporting the older adult through cancer treatment. Although the prevalence toward weight gain and obesity in older adults has increased nationally with an estimated 20.9 million obese elder Americans in 2010 (Arterburn, Crane, & Sullivan, 2004), a more common problem for older adults with cancer is weight loss. Older adults have a more prolonged response to acute malnutrition: once weight is lost, they are likely to take longer to regain the lost weight, remain undernourished longer, and be more susceptible to infections (Visvanathan & Chapman, 2009).

Weight loss leading to malnutrition diminishes an individual's ability to tolerate cancer treatment and causes more profound disease- and treatment-related toxicities (Adams, Shepard, et al., 2009). In a classic analysis of more than 3,000 patients with cancer enrolled in Eastern Cooperative Oncology Group protocols, weight loss was associated with lower response rates to chemotherapy and decreased survival (Dewys et al., 1980). In the study, loss of even 5% of baseline weight was associated with shorter survival times (Dewys et al., 1980).

Anorexia is the loss of appetite and a contributing factor to weight loss. The presence of anorexia has been shown to be a poor prognostic indicator in a recent meta-analysis of cancer clinical trials (Quinten et al., 2009). Older adults are susceptible to what is described as the "anorexia of aging," which is an age-associated reduction in appetite and food intake (Chapman, 2007). The ambulatory care oncology nurse must be aware of the complexity of the physical and physiologic changes of aging interacting with the cancer and treatment side effects.

Interrelatedness to Aging and Etiology

Anorexia in the older adult with cancer is influenced by physiologic changes in sensory function, including a diminished sense of smell and taste. This decline in sense of smell may decrease interest in food, influence the type of food eaten, and lead to decreased intake of food and nutrients (Chapman, 2007). Diminished smell may affect the ability to detect foods that are spoiled and increase the risk of foodborne infections (Gillman, 2009). A reduced sense of taste (hypogeusia) may lead to a less varied diet, putting the older patient at risk for micronutrient deficiencies (Ahmed & Haboubi, 2010). Dysgeusia (an altered sense of taste) and ageusia (the absence of taste) are common side effects of chemotherapy and have been reported in up to 77% of patients with cancer (Rehwaldt et al., 2009).

Changes in gastrointestinal motility associated with aging cause delays in emptying of the stomach after meals; this can lead to anorexia, decreased oral intake, and early satiety. Satiety is the feeling of fullness that persists after eating. Older adults in general are less hungry and more rapidly satiated after a meal than younger people (Clarkson et al., 1997). Changes in the concentrations of many central and peripherally acting hormones, neurotransmitters, and enzymes influence satiety. Circulating cytokines, such as interleukins 1 and 6 and tumor necrosis factor, that are released in response to stress or malignancy have been associated with anorexia, weight loss, and the development of cancer cachexia, a syndrome of profound weight loss and muscle wasting (Chapman, 2007).

Many social and psychological factors influence food intake in the older adult with cancer, including dietary preferences, culture, and religion. Older adults may be socially isolated and live on a fixed income, leaving limited financial and transportation resources for the purchase of food. Older adults who live alone may have decreased motivation for food preparation for just themselves. They may have decreased functional ability to independently access and prepare meals. Depression is a common psychological problem in the elderly and can be a significant cause of loss of appetite (Donini, Saina, & Cannella, 2003). Other factors, such as impaired cognition, fatigue, or pain, and the complex interaction between cancer- or treatment-related symptoms contribute to anorexia and weight loss.

Medications, including prescription and over-the-counter preparations, nutritional supplements, and herbal preparations, can cause a variety of symptoms such as nausea, vomiting, diarrhea, constipation, and early satiety that may contribute to anorexia and weight loss and potentiate malabsorption of nutrients (Ahmed & Haboubi, 2010; Visvanathan & Chapman, 2009). Preexisting conditions and comorbidities that potentially affect nutritional status, anorexia, and weight loss in older adults with cancer are listed in Figure 4-1.

Assessment

Screening and assessment of nutritional status, including the presence of anorexia and weight loss, should take place at the time of the cancer diagnosis to establish a baseline and identify risk factors and throughout treatment with reassessment corresponding to changes in physical, functional, and cognitive status (Furman, 2006). A multidisciplinary team with a geriatric nutritionist or registered dietitian who is knowledgeable of cancer and cancer treatments is essential to older adults at risk for anorexia and weight loss.

A variety of outpatient nutrition assessment and screening tools is available that can be used in older adults with cancer. The Patient-Generated Subjective Global Assessment (known as PG-SGA) is a tool that grades the nutritional risk of patients with cancer and includes sections for patient self-report and health provider assessment (Detsky et al., 1987). The Functional Assessment of Anorexia/Cachexia Therapy (known as the FAACT questionnaire) is widely used in cancer clinical trials and captures information on QOL aspects of anorexia and single-item patient ratings of appetite (Ribaudo et al., 2000). The Simplified Nutritional Appetite Questionnaire (known as SNAQ) is a quick and easy screening tool consisting of four questions on timing of eating, meal frequency, appetite, and taste. It has a high sensitivity and specificity in predicting weight loss in older outpatients (Neelemaata et al., 2008; Wilson et al., 2005).

Regardless of use of any specific tool, consistently monitoring weight is an easy assessment. Weight loss can be graded using the *Common Terminology Criteria for Adverse Events* (CTCAE) (National Cancer Institute [NCI] Cancer Therapy Evaluation Program, 2010). Rate of weight loss may also be a clinical consideration. Body mass index (BMI) is a calculation relating height to weight,

---

Figure 4-1. Comorbid Conditions That May Contribute to Anorexia and Weight Loss

- Endocrine: diabetes, thyroid and parathyroid abnormalities, hypoadrenalism
- Gastrointestinal: malabsorption syndromes, peptic ulcer disease, dysphagia, atrophic gastritis, colitis, constipation
- Neurologic: dementia, Alzheimer disease, Parkinson disease, stroke, motor neuron disease
- Psychological: depression, bereavement, alcoholism
- Oral: poor dentition, xerostomia, mucositis or esophagitis, oral infection
- Other: congestive heart failure, chronic obstructive pulmonary disease, renal failure, infection, malignancy, physical disability (arthritis)

Note. Based on information from Ahmed & Haboubi, 2010; Visvanathan & Chapman, 2009.

with a BMI of less than 22 kg/m^2 suggesting undernutrition, particularly if the BMI is less than 18.5 kg/m^2 and the weight is stable (Chapman, 2007). Changes that occur in aging, such as loss of height and changes in posture, can skew BMI measurements, and calculations may be inaccurate in the presence of conditions such as ascites and edema (Ahmed & Haboubi, 2010).

Assessment should include a physical examination and a review of laboratory test results. No single biochemical marker indicates malnutrition; rather, several tests are important nutritional status indicators, including serum albumin, prealbumin, hematocrit, lymphocyte count, serum folate, transferrin, and retinol-binding protein (Ahmed & Haboubi, 2010; Brown, 2002; Fuhrman, Charney, & Mueller, 2004). Various anthropometric measures, such as the skin fold test, may be used for weight loss and nutritional assessment but are more likely incorporated into the dietitian's full dietary assessment. Twenty-four-hour food intake recall and food diaries may be used to quantify intake; however, information collected may not be representative of typical intake, and altered cognition may affect accuracy.

Intervention and Management

Plans to address anorexia and weight loss in older adults with cancer should be individualized with the goal to maintain healthy weight and ambulatory lifestyle. A multidisciplinary team with physicians, nurses, geriatricians, registered dietitians, physical and occupational therapists, and oncology social workers can facilitate identification and treatment of underlying and contributing factors. Developing specific strategies for symptoms such as taste alterations may involve trial and error; little evidence exists to recommend specific suggestions such as adding or avoiding specific smells, foods, spices, or condiments. Patients should be encouraged to find what helps them. Some patients may find that smaller, more frequent meals are easier to manage and more palatable.

Management of anorexia and weight loss requires ongoing nursing support and encouragement. Target weight gains should be set with the goal of increasing nutritional food intake and preventing further weight loss. Dietary counseling has been shown to improve nutritional intake and body weight, decrease anorexia, and improve QOL and is recommended for practice (Adams, Cunningham, Caruso, Norling, & Shepard, 2009). A systematic review reported improved caloric intake from nutritional counseling and from oral liquid supplements (Brown, 2002). Oral supplements for older adults are best offered between meals to reduce appetite suppression at usual mealtimes (Chapman, 2007).

Many pharmacologic interventions have been investigated to treat anorexia and improve intake, but with the exception of corticosteroids and progestins, few have compelling evidence to support their use (Adams, Cunningham, et al., 2009; Brown, 2002; Yavuzsen, Davis, Walsh, Leggrans, & Lagman, 2005). Corticosteroids such as dexamethasone, methylprednisolone, and prednisolone are recommended as appetite stimulants (Adams, Cunningham, et al., 2009), but optimal dosing, scheduling, and duration of treatment has not been determined. Corticosteroids have a high side effect profile that will require close monitoring when used. Megestrol acetate has been extensively studied for appetite enhancement in patients with cancer and anorexia. Optimal dosing is 800 mg/day, but doses of 160 mg/day have stimulated appetite (Yavuzsen et al., 2005). Although usually well tolerated, megestrol can cause flushing, fluid retention, and an increased rate of deep vein thromboses (Chapman, 2007). Ongoing nursing assessment and evaluation of the plan to manage anorexia and weight loss in the older patient with cancer is necessary. Patient and family education of planned therapies, side effects, and self-care strategies is an important role for the ambulatory care oncology nurse.

Cognitive Impairment

Overview

Cognition is the act or process of knowing; it is our awareness of the world around us—our perception. In Latin, it means "to know, to conceptualize or recognize." Cognition commonly includes processes such as intelligence, memory, learning, language, attention, and orientation. Cognition also encompasses executive functioning, information processing, and visuospatial skill (Jansen, Miaskowski, Dodd, Dowling, & Kramer, 2005). Cognition is influenced greatly by education, acquired skills, heredity, and way of life. Memory is affected by aging. Most adults experience a gradual cognitive decline, typically with regard to memory. This mild memory loss usually does not compromise functional ability (Peterson, 2011).

Mild cognitive impairment (MCI) is cognitive decline greater than expected for an individual's age and education level but does not interfere notably with ADLs (Gauthier et al., 2006); it is a slight impairment in cognitive function (typically memory) with otherwise normal function. On the continuum of cognitive function, MCI lies between and overlaps normal aging and dementia, and it is now recognized as a risk factor for dementia (Levey, Lah, Goldstein, Steenland, & Bliwise, 2006).

Dementia is not a normal part of aging and indicates problems with at least two brain functions, such as memory loss along with impaired judgment or language. Often, this cognitive decline worsens over time, deteriorating functional capacity and impairing the ability to carry out ADLs. Dementia is a constellation of symptoms in which altered intellectual and social abilities manifest severely enough to interfere with daily functioning (Chertkow, 2008). Dementia can present as confusion, inability to remember people and names, and changes in personality and social behavior. The behavioral and psychological symptoms of dementia include psychological symptoms such as anxiety, depressed mood, delusion, and hallucinations as well as behavioral symptoms such as physical aggression, restlessness, agitation, wandering, and verbal insults (Ballard, Corbett, Chitramohan, & Aarsland, 2009). Behavioral changes increase in frequency and intensity as an individual progresses through the stages of dementia (Volicer & Hurley, 2003). Age is the strongest risk factor for dementia. Dramatic increases in the number of the "oldest old" (people older than 85 years) across all racial and ethnic groups will significantly impact the numbers of people experiencing dementia (Thies & Bleiler, 2011). Among the forms of progressive dementia are Alzheimer disease (AD), vascular dementia (VaD), and dementia with Lewy bodies (Fletcher, 2008).

AD is the most common form of dementia. AD onset is often steady and gradual, progressing over time. The loss of abilities in AD occurs over a period of months to years—from 2 to 20 years with an average of 10 years from the early stages until death (Hebert, Scherr, Bienias, Bennett, & Evans, 2003). Mild AD is associated with subtle changes such as depression, whereas moderate AD is associated with delusions, agitation, apathy, dysphoria, anxiety, and aberrant motor behavior (Howieson et al., 2008).

VaD is typically the result of multiple small strokes that occur at different times and tend to have a sudden onset and a course that is slower and more highly variable than AD (O'Brien et al., 2003). The loss of function is related to the part of the brain that sustains damage. The loss of abilities can follow a fluctuating course of sudden decline in ability, followed by a period with little change, followed by another rapid change. The person may have episodes of acute confusion or delirium following these small strokes. Risk factors for VaD are similar to those for other vascular disease, including hypertension, smoking, angina, and diabetes (O'Brien et al., 2003).

Dementia with Lewy bodies (also called Lewy body disease) is another dementia type. Lewy bodies are abnormal insoluble proteins that develop inside nerve cells and have long been associated with Parkinson disease. The main features of dementia with Lewy bodies are different from AD and involve symptoms similar to Parkinson disease, such as a blank facial expression, difficulty swallowing, shuffling gait, and stiff cogwheel rigidity. Compared to AD, patients with dementia with Lewy bodies have more fluctuation in cognitive impairment, visual hallucinations, behavior disturbance, and more pronounced attentional, executive, and visuospatial abnormalities (Aarsland, Londos, & Ballard, 2009).

Delirium is an acute-onset perceptual disturbance that is a common and serious condition in older adults with cancer (American Association of Neuroscience Nurses [AANN], 2007; Breitbart, Gibson, & Tremblay, 2002). It is defined as a disturbance of consciousness and attention with a change in cognition or perception (Centeno, Sanz, & Bruera, 2004). Delirium in advanced cancer is often poorly identified and inappropriately managed (Centeno et al., 2004). When delirium occurs, patients experience disturbing symptoms and suffering, and the family and caregivers experience fear and anxiety. Advanced age, dementia, sensory losses, advanced illness, complex cancer treatments, and pharmacotherapy increase the risk of delirium in older adults with cancer (Holroyd-Leduc, Khandwala, & Sink, 2010; Michaud et al., 2007). Precipitating factors in older adults can be acute stressors, such as sudden/severe illness (e.g., surgery, metabolic disorders, infection, sleep deprivation, drug reactions, or drug-drug interactions) (Galanakis, Bickel, Gradinger, von Gumppenberg, & Forstl, 2001; Holroyd-Leduc et al., 2010; Lipowski, 1989; Litaker, Locala, Franco, Bronson, & Tannous, 2001; Michaud et al., 2007). The ambulatory care nurse can be instrumental in the early recognition of delirium. It is the rapid onset of symptoms that distinguishes delirium from the other forms of cognitive impairment. The clinical features of delirium are listed in Figure 4-2.

The ambulatory care nurse is in an ideal position to provide ongoing education and support to patients with cognitive impairment and their loved ones. If the patient is in the home setting, the ambulatory care nurse can work collaboratively with homecare nursing services to coordinate care, provide for support services, and manage the cognitive changes.

Clinical Significance and Prevalence

Cognitive decline is a fear for many older adults. This decline can be devastating for patients and their loved ones, with behavioral changes and functional disability causing a potential loss of dignity and increasing dependence.

Epidemiologic studies estimate that 3%–19% of adults who are older than age 65 experience MCI, and dementia affects 5%–10% of Americans age 65 and older (Gauthier et al., 2006). Globally, dementia rates are projected to rise dramatically because of the aging of the population. Projected estimates of 35 million affected with dementia in 2010 to more than 65 million people by 2030 are staggering (Brodaty et al., 2011). The increase in the prevalence of dementia will generate substantial challenges

---

Figure 4-2. Clinical Features of Delirium

- Onset—acute (hours to days)
- Course—fluctuating emotional disturbances throughout the day, with escalation of disturbed behavior at night ("sundowning")
- Reversibility—can be reversed in some patients
- Level of consciousness—altered (reduced awareness of the surroundings)
- Attention—reduced ability to focus, sustain, or shift attention
- Alertness—fluctuates between lethargy and hypervigilance
- Thought processes—memory deficit, disorientation, and language disturbances
- Psychotic symptoms—hallucinations and delusions common
- Sensory impairment—diminished hearing and visual acuity
- Physical findings—physical weakness leading to functional decline
- Intervention—emergent evaluation essential

Note. Based on information from Caraceni & Simonetti, 2009; Centeno et al., 2004; Foreman et al., 2003.

to the healthcare system and the caregivers who typically provide the care that individuals with dementia need. The behavioral and psychological disturbances associated with dementia lead to increased suffering, early institutionalization, increased cost of care, and diminished QOL for the caregivers and family.

Delirium is associated with significant cognitive decline, functional decline, decreased QOL, and loss of independence (Inouye, 2006; Marcantonio et al., 2003; McCusker, Cole, Dendukuri, Belzile, & Primeau, 2001). In patients with advanced cancer, delirium independently predicts mortality (Caraceni et al., 2000; McAvay et al., 2006). Approximately one-third of patients with cancer who experience delirium have a poorer prognosis than patients in the general population who are diagnosed with delirium (Inouye, 2006). Delirium is associated with increased incidence of falls, impaired mobility, diminished capacity to perform ADLs, and disrupted communication (Tuma & DeAngelis, 2000). This disruption of communication makes the assessment, treatment, and management of the cancer and associated symptoms extremely complex (Caraceni et al., 2000). Under-recognition of delirium is a major issue (Centeno et al., 2004), and evidence suggests that early detection improves outcomes (Cole, 2004; Milisen et al., 2001).

Interrelatedness to Aging

Just as age-related degenerative changes can precipitate organ system decline, aging and other pathologic factors affect the brain and other structures of the central nervous system. These changes do not develop uniformly and are subject to individual risk factors, such as genetics, past experiences, educational background, and current living conditions (Timiras, 2007). Age-related physiologic changes, including decreased cerebral blood flow and atherosclerotic changes, increase cerebrovascular vascular resistance (AANN, 2007). Evidence suggests that cardiovascular disease and vascular risk factors may be important in the development of MCI and dementia. Risk factors collectively known as *metabolic syndrome,* including abdominal obesity, impaired fasting glucose, hypertension, low high-density lipoprotein, and high triglycerides, are potential independent risk factors for cognitive decline and dementia (Panza et al., 2008).

Cognitive function may be affected by changes in neuromuscular fibers and synapses that slow processing speed, response times, and reflex activity. Changes in the levels of neurotransmitters such as serotonin and dopamine may affect cognition by altering mood, including depression, and decreased acetylcholine levels are associated with memory impairment (AANN, 2007). Changes in sleep patterns, decreased quality of sleep, and changes in sleep-wake cycles may have a significant impact on alertness and functional status (AANN, 2007). Age-related sensory changes, such as changes in vision, hearing, touch, and sensation, may contribute to impaired cognition.

Interrelatedness to Treatment

Cognitive impairment is frequently observed in patients with primary brain tumors and brain metastases. Tumor location can affect cognition (Mulrooney, 2010). It would seem reasonable that patients with tumors in the frontal lobes are most affected because this is the area of the brain that controls reasoning, memory, problem solving, and judgment, but studies have reported conflicting results, and some cognitive functions were not altered by frontal tumor location (Kaleita et al., 2004). Patients who receive radiation to the brain are at increased risk for long-term complications, including radiation necrosis and diffuse cerebral atrophy, which can occur months to years after treatment (Schneck & Janss, 2011). Radiation necrosis causes focal tissue necrosis and persistent inflammation in the specific area of the brain that received radiation. Although the focal effects can be severe, this condition has become less common with advances in radiation and radiosurgery procedures (Ricard, Taillia, & Renard, 2009). A more generalized condition, diffuse cerebral atrophy, may also occur and is associated with cognitive decline, personality changes, and gait disturbances (Schneck & Janss, 2011). This progressive dysfunction is being increasingly reported after radiation therapy and is especially concerning for patients receiving prophylactic cranial irradiation and patients with primary brain tumors with extended survival, such as those with low-grade gliomas and primary central nervous system lymphoma (Ricard et al., 2009). Patients who receive whole brain radiation therapy may develop leukoencephalopathy that can occur 6–24 months after treatment (Mulrooney, 2010).

Certain chemotherapy or biotherapy agents, such as interleukin-2, cytosine arabinoside, and ifosfamide, are known to cause acute cognitive impairment and confusion; however, a growing body of evidence links a more subtle and latent cognitive impairment commonly referred to as *chemobrain* to chemotherapies as well. This impairment involves decline in memory, concentration, and organizational or multitasking skills (Mulrooney, 2010). For some patients, the alterations in cognitive function are transient and resolve after treatment is completed, whereas others may experience long-lasting changes in cognitive function. Cognitive impairment from chemotherapy is estimated to occur in 17%–75% of patients, and 17%–35% may suffer from long-term effects (Myers, Pierce, & Pazdernik, 2008). The exact percentage of patients who are vulnerable to these adverse side effects is unknown and is likely related to the type and dose of treatment a patient receives (International Cognition and Cancer Task Force, n.d.). Many medications used to treat comorbid conditions may affect cognitive status as well. Table 4-1 outlines some common medications that can affect cognition in older adults with cancer.

Assessment

In order to differentiate whether the cognitive impairment results from a potentially reversible condition or is a result of aging, a thorough assess-

Table 4-1. Drugs That Affect Cognition in the Older Adult With Cancer	
Category	**Examples**
Analgesics	Acetaminophen, salicylates
Antibiotics	Quinolones
Anticholinergics	Atropine, scopolamine
Anticonvulsants	Carbamazepine, phenobarbital, phenytoin
Antidepressants	Amitriptyline, doxepin
Antiemetics	Dronabinol, metoclopramide, prochlorperazine
Antihistamines	Chlorpheniramine, diphenhydramine
Antihypertensives	Clonidine, propranolol
Antiparkinsonians	Amantadine, levodopa
Antispasmodics	Belladonna alkaloids, hyoscyamine
Cardiac agents	Digoxin, dipyridamole
Chemotherapy/biotherapy	Bleomycin, carmustine, cytarabine, cisplatin, fluorouracil, ifosfamide, interferon, interleukin, L-asparaginase, methotrexate, mitomycin, prednisone, procarbazine, vincristine, vinblastine
Diabetic agents	Chlorpropamide
H_2 receptor antagonists	Cimetidine, ranitidine
Nonsteroidal anti-inflammatory drugs	Celecoxib, indomethacin
Opioids	Meperidine, pentazocine, propoxyphene
Sedatives, barbiturates	Diazepam, flurazepam

Note. Based on information from Cancelli et al., 2009; Centeno et al., 2004.

ment is required. Common reversible causes of cognitive impairment include metabolic alterations, vitamin deficiencies, thyroid dysfunction, infections, depression, drug reaction or drug-drug interaction, hypoxia, fluid balance disturbance, cerebrovascular disorders, brain lesions, and pain (Fletcher, 2008). The assessment for impaired cognition should include physical assessment and diagnostic studies to rule out potential contributing causes. Diagnostic tests include (Fletcher, 2008; Foy & Okpalugo, 2009)

- Serum electrolytes, creatinine (Cr), glucose
- Liver function tests, ammonia, complete blood count, folate

- B_{12} level and thyroid function
- Blood cultures, urinalysis, urine culture
- Drug levels for digoxin and lithium, if indicated
- Toxic screen of blood and urine when an overdose is suspected
- Imaging of the brain and evaluation of cerebrospinal fluid
- Electroencephalography testing to rule out seizure disorder.

Assessment should include history taking, which encompasses three important domains: functional, cognitive, and behavioral characteristics and observations. This involves interviewing the patient, followed by elaborating and clarifying statements with the family or caregivers (Fletcher, 2008). The oncology nurse is often dependent upon communication from family members about the condition of the patient. The family or caregiver is often the first to notice subtle changes in mood, behavior, and mental clarity. In older adults, any reports of changes in cognition should initiate a mental status evaluation. A structured process for screening should be established. The assessment should include a calm, orderly approach in a quiet, soothing environment. Adequate time should be allowed for questions to be answered, and family members and caregivers should be included to provide additional information or observations. Ensure that adaptive devices (e.g., hearing aids, glasses) are used (AANN, 2007).

A number of tools are available to measure functional assessment; however, Karnofsky Performance Status or Eastern Cooperative Oncology Group performance status ratings are frequently used in ambulatory assessments. The ability to perform instrumental ADLs can be assessed by the Functional Activities Questionnaire (known as the FAQ), which is an informant-based measure of functional capabilities and has been recognized for its capacity to distinguish the early onset of dementia (Pfeffer, Kurosaki, Harrah, Chance, & Filos, 1982). Cognitive status can be assessed in the framework of a broader evaluation of mental status. The components of a mental status evaluation include orientation to person, place, and time; attention and concentration ability; memory; judgment; executive control functions (ability to abstract, plan, and sequence); speech and language; mood and affect; and the presence of delusions or hallucinations (Fletcher, 2008). The Mini-Mental State Exam (MMSE) is a standardized 30-point tool used extensively to measure cognition (Folstein, Folstein, & McHugh, 1975). The MMSE can be used in clinical settings, is relatively easy to administer, and takes about 10 minutes to complete. It can be easily incorporated into the ambulatory assessment, and the scores can be trended over time to identify alterations to cognition (Folstein et al., 1975). Any score of 25 points or more (out of 30) is considered normal. Below this, scores can indicate severe (9 or less points), moderate (10–20 points), or mild (21–24 points) dementia (Mungas, 1991). A criticism of the MMSE had been that it is significantly influenced by age, level of education, language, and verbal ability (Braes, Milisen, & Foreman, 2008). Since 1993, the MMSE has been available with an attached table that enables patient-specific norms to be identified on the basis of age and education level (Crum, Anthony, Bassett, & Folstein, 1993). It is now available in multiple languages.

Another simple, reliable, and clinically useful tool in the detection of mild dementia is the Clock Drawing Test (CDT) (Sunderland et al., 1989). It has numerous variations, but all involve asking the patient to draw the face of a clock and then add the arms of the clock to denote a certain time (11:10 and 8:20 are commonly used). The instructions may be repeated, but no additional help may be given, and generally no time limit is set for the test but it should take only one to two minutes. The CDT is considered normal if all numbers are depicted in the correct sequence and position and if the hands display the requested time. The CDT requires a number of cognitive, motor, and perceptual functions required simultaneously for successful completion. Royall (1996) suggested that the executive function required for clock-drawing involves similar demands as independent living skills.

The Mini-Cog is another assessment tool that has the advantages of being administered quickly, requiring only paper and pencil, and being relatively uninfluenced by level of education or language of origin (AANN, 2007). It includes the CDT as a distracter with an uncued three-item recall test. The patient is asked to listen to the clinician say three unrelated items (e.g., pen, table, ring), and then the patient should repeat them aloud. The patient is then asked to perform the CDT; once completed, the patient is asked to recall the three words presented previously. The Mini-Cog is scored as 1 point for each recalled word (3 points total) with 2 points for normal clock and 0 points for abnormal CDT. The recall and CDT are combined to get the Mini-Cog score, with a score of 0–2 indicating a positive screen for dementia (AANN, 2007).

The Neuropsychiatric Inventory Questionnaire (NPI-Q) measures frequency and severity of behavioral symptoms in individuals with dementia and helps to distinguish the cause (Cummings et al., 1994). This questionnaire is a validated clinical instrument for evaluating psychopathology in dementia. The NPI-Q provides a brief, reliable, informant-based assessment of neuropsychiatric symptoms and associated caregiver distress that may be suitable for use in general clinical practice (see Figure 4-3). Many other neuropsychological tests are available that can provide comprehensive evaluation of cognitive functioning, but their administration requires specialized training and can be time-intensive (one to six hours), which may be especially difficult for older patients dealing with cancer and its treatment (Tannock, Ahles, Ganz, & van Dam, 2004). Even without the use of a specific tool, the ambulatory care oncology nurse can assess for cognitive impairment in the clinic setting or by telephone ascertaining if the patient is alert and oriented to time, person, and place; through a discussion of current events; and through assessment of behavior and judgment within present-day context. Assessment should always include evaluation for pain, fatigue, depression, and sleep disturbances, as all may affect cognition and functional status. Review of medications and prior medical history/comorbidity assessment is imperative to rule out contributing causes.

Figure 4-3. The Neuropsychiatric Inventory Questionnaire (NPI-Q)

Please answer the following questions based on <u>changes</u> that have occurred since the patient first began to experience memory problems.

Circle "Yes" <u>only</u> if the symptom(s) has been present <u>in the last month</u>. Otherwise, circle "No". For each item marked "Yes":

a) Rate the SEVERITY of the symptom (how it affects <u>the patient</u>):
        1 = **Mild** (noticeable, but not a significant change)
        2 = **Moderate** (significant, but not a dramatic change)
        3 = **Severe** (very marked or prominent, a dramatic change)

b) Rate the DISTRESS you experience due to that symptom (how it affects <u>you</u>):
        0 = **Not distressing at all**
        1 = **Minimal** (slightly distressing, not a problem to cope with)
        2 = **Mild** (not very distressing, generally easy to cope with)
        3 = **Moderate** (fairly distressing, not always easy to cope with)
        4 = **Severe** (very distressing, difficult to cope with)
        5 = **Extreme or Very Severe** (extremely distressing, unable to
           cope with)

Please answer each question carefully. Ask for assistance if you have any questions.

Delusions   Does the patient have false beliefs, such as thinking that others are stealing from him/her or planning to harm him/her in some way?

Yes   No   SEVERITY: 1 2 3   DISTRESS: 0 1 2 3 4 5

Hallucinations   Does the patient have hallucinations such as false visions or voices? Does he or she seem to hear or see things that are not present?

Yes   No   SEVERITY: 1 2 3   DISTRESS: 0 1 2 3 4 5

Agitation/Aggression Is the patient resistive to help from others at times, or hard to handle?

Yes   No   SEVERITY: 1 2 3   DISTRESS: 0 1 2 3 4 5

Depression/Dysphoria Does the patient seem sad or say that he /she is depressed?

Yes   No   SEVERITY: 1 2 3   DISTRESS: 0 1 2 3 4 5

(Continued on next page)

Figure 4-3. The Neuropsychiatric Inventory Questionnaire (NPI-Q) *(Continued)*

Anxiety   Does the patient become upset when separated from you? Doeshe/she have any other signs of nervousness such as shortness of breath, sighing, being unable to relax, or feeling excessively tense?

Yes   No   SEVERITY: 1 2 3   DISTRESS: 0 1 2 3 4 5

Elation/Euphoria   Does the patient appear to feel too good or act excessively happy?

Yes   No   SEVERITY: 1 2 3   DISTRESS: 0 1 2 3 4 5

Apathy/Indifference   Does the patient seem less interested in his/her usual activities or in the activities and plans of others?

Yes   No   SEVERITY: 1 2 3   DISTRESS: 0 1 2 3 4 5

Disinhibition   Does the patient seem to act impulsively, for example, talking to strangers as if he/she knows them, or saying things that may hurt people's feelings?

Yes   No   SEVERITY: 1 2 3   DISTRESS: 0 1 2 3 4 5

Irritability/Lability   Is the patient impatient and cranky? Does he/she have difficulty coping with delays or waiting for planned activities?

Yes   No   SEVERITY: 1 2 3   DISTRESS: 0 1 2 3 4 5

Motor Disturbance   Does the patient engage in repetitive activities such as pacing around the house, handling buttons, wrapping string, or doing other things repeatedly?

Yes   No   SEVERITY: 1 2 3   DISTRESS: 0 1 2 3 4 5

Nightime Behaviors   Does the patient awaken you during the night, rise too early in the morning, or take excessive naps during the day?

Yes   No   SEVERITY: 1 2 3   DISTRESS: 0 1 2 3 4 5

Appetite/Eating   Has the patient lost or gained weight, or had a change in the type of food he/she likes?

Yes   No   SEVERITY: 1 2 3   DISTRESS: 0 1 2 3 4 5

(Continued on next page)

Figure 4-3. The Neuropsychiatric Inventory Questionnaire (NPI-Q) *(Continued)*

NPI-Q SUMMARY

	No	Severity			Caregiver Distress					
Delusions	0	1	2	3	0	1	2	3	4	5
Hallucinations	0	1	2	3	0	1	2	3	4	5
Agitation/Aggression	0	1	2	3	0	1	2	3	4	5
Dysphoria/Depression	0	1	2	3	0	1	2	3	4	5
Anxiety	0	1	2	3	0	1	2	3	4	5
Euphoria/Elation	0	1	2	3	0	1	2	3	4	5
Apathy/Indifference	0	1	2	3	0	1	2	3	4	5
Disinhibition	0	1	2	3	0	1	2	3	4	5
Irritability/Lability	0	1	2	3	0	1	2	3	4	5
Aberrant Motor	0	1	2	3	0	1	2	3	4	5
Nighttime Behavior	0	1	2	3	0	1	2	3	4	5
Appetite/Eating	0	1	2	3	0	1	2	3	4	5
TOTAL										

Note. Copyright 1994 by J.L. Cummings. Used with permission. Permission for commercial use is required.

Intervention and Management

The goals in care planning and management of the individual who presents with alterations in cognitive functioning are to identify and resolve any potentially reversible conditions, control any comorbid conditions, and recognize and intervene early (Manning, 2004). Ambulatory care oncology nurses should encourage all patients to maintain a healthy lifestyle to prevent and control vascular risk factors, as effective management may delay onset of dementia syndromes and may prevent progression in patients with vascular dementia (Panza et al., 2008; Román, 2008). An ambulatory care nursing plan should be individualized to promote and optimize nutritional status of the older adult with cancer. A growing body of evidence indicates that deficiencies in essential micronutrients, such as antioxidants and B vitamins, are risk factors for MCI (Del Parigi, Panza, Capurso, & Solfrizzi, 2006), but additional research is needed before preventive dietary recommendations can be made.

The ambulatory care oncology nurse should encourage physical activity appropriate to the patient's functional and medical status. A recent meta-analysis confirmed that activities that improve cardiopulmonary fitness are beneficial for cognitive function in older adults (Angevaren, Aufdemkampe, Verhaar, Aleman, & Vanhees, 2008). Encouraging physical fitness in the older adult with cancer has many benefits as well. Other self-care strategies for the older adult with cancer with MCI may include continued mental and social stimulation, as studies suggest that lifelong learning, mental exercise, continuing social engagement, and stress reduction may be important factors in promoting cognitive vitality in aging (Fillit et al., 2002).

Cognitive-behavioral therapy, brain exercises, memory games, relaxation and stress reduction activities, and organizational and note-taking strategies are all useful suggestions, but few studies have proved their effectiveness. A relationship between social support and coping ability has been demonstrated (Mulrooney, 2010). The ambulatory care oncology nurse can work with a social worker for referral and needs assessment to identify coping methods and promote social support (family, friends, or referral to a group) resources and programs as needed.

Medications

Two medication classes are approved for the treatment of AD. Cholinesterase inhibitors (ChEIs) are indicated for the treatment of mild to moderate AD and include donepezil (Aricept®), galantamine (Reminyl®), tacrine (Cognex®), and rivastigmine (Exelon®). Because early treatment of mild to moderate AD is associated with a better response than delayed treatment (Levey et al., 2006), the use of ChEIs in MCI is currently being studied. ChEI use was not associated with any delay in the onset of AD or dementia, and the safety profile showed significant risks associated with ChEIs. It is recommended that ChEIs be used with caution in patients with cardiovascular risk factors (Raschetti, Emiliano, Vanacore, & Maggini, 2007). Other types of agents have been investigated such as antioxidants, estrogen replacement therapy, and cyclooxygenase-2-selective inhibitors, although none have shown significant beneficial effects in delaying cognitive decline or progression to AD (Levey et al., 2006).

Research targeting new drugs to improve symptoms and delay progression to AD is needed. No evidence shows the long-term efficacy of currently approved pharmacologic treatments in MCI or in MCI associated with chemotherapy (Winblad et al., 2004). Small studies looking at the benefit of medications such as modafinil to improve cognitive performance have been shown to enhance memory and attention skills in cancer survivors (Kohli, Fisher, Tra, Wesnes, & Morrow, 2007), but further research is needed before generalizing these findings to older adults with cancer. Memantine (Ebixa®), an N-methyl-D-aspartate antagonist, is the only treatment approved for the management of moderate to severe dementia. For patients diagnosed with dementia with Lewy bodies, neuroleptics (antipsychotics) should be avoided because of an increased risk for a life-threatening illness called neuroleptic malignant syndrome, which is characterized by muscle rigidity, fever, autonomic instability, delirium, and elevated creatine phosphokinase. Medications to avoid include antipsychotics (e.g., haloperidol), drugs for urinary incontinence, and diphenhydramine, an antihistamine (Neef & Walling, 2006).

The mainstay of treatment for the behavioral and psychological symptoms of dementia has been antipsychotic agents. However, the U.S. Food and Drug Administration (FDA) Psychopharmacologic Drugs Advisory Committee (2008) issued a black box warning on all conventional and atypical antipsychotic agents on the basis of evidence that their use leads to increased mortality for elderly patients. This has made the need for other agents compelling. A recent study based on the National Institute of Mental Health Clinical Antipsychotic Trials of Intervention Effectiveness—Alzheimer's Disease suggested that risperidone and olanzapine, but not quetiapine, had greater improvement than placebo on selected psychosis symptoms and global measures of behavior, although worsening depression occurred in the olanzapine-treated group (Sultzer et al., 2008).

Antipsychotic medications are the medication of choice for the treatment of delirium, and the indications for its use should be documented. The family/caregiver should understand that antipsychotic medications are indicated to treat agitation, fear, and hallucinations. Sedating drugs may be ordered to manage severe agitation to allow the patient to rest or at the end of life for the patient to die a peaceful death. Table 4-2 outlines the pharmacologic agents used to manage delirium.

Supportive Interventions

Support, education, and counseling should be provided to all families and caregivers of patients with cognitive impairment. The ambulatory care oncology nurse should facilitate caregiver support with both education and assistance in obtaining appropriate referrals and support. The burden experienced by the family/caregiver is the primary determinant of how long the patient will be able to remain at home (Etters, Goodall, & Harrison, 2008). Hall and Buckwalter (1987) first proposed a theoretical framework for nursing interventions for people with dementia called the progressively lowered stress threshold model (PLST). The model proposes the following nine actions that nurses can model and teach to caregivers who are managing and coping with an individual with cognitive changes (Hall & Buckwalter, 1987).

1. Maximize safety by modifying the environment to compensate for cognitive losses.
2. Control any factors that increase stress such as fatigue; physical stressors; competing or overwhelming stimuli; changes in routine, caregiver, or environment; and activities or demands that exceed the person's functional status.
3. Plan and maintain a consistent routine.

Table 4-2. Pharmacologic Intervention for the Management of Delirium

Drug	Starting Dose	Comment
Haloperidol	0.5–2 mg by mouth every 8–12 hours	Can be given IV, SC, or IM
Chlorpromazine	25–50 mg by mouth or IM every 6–8 hours	Sedating May cause hypotension
Risperidone	0.5–1 mg by mouth every 8–12 hours	–
Olanzapine	5–10 mg by mouth or oral dissolvable tablet every 8–12 hours	–
Lorazepam	0.5–1 mg by mouth every 1–4 hours for severe agitation	First-line treatment in delirium or seizures associated with alcohol or sedative withdrawal only Use with haloperidol to control agitation. If used alone, may worsen delirium.

IM—intramuscular; SC—subcutaneous

Note. Based on information from Centeno et al., 2004; Fong et al., 2009; Inouye, 2006; Lonergan et al., 2007.

4. Implement regular rest periods to compensate for fatigue and loss of reserve energy.
5. Provide unconditional positive regard.
6. Remain nonjudgmental about the appropriateness of all behaviors except those that present a threat to safety.
7. Recognize individual expressions of fatigue, anxiety, and increasing stress, and intervene to reduce stressors as soon as possible.
8. Modify reality orientation and other therapeutic interventions to incorporate only the information needed for safe function.
9. Use reassuring forms of therapy, such as music or reminiscence.

Intervening to reduce risk factors can be the most successful delirium prevention strategy. Recommendations include geriatricians on the patient care team, maintenance of hydration, maintenance of adequate oxygen saturation levels, treatment of pain, elimination of unnecessary medications, and promotion of activity (Milisen et al., 2001). The patient's goals of care, extent of disease, and the potential to address reversible causes should guide the treatment course (Cole, 2004). Once delirium is recognized, it must be treated. Interventions to relieve distress and suffering should be implemented and include reorienting the patient, protecting the patient and others, and identifying any potentially reversible causes of delirium. It is important to establish and maintain open communication and a supportive relationship with the patient and family in order to provide reassurance and educate the family and caregivers about the course, expected outcomes, and what they can do to support the patient. Some supportive interventions to manage delirium are listed in Table 4-3.

Table 4-3. Supportive Interventions to Manage Delirium	
Clinical Issue	**Intervention**
Visual impairment	Provide eyeglasses, magnifiers, and night lights.
Hearing loss	Provide amplifying devices.
Sleep deprivation	Provide back rub, progressive relaxation, music therapy, and reflexology. Limit noise at night.
Disorientation	Provide verbal reorientation, and have a clock, calendar, and familiar items from home visible.
Sensory overload	Ask simple, direct questions; speak clearly and slowly. Maintain routines; avoid change.
Pain	Conduct frequent pain assessment. Provide adequate analgesia. Implement nonpharmacologic interventions, including change of position, heat, and massage.
Inactivity and immobility	Provide for daily ambulation and periods out of bed. Provide for physical therapy.

Note. Based on information from Foreman et al., 2003; Inouye, 2006; Michaud et al., 2007.

Constipation

Overview

Constipation is decreased or difficult evacuation of feces. This alters what is considered an individual's normal bowel pattern, which is usually no less than three stools per week and no more than three per day (NCI, 2010). Patients often describe it as straining, hard stool, feeling of incomplete evacuation, and nonproductive urge (Bouras & Tangalos, 2009). For older patients with cancer, constipation can be secondary to the disease, a side effect of treatment, or secondary to preexisting conditions. Dysmotility causing delay in transit within the colon is a frequent nonobstructive cause of constipation (McCrea, Miaskowski, Stotts, Macera, & Varma, 2008). Many factors can alter colonic motility, including endocrine abnormalities, neurogenic causes, and medical therapies, including anticancer and pain medications. Multiple factors may cause constipation in an individual (Rao & Go, 2010) (see Figure 4-4).

Figure 4-4. Factors Contributing to Constipation in the Older Adult

Endocrine/Metabolic Disorders
- Hypothyroidism
- Hyperparathyroidism
- Hypercalcemia
- Hypomagnesemia
- Hypokalemia
- Diabetes mellitus
- Chronic renal disease

Neurogenic/Neurologic Disorders
- Cerebrovascular events
- Parkinson disease
- Spinal cord tumors
- Trauma
- Multiple sclerosis
- Autonomic neuropathy
- Impaired cognition

Myopathic Disorders
- Scleroderma
- Amyloidosis

Psychological Disorders
- Depression
- Anxiety

Other
- Diet
- Dehydration
- Immobility
- Medications (see Figure 4-5)

Note. Based on information from Leppert, 2010; McCrea et al., 2008; National Cancer Institute, 2010; Rao & Go, 2010.

Pelvic floor dysfunction, common in patients with history of anorectal surgery, or changes in pelvic muscles may disrupt adequate propulsion, thus affecting bowel movements. In addition to advanced age, risk factors for chronic constipation include frailty, decreased mobility or physical inactivity, depression, low income and educational level, medications, poor nutrition, decreased hydration, non-White race, and female (Bouras & Tanglaos, 2009). For patients with cancer, constipation is more than an annoying problem. It can be a major source of discomfort and psychological distress and can affect nutritional intake and socialization (Mercandante, Ferrera, & Casuccio, 2010). Constipation from reduced fluid intake is a commonly recognized symptom in older adults and can contribute to decreased QOL (Bosshard, Dreher, Schnegg, & Bula, 2004).

Clinical Significance and Prevalence

Constipation affects almost one in six adults and is even more problematic in the elderly (Camilleri & Bharucha, 2010). Adult prevalence rates are estimated at 2%–27% (Bouras & Tangalos, 2009). Severe chronic constipation is seen almost exclusively in women, and elderly women have rates of constipation two to three times higher than their male counterparts (Bouras & Tangalos, 2009). For patients with cancer, constipation constitutes a significant clinical problem affecting QOL, with up to 90% of patients on opioids experiencing chronic constipation (Clemens & Klaschik, 2010; Leppert, 2010). This may lead to inappropriate opioid dosing and, consequently, inadequate analgesia (Überall & Müller-Schwege, 2006). In older adults, constipation has been linked to acute states of confusion (Young & Inouye, 2007), urinary tract infection (Thomas, 2007), and intestinal obstruction and bowel perforation (Gallagher & O'Mahony, 2009).

Interrelatedness to Aging

In the elderly, diminished sensitivity to thirst may lead to decreased fluid intake and subsequent constipation. Some studies have shown slowing of colonic transit and reduced propulsive efficacy in older adults, whereas others have detected no significant differences between young and old patients (Bouras & Tangalos, 2009). Changes in both the release and uptake of calcium affecting muscle contraction may contribute to lengthened colonic transit time, as could a decrease in enteric neurons that occurs with aging (McCrea et al., 2008; Sykes, 2006). Age-related alterations in the colon's mechanical properties, such as loss of plasticity and compliance as well as structural changes seen with diverticulosis, may affect bowel function (Camilleri, Lee, Viramontes, Bharucha, & Tangalos, 2000). Despite these age-related changes, constipation in the older adult with cancer is more likely to be attributed to altered dietary intake, medications, chronic illness, and immobility (McCrea et al., 2008). Psychosocial factors such as distress, lack of privacy, and dependency on others have been associated with constipation (Candy, Jones, Goodman, Drake, & Tookman, 2011). The older adult may ignore the impulse to defecate, which can lead to fecal retention. Chronic retention can lead to suppression of rectal sensation and decreased urge to defecate. Ultimately, only large stool volumes may be perceived, and difficulties with evacuation may occur (Bouras & Tangalos, 2009).

Interrelatedness to Treatment

Cancer-related causes of constipation include colon obstruction due to tumor, enlarged lymph nodes, or adhesions caused by abdominal or pelvic surgery. Liver metastasis or peritoneal or mesenteric spread of disease can also increase risk of constipation (Woolery et al., 2008). Impingement of nerves from spinal cord compression may affect bowel function as well as metabolic abnormalities, particularly hypercalcemia and hypokalemia. Patients with small cell lung cancer and carcinoid tumors may experience constipation from paraneoplastic chemical mediators that inhibit peristalsis (Sykes, 2006).

For older adults undergoing cancer treatment, maintaining adequate fluid intake may be problematic and may increase their vulnerability for the development of constipation. The most common cause of constipation for patients with cancer is medications, such as chemotherapy, pain medications, and serotonin-based drugs that relieve nausea and vomiting (Solomon & Cherny, 2006). Medications used to manage comorbid conditions in the older adult also cause constipation. Figure 4-5 lists medication types that may contribute to constipation.

Figure 4-5. Medications That Contribute to Constipation	
• Analgesic drugs • Chemotherapy agents • 5-HT$_3$ receptor agonists • Calcium and aluminum antacids • Calcium supplements • Diuretics • Anticholinergic drugs • Antidepressant drugs • Antihistamines	• Anticonvulsants • Antiparkinsonian medications • Lithium • Antidiarrheals • Antihypertensive and antiarrhythmic drugs • Calcium channel blockers • Bile acid resins • Iron preparations

Note. Based on information from Bouras & Tangalos, 2009; Rao & Go, 2010.

For chemotherapy agents such as the vinca alkaloids (vincristine, vinblastine, and vinorelbine) and the platinums (carboplatin and oxaliplatin), constipation is a well-known side effect. Thalidomide and temozolomide can also cause constipation. Antiemetic medications administered concurrently may contribute to or potentiate the symptom as well. The mechanism by which these drugs cause constipation is most often associated with neurotoxic effects on enteric neurons that innervate the intestines (Sykes, 2006).

Opioid drugs affect bowel function by targeting mu-opioid receptors inhibiting neural pathways that coordinate motility. This leads to decreased peristalsis and slowed intestinal transit time (Leppert, 2010). Patients receiving chronic opioid therapy do not develop tolerance to the constipating effects (Ballantyne, 2007). Symptoms of opioid-induced bowel dysfunction include dry, hard stools, straining, bloating, abdominal cramping, distension, and gastric reflux (Pappagallo, 2001). The physical discomfort, pain, and interference with QOL often force patients to decrease their dose, refuse dose escalation, or stop opioids completely. Approximately 80%–90% of all opioid-treated patients experience constipation (Kurz & Sessler, 2003; Leppert, 2010).

Assessment

The process of defecation is person-specific, and an individualized assessment and plan of care is essential (Candy et al., 2011). Inconsistency in the assessment of constipation in patients with cancer can lead to the symptom being poorly managed. Several tools are available to assess a patient's individual risk for developing constipation, but few have been validated specifically for patients with cancer. The Constipation Assessment Scale (McMillan & Williams, 1989) is an easy-to-use, eight-item tool that provides a reliable indicator for the presence and severity of constipation in patients with cancer. It is also helpful to use one grading system when assessing the severity of constipation. The NCI CTCAE (2010) defines constipation as a disorder characterized by irregular or difficult evacuation of the bowels; constipation is graded on a scale of one to four (see Figure 4-6).

Figure 4-6. National Cancer Institute Cancer Therapy Evaluation Program Criteria for Constipation			
Grade 1	Grade 2	Grade 3	Grade 4
Occasional or intermittent symptoms with occasional use of stool softeners, laxatives, dietary modification, or enemas	Persistent symptoms with regular use of laxatives or enemas, affecting or limiting instrumental ADL	Obstipation with manual evacuation indicated, limiting self-care ADL	Life-threatening consequences with urgent intervention indicated

ADL—activities of daily living

Note. From *Common Terminology Criteria for Adverse Events* [v.4.03], by National Cancer Institute Cancer Therapy Evaluation Program, 2010. Retrieved from http://evs.nci.nih.gov/ftp1/CTCAE/CTCAE_4.03_2010-06-14_QuickReference_8.5x11.pdf.

Managing constipation in the older adult involves a comprehensive assessment. The assessment should include inquiry of stool frequency, stool consistency, stool size, ease of passing stool, and degree of straining. The ambulatory care oncology nurse should determine if there is oozing of stool, sensations of incomplete emptying, and presence of associated symptoms, including nausea, vomiting, bloating, abdominal or rectal fullness, bleeding, tenesmus, pain, or urinary incontinence. The onset and duration of the constipation should be determined, as well as the history of the patient's normal bowel pattern, including when the last bowel movement occurred. Questions the nurse should ask the patient to assess the level of constipation include (NCI, 2010)

- What is normal for you (frequency, amount, and timing)?
- When was the last bowel movement? What were the amount, consistency, and color? Was blood passed with it?
- Have you been having any abdominal discomfort, cramping, nausea or vomiting, pain, excessive gas, or rectal fullness?
- Do you regularly use laxatives or enemas? What do you usually do to relieve constipation? Does it usually work?
- What type of diet do you follow? How much and what type of fluids are taken on a regular basis?
- What medication (dose and frequency) are you taking?
- Is this symptom a recent change?
- How many times a day is flatus passed?

The patient's activity level should be assessed for the predisposing factors of immobility or sedentary lifestyle.

A social history should be structured to determine:

- Living arrangements
- Available support systems
- Ability to perform ADLs
- Ability to get to and use the bathroom (NCI, 2010)

- Ability to obtain and prepare food
- Ability to chew and swallow.

The ambulatory care oncology nurse should review all medications, including prescription and over-the-counter medications, supplements, herbal preparations, and laxatives, and confer with a pharmacist for assistance in identifying those that may cause constipation.

Physical Assessment

The abdomen should be inspected for pain, distension, or bloating. Bowel sounds should be auscultated for their presence or absence, frequency, and quadrant location. A complete pain assessment should be performed on all patients who indicate they have pain. Diagnostic tests that may be ordered include a metabolic panel to assess for dehydration, metabolic abnormalities, and thyroid function. An x-ray of the abdomen should be performed to determine evidence of an excessive amount of retained stool in the colon. Barium studies and additional specialized tests may be ordered to help determine the etiology of constipation (Camilleri & Bharucha, 2010).

Interventions and Management

The goal for managing constipation in older adults with cancer should focus on prevention. Ambulatory care oncology nurses should understand individual patient risk factors for constipation and plan interventions based on assessment, comorbidities, and anticipated treatment. Older adults should be educated about their individualized risk for constipation and preventive measures that they can implement.

Fluid and dietary interventions: Increasing dietary fiber is often recommended to older patients to promote good bowel function, as most adults consume only 10–20 g of the recommended 30–40 g of fiber daily (Bisanz, 2005). Both water-soluble and bulk-forming fiber is needed and can be found in foods such as oat products, fruits, legumes, and pectin (water soluble) and also wheat, vegetables, and bran (bulk forming). For patients experiencing bowel difficulties, medicinal fiber, such as psyllium and methylcellulose, is usually prescribed instead of nutritional fiber from foods. Regardless of the source of fiber, patients should be instructed to gradually increase the amount along with increasing fluids. The effective and safe use of fiber supplements requires at least 1.5 L of fluid daily (Librach et al., 2010). In patients with advanced cancer, increasing fiber without increasing fluids can worsen constipation and result in impaction and obstruction (Leppert, 2010). Although dietary modifications alone may not be successful and fiber supplements require additional fluid, older adults can be encouraged to slowly increase their intake of fiber-rich foods such as bran, fruits, vegetables, and nuts as a preventive strategy (Solomon & Cherny, 2006).

Adequate fluid consumption has been associated with decreased constipation and decreased use of laxatives (Robinson & Rosher, 2002). The current recommendation based on expert opinion for fluid intake for adults to manage constipation is eight 8-ounce glasses of water daily (Bisanz et al., 2009). A warm or hot drink approximately a half-hour before the time of the patient's usual defecation may also be helpful (NCI, 2010). In older patients with cancer who have renal or cardiac disease, increasing the individual's fluid intake should be monitored carefully to avoid fluid overload.

Physical activity and exercise: Physical activity affects colonic motor function, and epidemiologic data support the notion that those who are more physically active are less constipated. In the elderly, constipation correlates with decreased physical activity (Müller-Lissner, Kamm, Scarpignato, & Wald, 2005). Although the evidence supporting the effectiveness of exercise to treat constipation is lacking (Woolery et al., 2008), nurses can encourage moderate physical activity as an overall recommendation for health.

Pelvic floor rehabilitative exercises may be useful for patients with pelvic floor dysfunction. Therapy focuses on sensory and muscular retraining of the rectum and pelvic floor muscles. Patients are taught to use their abdominal muscles to increase intra-abdominal pressure and to keep pelvic floor muscles relaxed to facilitate evacuation of stool (Bouras & Tangalos, 2009).

Behavioral modifications: Patients can be educated to establish bowel or timed toilet training to "train" the bowel to move at a specific time each day. The most powerful gastrocolic reflex occurs in the morning after a meal (Librach et al., 2010; Rao & Go, 2010), so the patient should be instructed to sit on the toilet and attempt to move bowels in the morning after breakfast. Correct positioning and sitting upright while toileting can facilitate movement of bowels. The use of a footstool, a raised toilet seat, or a toilet seat with arms may be helpful to maintain positioning and to bear down. Patients should avoid straining for longer than five minutes (Rao & Go, 2010).

Pharmacologic interventions: For the older adult with cancer, use of laxatives must be individualized with special attention to the patient's medical history, including cardiac and renal comorbidities, drug interactions, planned cancer treatment, and potential side effects. Medications should be prescribed based on the underlying etiology. Table 4-4 outlines common pharmacologic agents used in the management of constipation in the older adult.

Key Points

- In patients with myelosuppression, rectal examinations, suppositories, and enemas should be avoided. These interventions may produce discomfort, bleeding, anal fissures, abscesses, or infection (National Comprehensive Cancer Network [NCCN], 2011b). In patients with healthy immune systems, manual disimpaction, enemas, and suppositories may be used (Bisanz, 2005; Librach et al., 2010).
- In patients with abdominal pain associated with large tumor burden, osmotic laxatives are encouraged because they produce a milder peristalsis than stimulants (Bisanz, 2005).

Table 4-4. Common Medications Used to Manage Constipation in the Older Adult

Type	Example	Comments
Bulk-forming laxatives	Psyllium Methylcellulose	Use cautiously in older adults. Oral hydration required. Gas and bloating at initiation of therapy. Not recommended in immobile adults or at end of life.
Osmotic laxatives	Lactulose, sorbitol Polyethylene glycol (PEG)	Generally safe to use in older adults. Bloating and gas may limit their use. Sweet taste may exacerbate nausea.
Saline laxatives	Magnesium citrate Magnesium hydroxide	May increase sodium and magnesium; use with caution in patients with renal disease.
Stimulants	Bisacodyl Senna Cascara	Cramping may limit its use in older adults. Recommended along with a stool softener in patients with cancer as prevention in opioid-induced constipation (Bisanz et al., 2009).
Softeners/surfactants	Docusate	Higher doses may stimulate peristalsis. Often used in combination with senna.
Lubricants	Mineral oil Glycerin suppositories	Risk for aspiration pneumonia and malabsorption of fat-soluble vitamins. May be helpful for relief of excessive straining.
Prokinetics	Metoclopramide	Used for severe constipation or in patients who do not find relief from bowel programs (Bisanz et al., 2009). Contraindicated in suspected or documented cases of bowel obstruction.
Opioid antagonists	Naloxone	Mixed results with oral and enteral routes for management of opioid-induced constipation. Potential adverse effects include loss of analgesia and opioid withdrawal.
Mu antagonists	Methylnaltrexone	Recommended for refractory opioid-induced constipation that has failed optimal laxative therapy in patients with advanced illness and receiving palliative care (Bisanz et al., 2009).

- Mineral oil by mouth can be effective for softening stool but should not be routinely used because of potential malabsorption of nutrients (Bisanz, 2005). Patients with dysphagia should not use oral mineral oil because of the risk of lipoid aspiration pneumonia.

- Routine administration of laxatives after diagnostic procedures using barium can prevent constipation with impaction (Bisanz, 2005).
- Fecal impaction, incontinence, colonic dilatation, and even perforation can complicate constipation, creating the need for surgical intervention. However, unless constipation is caused by a malignant bowel obstruction, surgery has little role in the management of constipation in the older adult (NCCN, 2011b).
- The NCCN guidelines and expert opinion supports the use of a stimulant laxative plus a stool softener in preventing and managing constipation in patients with cancer at the end of life (NCCN, 2011b).

Opioid-Induced Constipation

Evidence and expert opinion support the initiation of a prophylactic bowel regimen when prescribing opioids in patients with cancer (Bisanz, 2005; Bisanz et al., 2009; Kalso, Edwards, Moore, & McQuay; 2004; Miaskowski et al., 2005; NCCN, 2011b). In the older patient, opioid-induced constipation should be anticipated and a prophylactic bowel regimen initiated with frequent monitoring. The recommended bowl regimen based on expert opinion is docusate sodium (100–300 mg/day) plus senna (two to six tablets twice daily) (Bisanz et al., 2009). Expert opinion also supports using bowel function and not opioid dosing as a guide for individually titrating the laxative dose for effectiveness (Bisanz et al., 2009). Poorly hydrated patients with opioid-induced constipation may develop a bowel impaction; therefore, the use of bulk laxatives is not recommended (Miaskowski et al., 2005).

In the ambulatory setting, nurses should assess patients being treated with opioids at least every other day for bowel activity. The use of opioid rotation to manage opioid-induced constipation is another strategy that has been used with effectiveness (Bisanz et al., 2009). For example, rotating sustained-release morphine to transdermal fentanyl patch has demonstrated a significant decline in constipation (Ahmedzai & Brooks, 1997; Miaskowski et al., 2005; Radbruch et al., 2000).

The FDA approved methylnaltrexone in 2008 for refractory opioid-induced constipation in patients who are receiving palliative care (Bisanz et al., 2009). Methylnaltrexone, given subcutaneously at doses of 5–20 mg, induced a bowel movement within four hours (Becker, Galandi, & Blum, 2007; Portenoy et al., 2008). The ambulatory care oncology nurse is responsible for assessing readiness to learn and teaching the patient or family member to administer the daily subcutaneous injection.

Naloxone is an opioid receptor antagonist. When administered to opioid-tolerant patients, both oral and parenteral routes have shown mixed results for managing opioid-induced constipation. The potential risks in opioid-tolerant patients include withdrawal symptoms such as nausea, sweating, abdominal pain and cramps, and restlessness (Friedman & Dello Buono, 2001).

The management of constipation in older adults with cancer is challenging for both patients and healthcare clinicians. Constipation symptoms can be severe, affect function and QOL, and lead to hospitalization. In the older adult, constipation usually has multiple etiologies, including age-related issues, disease, comorbidities, medications, and treatment. The prevention and management of constipation should be essential components of ambulatory nursing practice. Interventions should be specifically targeted at the etiology, and both nonpharmacologic and pharmacologic interventions should be used.

Dehydration

Overview

Dehydration occurs as a result of decreased fluid intake or increased fluid losses that can be acute from diarrhea, vomiting, or blood loss or chronic from persistent anorexia. Older adults are vulnerable to chronic dehydration, usually caused by insufficient fluid intake (Bennett, Thomas, & Riegel, 2004). Older people are also more vulnerable to shifts in fluid balance, both overhydration and dehydration, and advanced age is associated with an increased likelihood of dehydration (Mentes, 2008). Side effects from cancer and cancer treatment such as mucositis and chemotherapy- or radiation-induced diarrhea can contribute to dehydration. Therefore, maintaining adequate fluid balance is an essential aspect of care management of the older adult during cancer treatment.

Ambulatory care oncology nurses must accurately assess older adults with cancer and their individual risk for dehydration and incorporate the knowledge of aging and comorbidities to proactively plan interventions to promote enhanced tolerance of cancer treatment and improved QOL.

Clinical Significance and Prevalence

Consequences of dehydration can be severe and include renal failure, electrolyte imbalance, medication toxicity, constipation, urinary tract and respiratory infections, delirium, falls, and seizures (Mentes, 2006; Mukand, Cai, Zielinski, Danish, & Burman, 2003). Dehydration increases the likelihood of thromboembolic events and kidney stones (Schols, de Groot, van der Cammen, & Rikkert, 2009) and complicates the treatment of many other illnesses, including cancer. Dehydration is the most common precipitant of electrolyte imbalances (Gillman, 2009).

Interrelatedness to Aging and Etiology

Changes occur with aging that increase the risk for dehydration. Total body fluid decreases with age, comprising only 40% water compared to 60% water for younger individuals (Gillman, 2009). Muscle mass is lost with age, thus increasing the proportion of fat cells, which contain less water than muscle cells. This leads to decreased intracellular volume (Metheny, 2000). In comparison to males, females have less total body water because of a higher percentage of body fat and less muscle mass.

As individuals age, a decreased perception or sensation of thirst exists; this can lead to decreased fluid intake. Physiologic kidney changes that occur with aging include a decreased ability to concentrate urine and a decrease in the function of antidiuretic hormone, which helps the body conserve water (Luckey & Parsa, 2003). Although these changes themselves do not cause dehydration, they do contribute to the increased vulnerability of the older patient to changes in fluid balance.

Psychosocial factors causing decreased intake and comorbidities can contribute to dehydration in the older adult. Cognitive impairment may cause forgetfulness, resulting in the inability to remember to consume fluids. Some older adults may purposefully withhold fluids because of fear of incontinence. Depression can affect intake of both foods and fluids. Physical disabilities or limitations may prevent or reduce access to fluids.

Polypharmacy, especially the use of more than four medications, with severe dehydration has been historically reported in nursing home patients (Lavizzo-Mourey, Johnson, & Stolley, 1988). Medications that affect kidney function, including diuretics, laxatives, angiotensin-converting enzyme inhibitors, and psychotropic drugs, such as antipsychotics and anxiolytics, and especially those with anticholinergic effects, can affect hydration status (Mentes, 2006). Medications, particularly antibiotics, can cause diarrhea, and adults older than age 65 are at increased risk for antibiotic-associated diarrhea (Kale-Pradham, Jassal, & Wilhelm, 2010).

Comorbidities such as cardiac disease, congestive heart failure, diabetes mellitus, and acute infections (pneumonia, upper respiratory, urinary tract, or skin infections and gastroenteritis) can contribute to the development of dehydration (Gillman, 2009; Mentes, 2006). Chronic conditions that affect the bowel such as irritable bowel syndrome, spastic colon, and celiac disease may also affect fluid status.

Interrelatedness to Cancer and Treatment

Side effects from cancer and cancer treatment contribute to altered fluid balance. Anorexia, nausea, taste changes, dysphagia, vomiting, constipation, diarrhea, and fatigue can affect intake and output, increasing the risk of dehydration. Cancers associated with an increased risk of dehydration include head and neck cancers, those requiring chest or mediastinal radiation, those causing significant dysphagia such as esophageal or gastric cancers, and cancers known to cause abdominal obstruction such as ovarian cancer (Price, 2010). Hyponatremia (low sodium) and volume depletion can result from third space fluid accumulation associated with ascites, hypoalbuminemia, and lymphatic and venous obstruction. Cancer treatment–induced diarrhea is a common side effect of some treatments. If persistent or severe, it can have serious consequences, including life-threatening electrolyte abnormalities and dehydration, and may contribute to cardiovascular morbidity (Benson et al., 2004). Dehydration can occur as an acute effect from common chemotherapy and targeted agents, especially those listed in Figure 4-7. Radiation therapy to the abdomen, pelvis, or lumbosacral areas can cause acute or chronic diarrhea depending on total dose, location, and amount of bowel within the radiation field (Coleman, 2009).

Assessment

Monitoring intake and output is commonplace in the hospital and inpatient settings. Accurately quantifying intake for ambulatory patients is more challenging, as patients may not remember to record intake and may have difficulty quantifying the amount of urine or stool, especially with diarrhea. Emphasis should be placed on establishing the severity of fluid intake and loss in addition to presence of symptoms and clinical assessment (Lawlor, 2002).

The ambulatory care oncology nurse should assess for signs and symptoms of dehydration (see Figure 4-8). Not all patients will exhibit the classic signs of dehydration on clinical examination. Older adults with chronic dehydration may not display some common clinical signs such as elevated heart rate or high urine specific gravity (Bennett et al., 2004). Dry mucous membranes and longitudinal furrows on the tongue are among the more sensitive clinical indictors of dehydration (Price, 2010), so assessment of the older adult's oral mucosa is especially important. Absence of sweat

---

Figure 4-7. Common Anticancer Agents That Cause Diarrhea

- Capecitabine
- Cetuximab
- Docetaxel
- Erlotinib
- Fluorouracil
- Gefitinib
- Irinotecan
- Lapatinib
- Oxaliplatin
- Paclitaxel
- Topotecan

Figure 4-8. Signs and Symptoms of Hypovolemic Dehydration

- Dry oral mucosa
- Decreased saliva
- Dry axilla
- Poor skin turgor
- Headache
- Decreased urine output
- Dark, concentrated urine
- Speech incoherence
- Sunken eyes
- Tongue furrows
- Extremity weakness
- Tachycardia
- Orthostatic hypotension

in the axilla was reported to suggest dehydration, especially in patients with vomiting, diarrhea, or decreased oral intake (McGee, Abernethy, & Simel, 1999), although the sensitivity of axilla moisture as an indicator for dehydration may not be reliable (Hodgkinson, Evans, & Wood, 2003). Presence of orthostatic hypotension and poor skin turgor on assessment are common clinical indicators of dehydration (Price, 2010). When the nurse is assessing for orthostatic changes, the patient should be supine for at least two minutes before blood pressure and pulse are measured and should stand for one to two minutes before upright vital signs are measured. A drop in systolic blood pressure upon standing is associated with dehydration in older adults (Vivanti, Harvey, Ash, & Battistutta, 2008). Skin turgor assessment may not be a reliable indicator of dehydration in older adults because skin loses elasticity with age. Cachexia may alter skin turgor assessment (Lawlor, 2002). Weight monitoring is essential, as short-term fluctuations in weight are more likely to be attributable to fluid imbalance (Price, 2010). Caution should be taken when using weight as a measurement for dehydration in a patient with third space losses, such as ascites, because overall weight may not change.

Laboratory Assessment

The most reliable indicators of dehydration include increased serum sodium, increased serum osmolality, and increased ratio of blood urea nitrogen (BUN) to serum Cr (Mentes, 2008). BUN/Cr ratio greater than 25 signifies dehydration, and a ratio of 20–24 implies impending dehydration (Mentes, 2008). Elevations in serum Cr level should be evaluated against the patient's baseline serum Cr level. Muscle mass influences Cr levels and is usually lower in patients with advanced disease and elevated in the setting of acute and chronic renal impairment (Lawlor, 2002). BUN level can be a marker for dehydration but may be elevated for other reasons such as blood loss with gastrointestinal tract infection, renal disease, and diabetes (Daniels, 2010). In a patient who is dehydrated, the hematocrit may be elevated and should be monitored within the context of the patient's disease and treatment.

Monitoring urine studies, such as osmolarity, specific gravity, and urine color, may provide additional data. Urine sodium of less than 25 mEq/L is usually associated with fluid deficit (Lawlor, 2002). Urine color has been shown to be a reliable indicator of hydration status and correlated with urine specific gravity in older adults with adequate renal function in nursing homes and long-term care facilities (Mentes, 2006; Mentes, Wakefield, & Culp, 2006; Wakefield, Mentes, Diggelmann, & Culp, 2002). The nurse should keep in mind that certain foods (e.g., beets, blackberries, asparagus, carrots) and medications (e.g., warfarin, multivitamins, certain chemotherapy drugs) can discolor urine. The ambulatory care oncology nursing assessment should always include a review of all patient medications, including prescription, over-the-counter, and herbal preparations.

Intervention and Management

The best treatment for dehydration in the older adult is prevention. Patient and caregiver education should include the importance of adequate hydration and potential signs and symptoms of dehydration. Fluid requirements for an average adult is 1.5 liters daily, and if active, up to 3 liters (Price, 2010). Medications and comorbidities may influence this amount. Patients should be educated about their personal risk for dehydration based on their disease, comorbidities, and planned cancer treatment. Fluid needs may increase if side effects cause decreased intake or increased output. Patients should be instructed to monitor intake and output and taught the importance of taking fluids even if not thirsty. A simple suggestion to encourage adequate intake is to have the patient or caregiver fill an empty container or milk jug with water equal to the amount of the daily fluid requirement. As fluids are consumed, equal amounts of water can be emptied from the jug. This provides a visual representation of the daily requirements for the older adult. Motivated older adults who are at risk for chronic dehydration can be taught to monitor daily weights and urine color.

If the older adult does experience dehydration, the goals are to rehydrate quickly but safely and to avoid overhydration. IV fluids, with electrolyte replacement if necessary, administered in the ambulatory infusion unit may prevent the need for hospitalization. Oral fluids should be encouraged, including water, soups, gelatins, juices, and sports drinks, and the consumption of alcohol and caffeine should be discouraged. Weight and electrolytes should be closely monitored.

Prompt recognition and aggressive evidence-based management of side effects that impact hydration is critical. Older adults who experience diarrhea with chemotherapy or radiation are at high risk for experiencing repeat episodes of diarrhea with subsequent cycles. Strategies to prevent or reduce diarrhea can reduce the need for dose delays or reductions and can influence survival (Anthony, 2003; Muehlbauer et al., 2009). Anorexia, dysphagia, and other side effects that affect oral intake should be frequently assessed, and evidence-based management strategies should be promptly implemented. For patients with head and neck cancer undergoing chemoradiation, discussion with the multidisciplinary team about the use of percutaneous feeding tubes may be indicated. Early nutritional intervention has been shown to reduce dehydration and weight loss in patients with head and neck cancer who are undergoing radiation therapy (Piquet et al., 2002).

Dysphagia

Overview

Dysphagia is difficulty swallowing. Although it is a commonly recognized symptom associated with esophageal and head and neck cancers, nearly 40%

of all adults age 65 and older report difficulty swallowing (Rofes et al., 2011). Age-related changes place the older adult at increased risk for alterations in swallowing that can be further complicated by cancer and cancer treatments. Dysphagia can have a profound effect on nutritional status with consequences including weight loss, dehydration, fatigue, and aspiration pneumonia as well as a general decline in functional status and decreased QOL (Ney, Weiss, Kind, & Robbins, 2009). Ambulatory care oncology nurses need to be aware of dysphagia as an often unrecognized and underdiagnosed symptom in the older adult that can significantly affect cancer treatment and QOL. Understanding the etiology, signs, symptoms, and implications of dysphagia will help develop individualized management strategies. Early detection and proactive management of dysphagia is crucial and can reduce morbidity (White, O'Rourke, Ong, Cordato, & Chan, 2008).

Clinical Significance and Prevalence

Dysphagia can contribute to weight loss, dehydration, malnutrition, and respiratory infection. It is the major factor leading to aspiration pneumonia in the older adult (Rofes et al., 2011). Dysphagia has social and psychological consequences as well. Eating and drinking for many older adults is viewed as a social event, such as sharing meals with family and friends. Difficulty swallowing can lead to anxiety and distress at mealtimes, social isolation, depression, and decreased QOL (Ekberg, Hamdy, Woisard, Wuttg-Hannig, & Ortega, 2002; Nguyen et al., 2005). Dysphagia is a significant morbidity associated with head and neck cancer, with post-treatment dysphagia occurring in 50%–60% of patients (Kuhlbersh et al., 2006).

Interrelatedness to Aging and Etiology

Anatomic and physiologic changes associated with aging cause alterations in swallowing. Reduced tongue pressures affect propulsion of food, and delayed sensory relays contribute to slowed swallowing seen in older adults (Ney et al., 2009; Rofes et al., 2011). Decreased saliva-producing acinar cell reserves may contribute to dysphagia, especially in the presence of xerostomia or dry mouth. Many medications commonly prescribed to older adults can cause xerostomia, including anticholinergics, opioids, and diuretics. The effects of sedative, neuroleptic, and antidepressant medications can also contribute to impaired swallowing (Rofes et al., 2011). Comorbid neurologic and neuromuscular conditions such as stroke, Parkinson disease, Alzheimer disease, and other dementia syndromes can alter coordination of swallowing and contribute to dysphagia (Ney et al., 2009).

Cancer-related causes of dysphagia can be associated with tumor obstruction or lymph node involvement in the head and neck, esophageal, or lung regions. Damage to the laryngeal nerve and structural changes with head and neck, thyroid, and spinal cord surgeries can potentially affect swallowing. Side effects from radiation therapy and chemotherapy causing xerostomia and stomatitis and the long-term effect of tissue fibrosis are also causal factors. Older adults with cancer are at increased risk for developing mucositis, which can contribute to dysphagia (Bond, 2006).

Assessment

Clinical assessment of the older adult with cancer should include evaluation for the signs and symptoms of dysphagia listed in Figure 4-9. The ambulatory care oncology nurse can conduct a simple swallow test in the office by observing the patient swallowing food or water. After the patient swallows, the patient should be observed for a minute or more to monitor for delayed swallow initiation, excessive saliva, drooling, coughing, throat clearing, or a change in voice quality. A delayed cough response may also indicate problem (Paik, 2011). Presence of the gag reflex should not be used as a screening tool for dysphagia, as patients may have a normal gag reflex and still be experiencing dysphagia (Marik & Kaplan, 2003). Including observations from family members and caregivers about mealtime behaviors, such as changes in head positioning while swallowing or constant throat clearing, may be helpful. Evaluating food intake and noting specific food items that patients select or avoid may provide additional information when assessing for swallowing problems. Patients may have difficulty with thin fluids or thick bolus foods, and some foods or fluids may be avoided due to stomatitis or xerostomia. Patient weight and general nutritional status, as well as medications and comorbid conditions, should be noted in the ambulatory care nursing assessment. If a swallowing dysfunction is suspected, discussion with the oncologist regarding a formal evaluation and referral for a videofluoroscopy swallowing study or modified barium swallow is warranted.

Interventions and Management

Management of dysphagia in the older adult with cancer should be multidisciplinary and individualized. Using the expertise of registered dietitians, geriatricians, and speech and swallowing pathologists can be helpful for the nurse to individualize interventions, including dietary modifications, oral hygiene, postural adjustments, and swallowing exercises.

Figure 4-9. Signs and Symptoms of Dysphagia

- Food "sticking" in throat
- Multiple swallows per mouthful
- Pain or discomfort with swallowing
- Neck, chest pain, or heartburn with or after eating
- Food spillage from mouth
- Excessive drooling or difficulty managing secretions

- Choking, coughing, or constant throat clearing while eating
- Difficulty initiating swallow
- Pocketing of food in mouth
- Change in voice, "wet" voice with eating

Dietary Modifications

Patients will vary in their ability to swallow. The consistency of food should be individualized according to the findings from the swallowing evaluation. Recommendations, such as alternating liquids and solids to help wash down residual food and avoiding mixing foods and fluids in the same mouthful, may be helpful as single textures are easier to swallow than multiple textures (Ney et al., 2009). Avoiding very hot, dry, spicy, hard, or scratchy foods can be suggested, as well as eating six to eight small meals a day rather than three large meals (Grant & Rivera, 1995). The ambulatory care oncology nurse can work with the registered dietitian to encourage acceptable dietary items that provide adequate fluid and nutrition. Oral supplementation may be suggested to increase weight and improve nutritional status.

Percutaneous endoscopic gastrostomy (PEG) tubes for enteral feeding may be inserted prior to the start of treatment and be used during cancer treatment to help supplement and maintain adequate nutritional intake.

Oral Hygiene

Systematic reviews have demonstrated that enhanced oral hygiene decreases respiratory complications in elderly patients in hospitals and nursing homes (Azarpazhooh & Leake, 2006; Sjögren, Nilsson, Forsell, Johansson, & Hoogstraate, 2008). Because of the increased risk for aspiration pneumonia in patients with dysphagia, an aggressive and proactive oral hygiene regimen should be instituted, including brushing of teeth and dentures after meals. Periodic dental examinations and professional cleanings are encouraged, provided the patient's blood counts are adequate (Sjögren et al., 2008). Surveillance and management of xerostomia and stomatitis are required for rapid recognition and early intervention to reduce compounding dysphagia.

Postural Maneuvers and Exercise Strategies

Minimizing distractions during eating and careful, slow swallowing should be encouraged. A general postural rule to facilitate safe swallowing is to eat upright in a seated position (Ney et al., 2009). A swallowing specialist may suggest specific postural maneuvers such as anterior neck flexion (the chin tuck), posterior flexion (chin raise), and head rotation with swallowing based on the patient's assessment. Rehabilitative exercises aimed at increasing strength and range of motion of the head and neck muscles, including the tongue, are frequently prescribed for dysphagia. One such exercise is the tongue-hold, in which the patient swallows while holding the tip of the tongue between the teeth. Evidence has shown such exercises can improve swallowing and dietary intake of older adults after stroke (Ney et al., 2009; Rofes et al., 2011). Compelling evidence suggests that beginning swallowing exercises prior to chemoradiation improves swallowing and QOL for patients with head and neck cancer (Carroll et al., 2008; Kuhlbersh et al., 2006; Manikantan et al., 2009). Further research is needed to confirm regular use of swallowing exercises to prevent dysphagia associated with aging. The ambulatory care oncology nurse can suggest swallowing exercises as a proactive self-care strategy, as these exercises are simple and easy to do. Providing information, education, and encouragement to the older adult for both preventive and treatment-related interventions should be ongoing. Education of the patient and significant others about the risks of aspiration, the signs of choking, and performing the Heimlich maneuver is essential (Ney et al., 2009).

Dyspnea

Overview

Patients older than age 65 bear a disproportionate burden of cancer as well as an increased prevalence of medical problems such as chronic obstructive pulmonary disease, heart disease, diabetes, and hypertension. Dyspnea is experienced as limited or difficult respiration greater than expected given the current level of activity. Dyspnea occurs frequently in older adults, is associated with poor health, interferes with daily functioning, and contributes to mortality. Dyspnea is a common symptom of lung cancer and numerous advanced cancers (Yancik, Ganz, Varricchio, & Conley, 2001). It can be multifactorial in origin and is often an underrecognized and undertreated symptom in cancer ("Dyspnea in Cancer Patients Needs More Attention," 2006). Optimal treatment and management requires an understanding of the etiology of the disorder as well as the impact on the patient's QOL in order to direct appropriate treatment of malignant conditions.

Clinical Significance and Prevalence

No precise data exist on the prevalence of dyspnea in the older adult population. Rates vary among clinical settings and underlying diseases, and the morbidity associated with dyspnea can range from minor to disabling (Hooshiaran et al., 2010). Smoking history is very important, as 20% of all smokers develop chronic obstructive airway disease ("Dyspnea in Cancer Patients Needs More Attention," 2006). For patients with lung cancer, dyspnea is the most frequently distressing and burdensome symptom with a prevalence of 55%–90% (Xue & Abernethy, 2010). Approximately 25% of patients with any type of terminal cancer have symptoms of dyspnea either at rest or on exertion ("Dyspnea in Cancer Patients Needs More Attention," 2006).

Interrelatedness to Aging and Etiology

Patients' perceptions of dyspnea are affected by their previous experience, activity tolerance, and physical status. Dyspnea in the older adult can be related to debility secondary to anemia, atelectasis, pulmonary embolism, pneumonia, emphysema, cachexia-anorexia syndrome, or weakness. Concurrent diseases such as chronic obstructive pulmonary disease, asthma, congestive heart failure, acidosis, angina, and respiratory infection contribute to dyspnea, as well as psychological disruptions such as anxiety, depression, and panic disorders (Dickerson et al., 2001).

Conditions caused by cancer that can contribute to dyspnea are listed in Figure 4-10. Symptoms of dyspnea can manifest gradually or acutely if a cancer progresses and compromises the respiratory system. Cancer treatment–related causes of dyspnea include congestive heart failure, anemia secondary to chemotherapy, radiation-induced fibrosis and constrictive pericarditis, and hypothyroidism (Pan, 2003). The ambulatory care oncology nurse should perform assessments based on knowledge of this significant symptom and its association with cancer and treatment, comorbidities, and the process of aging.

Figure 4-10. Disease-Related Conditions Contributing to Dyspnea

- Pleural effusions
- Bronchial obstruction
- Mediastinal obstruction
- Superior vena cava syndrome
- Pericardial effusion
- Metastasis
- Lymphangitis
- Carcinomatosis
- Tumor replacing lung tissue
- Massive ascites
- Abdominal distention

Assessment

Dyspnea is a subjective experience described as an uncomfortable awareness of breathing, breathlessness, or severe shortness of breath (Hospice & Palliative Nurses Association, 1996). Like pain, the patient should be asked to rate dyspnea to establish a baseline; this will help the nurse to assess the response to specific therapies (Mahler et al., 2010). Assessment should start with using the patient's descriptor of how he or she is feeling, such as breathlessness, need to gasp or pant, unable to get enough air, or a feeling like suffocation (Kazanowski, 2003; Pan, 2003). Sample questions to assist the nurse in patient assessment are listed in Figure 4-11.

Multiple assessment tools have been developed, including the visual analog scale (Gift, 1989) and the Cancer Dyspnea Scale, which includes 12 items that assess the patient's sense of effort, anxiety, and discomfort (Tanaka, Akechi, Okuyama, Nishiwaki, & Uchitomi, 2000). Newer scales such as the Dyspnea-12 (Yorke, Moosavi, Shuldham, & Jones, 2010) have been developed to include the physical and affective aspects of dyspnea. The Respiratory Distress Observation Scale (Campbell, Templin, & Walch, 2010) is designed for patients who are unable to self-report. There have been no comparative trials demonstrating superior performance of one scale over another. Use of these questionnaires is valuable in the assessment of dyspnea, but the nurse should

---

Figure 4-11. Eliciting Patient Descriptors for the Assessment of Dyspnea

- When did it start? Onset (days, weeks, hours), acute versus chronic
- What makes it better or worse?
- What does it feel like?
- Are there other symptoms occurring with it (pain, chest tightness, palpitations, cough, fever, light-headedness)?
- How severe is it? (Use a scale such as visual analog scale of 1–10.)
- How much does it interfere with daily life and function?
- When is it at its worst?
- Is it persistent or intermittent?

---

ask the patient to describe the shortness of breath, keeping in mind that the patient's descriptors may help identify the underlying etiology. Obtaining the past medical history and social history is important in identifying factors that may have contributed to the development of dyspnea.

Interventions and Management

Optimal treatment of dyspnea starts with identification of the underlying etiology and addressing any reversible causes of the condition. The goal of care is to improve the subjective sensation as the patient describes. Patient and caregiver education should include the balance of energy expenditure with energy conservation, symptom monitoring, prompt healthcare seeking, and principles of dyspnea management, including
- Physical therapy to increase endurance
- Oxygen therapy: O_2 saturation greater than 90%
- Positioning to facilitate lung expansion
- Relaxation exercises
- Assistive devices such as a wheelchair to decrease physical activities that induce dyspnea (DiSalvo, Joyce, Culkin, Tyson, & Mackay, 2009)
- Providing cooler temperatures (DiSalvo et al., 2009).
  Medications that help alleviate dyspnea include the following.
- Steroids have demonstrated efficacy in lymphangitic carcinomatosis and superior vena cava syndrome ("Dyspnea in Cancer Patients Needs More Attention," 2006).
- Oral or parenteral opioids reduce ventilator demand by decreasing central respiratory drive; evidence supports their use in the management of dyspnea (DiSalvo et al., 2009).
- Beta agonists or anticholinergics may be helpful to reverse airway obstruction, especially with former smokers who may also have chronic bronchitis or emphysema (Cheung & Zimmermann, 2011).
- Benzodiazepines and phenothiazines have been found to help relieve dyspnea exacerbated by concomitant anxiety (Cheung & Zimmermann, 2011).

Fatigue

Overview

Cancer-related fatigue (CRF) is a persistent subjective sense of physical, emotional, and/or cognitive tiredness that interferes with usual functioning and is not proportional to recent activity (NCCN, 2011a). This fatigue is a common and distressing symptom, which presents as a continuum occurring throughout the spectrum of cancer diagnosis and involves therapy that frequently persists beyond the end of treatment (Broeckel, Jacobsen, Horton, Balducci, & Lyman, 1998; Mock et al., 2007). Compared with fatigue experienced by healthy adults, CRF is more distressing, more severe, and less likely to be relieved by rest (NCCN, 2011a). In the older adult with cancer, multiple physical and psychosocial factors may increase susceptibility. There often are complex interactions among the disease, treatment, and the use of central acting drugs for controlling symptoms or side effects of treatment that may potentiate the experience of fatigue (Wang, 2008). The ambulatory care oncology nurse should conduct focused assessments based on the knowledge of this common and significant symptom, its association with the treatment of cancer, and the complexity of its presentation in the older adult. Care goals are prompt recognition and intervention to prevent compromise of the treatment regimen and deterioration of the patient's functional status and to maintain pretreatment levels of independence.

Clinical Significance and Prevalence

Fatigue is a common experience in people with cancer, with studies reporting prevalence rates of 80%–100% (Campos, Hassan, Riechelmann, & Del-Giglio, 2011; Lawrence, Kupelnick, Miller, Devine, & Lau, 2004; Prue, Rankin, Allen, Gracey, & Cramp, 2006; Servaes, Verhagen, & Bleijenberg, 2002). Prolonged fatigue has been consistently reported among cancer survivors for months up to 10 years following primary cancer treatment (Campos et al., 2011; Gielissen, Wiborg, Verhagen, Knoop, & Bleijenberg, 2011; Harrington, Hansen, Moskowitz, Todd, & Feuerstein, 2010). Fatigue is associated with decreased physical functioning, deconditioning, and increased frailty and falls risk (Orre et al., 2008). Coexisting factors, such as pain, emotional distress, anemia, insomnia, dehydration, and nutritional issues, potentiate the fatigue experience, and comorbid conditions add to the complexity of treatment. Severe CRF may lead to dose reductions, delays, or withdrawal from the prescribed treatment regimens and can reduce the chance of remission or cure and significantly impair QOL (Curt et al., 2000; Morrow, Andrews, Hickok, Roscoe, & Matteson, 2002; Potter, 2004).

Interrelatedness to Aging

More than 10 million visits per year are made to a primary care provider for problems related to fatigue in the older adult, with approximately 50% of the U.S. population reporting being fatigued for at least part of the day (Gambert, 2005). Sarcopenia, the degenerative loss of muscle mass and strength that occurs with aging, can lead to decreased physical functioning, increased frailty and falls risk, mobility disorders, and loss of independent living and should be critically considered during the cancer treatment decision-making process. Additionally, metabolic disturbances secondary to insufficiency of organ systems (e.g., renal, hepatic, hematopoietic), compromised physical, social, and economic well-being (Given, 2008), mental and cognitive alterations (Lynch, 2005), and distress and depression (Raison, Capuron, & Miller, 2006) are common conditions in the older adult that could affect fatigue and the treatment course or outcomes.

Interrelatedness to Treatment

The fatigue symptoms that emerge secondary to a cancer diagnosis or during cancer treatment may be physical, psychological, or emotional. Older patients with cancer who are experiencing fatigue may withdraw from family and friends, need more sleep, and, in some cases, may not be able to think clearly or perform any physical activities. Fatigue related to cancer and cancer treatment is associated with significant and concerning outcomes in the older adult (see Figure 4-12).

Assessment

Fatigue should be assessed systematically using the patient's self-report or perception (Mock et al., 2007), capturing physical, emotional, and psychological aspects of distress. Patients should be screened for fatigue and potentially contributing factors, such as pain, medications, anemia, and sleep disturbances, at their initial visit and at regular intervals during and

---

Figure 4-12. Outcomes Associated With Cancer-Related Fatigue in the Older Adult

- Delay of recovery following surgery
- Increased risk of compromised organ function secondary to antineoplastic therapy (e.g., sepsis, SIADH, TLS)
- Pain and sleep disturbance
- Distress (may include anxiety and depression)
- Distress interfering with sleep, worsening fatigue
- Dose reductions, delays, or discontinuation of prescribed therapies
- Diminished functionality and loss of independence
- Loss of productivity and self-esteem
- Significant reductions in physical functioning and quality of life

SIADH—syndrome of inappropriate antidiuretic hormone secretion; TLS—tumor lysis syndrome

Note. Based on information from Berger & Farr, 1999; Luctkar-Flude et al., 2007; Mock et al., 2007; National Comprehensive Cancer Network, 2011a; Rubin et al., 2004.

following cancer treatment (NCCN, 2011a). Both one-dimensional and multidimensional tools are available for the assessment of fatigue, although not all are suited for the older adult. The Visual Analog Fatigue Scale is a simple, single-item tool designed to assess the presence and severity of CRF (Glaus, 1993). It can be used at multiple times throughout the course of a day or a course of therapy to help understand individual variation of fatigue (Rao & Cohen, 2008). The Brief Fatigue Inventory is also an easy to use, validated, unidimensional tool that uses a 0–10 numerical scale characterizing mild fatigue as 1–3, moderate fatigue as 4–6, and severe fatigue as 7–10 (Mendoza et al., 1999). The simple wording of the Brief Fatigue Inventory makes it easy to understand and translate.

Multidimensional tools have also been used to assess fatigue based on the belief that CRF is a multidimensional symptom affecting cognitive, behavioral, somatic, and affective domains of functioning (Rao & Cohen, 2008). The Functional Assessment of Cancer Therapy–Fatigue (FACT-F) is a well-known, validated tool designed to measure the fatigue symptoms of patients with cancer who have anemia (Yellen, Cella, Webster, Blendowski, & Kaplan, 1997). It contains the 28 items of the FACT-General (FACT-G) tool that assess general health-related quality of life and an additional 13 items to assess fatigue. Patients read through fatigue-specific statements, such as "I have energy" and "I am frustrated by being too tired to do the things I want to do" and rate them on a five-point Likert scale ranging from 0 (not at all) to 4 (very much so). A main disadvantage of the FACT-F is that its length may be too burdensome for an older adult with cancer to complete. The 13-item fatigue subscale, however, can be used alone and is easier and faster to complete. The Multidimensional Fatigue Symptom Inventory–Short Form (MFSI-SF) (Hann et al., 1998) is a 30-item tool also designed to assess the multidimensional nature of fatigue. It can be completed in a wide variety of settings in approximately five minutes and may facilitate assessment of the older adult. The MFSI-SF consists of 30 statements; patients indicate the extent to which they have experienced each symptom during the preceding week. Items are rated on a five-point scale indicating how true each statement was for the respondent during the past week (0 = not at all, 4 = extremely). The utility of the MFSI-SF is further increased by the use of a single response format for all 30 items (i.e., all items are answered on the same five-point scale) and the brief wording of the items being explored. As a result, the MFSI-SF may be easier to complete and less burdensome on fatigued patients than other multidimensional fatigue scales.

Intervention and Management

A multidisciplinary biopsychosocial approach with physicians, nurses, geriatricians, registered dietitians, physical and occupational therapists, and oncology social workers can facilitate identification and treatment of underlying and contributing causes of cancer-related fatigue, such as pain, emotional distress, sleep disturbance, anemia, and hypothyroidism. A review and reconciliation of all medications being taken by the patient should eliminate nonessential centrally acting drugs (Mock et al., 2000).

Nonpharmacologic interventions: Fatigue is an often neglected and under-reported symptom in the elderly, who may consider fatigue to be the usual course of aging (Rao & Cohen, 2008). Older adults may benefit from education about common patterns of fatigue associated with cancer treatments, such as cumulative fatigue during radiation therapy and cyclical fatigue with chemotherapy. This may help the patient understand and interpret fatigue, for example, as a treatment side effect rather than a symptom of progressive disease (Cope, 2006) or aging. NCCN recommends that patients and their families be informed that the management of fatigue is an integral part of the total health care (NCCN, 2011a).

A strong association exists between fatigue and insomnia, but whether CRF experienced during the day is related to the amount and quality of sleep obtained at night is unclear (Rao & Cohen, 2008). As normal aging is associated with changes in sleep (see Chapter 2), and some components of CRF (e.g., physical, emotional, cognitive) are thought to be influenced by disrupted sleep (Rao & Cohen, 2008), it is reasonable to encourage good sleep hygiene as a nursing intervention. Educating the patient about setting and maintaining regular sleep and wake times, avoiding long or late afternoon naps, and avoiding caffeine, alcohol, and nicotine within several hours of bedtime are all positive suggestions.

Evidence supports exercise several times per week as an effective intervention for reducing fatigue in patients during and after treatment (Mitchell, Beck, Hood, Moore, & Tanner, 2009). The patient and caregiver should be educated to balance energy expenditure with energy conservation and to maintain or increase current levels of functioning. The use of assistive energy-saving devices may be suggested. Other interventions likely to be effective include activity management, relaxation, massage, healing touch therapy, polarity therapy, and haptotherapy (Mitchell et al., 2009).

Pharmacologic interventions: Although medications play a role in managing CRF, no consensus has been established about which drugs are useful. Psychostimulants have been found to enhance alertness and reduce fatigue in people with nonmalignant disorders, and research is under way to address the question of whether these drugs could be effective in treating CRF. Common side effects include irritability, anorexia, insomnia, nausea, and rapid heart rate. Two antidepressants have been studied in CRF: paroxetine (Paxil®) and bupropion (Wellbutrin® SR). Paroxetine is a selective serotonin reuptake inhibitor (SSRI) that appears to improve mood but does not reduce CRF in those receiving chemotherapy. Further research through randomized controlled trials is needed to better understand the relationship between depression and fatigue in people with cancer, as well as the usefulness of antidepressants in CRF (Carroll, Kohli, Mustian, Roscoe, & Morrow, 2007). Low-dose corticosteroids have been thought to provide a benefit in managing fatigue; however, a review of four studies using progestational steroids found no benefit to patients with

CRF after eight weeks of treatment with these agents (Minton, Richardson, Sharpe, Hotopf, & Stone, 2008).

Pain

Overview

Persistent pain is one of the most common reasons older people seek medical care. The most common causes of pain in older adults are those related to musculoskeletal disorders such as back pain, arthritis, or neuropathic pain syndromes (Potter, Hami, Bryan, & Quigley, 2003). Treatment of pain in older adults with cancer may be more complex because of comorbid conditions or chronic nonmalignant pain disorders and disability. Older adults have been identified as an at-risk group for inadequate pain treatment. Older adults are at increased risk for adverse reactions to pain medications, likely because of pharmacokinetic changes, such as reduced renal excretion and hepatic metabolism, as well as age-related pharmacodynamic changes, such as an increased sensitivity to certain analgesics (Wynne, 2005). Effective pain management in older adults with cancer requires skill in pain assessment, recognition of the importance of a holistic interdisciplinary team approach to care, and knowledge of both pharmacologic and nonpharmacologic approaches to management.

Incidence and Prevalence

The incidence of pain in older adults living in the community ranges from 25% to 60% (Donald & Foy, 2004; Gibson & Helme, 2001). Miaskowski (2005) reported that 50% of patients undergoing cancer treatment and 80%–90% of patients with advanced cancer will experience moderate pain. Studies suggest that many patients undergoing active treatment for cancer experience pain, and 70%–90% of patients at the end of life experience unrelieved pain (Potter et al., 2003). In the older adult with cancer, pain can be related to disease, treatment, comorbid conditions, or to a combination of all of these.

Clinical Significance

Inadequate pain treatment may have serious consequences, including depression, anxiety, cognitive changes, sleep disturbances, and an inability to perform ADLs. In addition, poorly controlled pain contributes to diminished QOL, functional decline, recurrent falls, social isolation, polypharmacy, caregiver distress, and increased healthcare costs (American Geriatrics Society Panel on the Pharmacological Management of Persistent Pain in Older Persons, 2009; Foley, 2004).

Interrelatedness to Aging and Etiology

Older adults most vulnerable for inadequate treatment of pain are those who (Herr et al., 2010; Sawyer, Lillis, Bodner, & Allman, 2007)
• Are among the oldest-old (older than age 85)
• Have postoperative pain
• Present with a history of substance abuse
• Have cognitive impairment, delirium, or dementia
• Have severe psychological distress (depression, anxiety) or major psychiatric disorders
• Hold specific beliefs about pain management
• Do not speak English or have disease-related barriers to communication, such as laryngectomy or head and neck cancer
• Are living in a setting in which the caregivers are not trained in the assessment and management of pain.

Pain is classified by its duration (acute or chronic) and by its underlying pathophysiologic mechanisms (American Pain Society, 2008; Coda & Bonica, 2001; Turk & Okifuji, 2001). *Nociception* refers to the process by which information about tissue damage is conveyed to the central nervous system (Byers & Bonica, 2001; Urch, 2009). Nociceptors are sensory receptors that are the free endings of nerve fibers that are stimulated when there is pain. Nociceptive pain can further be divided into somatic or visceral pain (Byers & Bonica, 2001). Somatic pain may be classified as deep or superficial and includes pain originating from the skin, muscle, joint, or bone. Visceral pain is pain originating in the visceral organs, such as in the abdomen. Neuropathic pain is the result of injury in the peripheral or central nervous system, in which nerves have been infiltrated or compressed by tumors or inflamed by infection (Backonja, 2001; Galer, Schwartz, & Allen, 2001; Tasker, 2001). Neuropathic pain is frequently chronic and tends to be less responsive to treatment with opioids (Dworkin et al., 2010). The pain frequently has burning, lancinating, or electric-shock qualities (Oaklander, 2008). Mixed pain syndrome is a combination of both nociceptive and neuropathic pain. Breakthrough pain is pain that is incidental or related to movement or procedures (Haugen, Hjermstad, Hagen, Caraceni, & Kaasa, 2010).

Patients with cancer often have both nociceptive and neuropathic pain simultaneously, with breakthrough pain intermittently, and most have pain at multiple sites (Payne & Gonzales, 2004). The ambulatory care oncology nurse should be aware of the disorders associated with neuropathic pain (see Figure 4-13), as it leads to increased complexity in the management of pain in the older adult with cancer. In the ambulatory care setting, the nurse should consider chronologic age, the impact of comorbid conditions, and the cancer diagnosis when evaluating pain in the older adult. Understanding these factors, as well as the goals that the patient has for his or her life, will enable the nurse to intervene more effectively (Bourbonniere & Kagan, 2004).

Figure 4-13. Neuropathic Pain Syndromes

Peripheral Neuropathic Pain Syndromes	Central Pain Syndromes
• Chemotherapy-induced neuropathy • Complex regional pain syndrome • Diabetic neuropathy • Phantom limb pain • Plexopathies • Postherpetic neuralgia • Postmastectomy pain • Post-thoracotomy pain • Radiation therapy • Spinal cord compression • Trigeminal neuralgia • Tumor infiltration	• Alcohol-related neuropathy • Carpal tunnel pain • Guillain-Barré disease • Multiple sclerosis pain • Parkinson disease pain • Post-stroke pain • Sarcoidosis • Spinal cord injury

Note. Based on information from Dworkin et al., 2003.

Assessment and Screening

Assessment of pain should be performed consistently. Self-report is encouraged in patients with normal mentation or with mild to moderate cognitive impairment; a simple numeric rating scale of 0–10 may be used with 0 indicating no pain and 10 indicating the worst possible pain. The Brief Pain Inventory (BPI) also uses a numeric rating scale and has been used successfully to assess the severity and impact of cancer pain (Cleeland, 1989). The simple wording of the BPI makes it easy to understand as well as easy to translate. The level of pain assessed by the BPI can be divided into categories of mild (1–4), moderate (5–6), and severe (7–10) based on the amount of pain-related interference with function (Serlin, Mendoza, Nakamura, Edwards, & Cleeland, 1995). For patients with severe to moderate cognitive changes, the Pain Assessment in Advanced Dementia scale (often referred to as PAINAD) is a validated tool (Warden, Hurley, & Volicer, 2003) (see Table 4-5).

The goals of the clinical assessment are to determine the pain etiology, identify any comorbid conditions that may be causing or contributing to the pain, evaluate the patient's level of function, and identify care goals and personal priorities. Once these aspects are determined, a treatment and care plan can be developed to address the pain condition in a method congruent with the patient's individual goals. Essential components and questions included in a pain assessment are

- Location(s) and appearance of the painful site
- Intensity: Using a consistent pain rating scale, patients rate their pain presently and over the past seven days. Use of a consistent rating scale could include a numeric rating scale (0–10), a categorical scale (none, mild, moderate, severe), or an observational tool in patients who cannot self-report (Taylor & Herr, 2003).

- Quality: What does the pain feel like? Is it sharp, dull, burning, stabbing, or electric shock–like?
  - Nociceptive: aching, throbbing
  - Visceral: squeezing, cramping
  - Neuropathic: burning, tingling, electrical, painfully numb
- Temporal patterns: Is it intermittent or continuous? Are there precipitating, aggravating, and alleviating factors?
- Meaning of pain: How does your pain affect your ability to work, sleep, and function?
- Cultural factors: Is it acceptable to express that you are in pain? Do you use over-the-counter or home remedies for pain?
- Medication history: Obtain a pain treatment history and responses to previous pharmacologic interventions, including prior opioid use, analgesic effects, and why medications were stopped. In patients who have moderate to severe cognitive impairment, objective behaviors should be assessed that

Table 4-5. Pain Assessment in Advanced Dementia (PAINAD) Scale

Items*	0	1	2	Score
Breathing independent of vocalization	Normal	Occasional labored breathing. Short periods of hyperventilation.	Noisy labored breathing. Long period of hyperventilation. Cheyne-Stokes respirations.	
Negative vocalization	None	Occasional moan or groan. Low level speech with a negative or disapproving quality.	Repeated troubled calling out. Loud moaning or groaning. Crying.	
Facial expression	Smiling or inexpressive	Sad. Frightened. Frown.	Facial grimacing	
Body language	Relaxed	Tense. Distressed pacing. Fidgeting.	Rigid. Fists clenched. Knees pulled up. Pulling or pushing away. Striking out.	
Consolability	No need to console	Distracted or reassured by voice or touch.	Unable to console, distract, or reassure.	
			Total**	

*Five-item observational tool (see descriptors for each item)

**Total score ranges from 0–10 (based on a score of 0–2 for five items, with a higher score indicating more severe pain). 0 = "no pain," 10 = "severe pain."

Note. From "Development and Psychometric Evaluation of the Pain Assessment in Advanced Dementia (PAINAD) Scale," by V. Warden, A.C. Hurley, and L. Volicer, 2003, Journal of the American Medical Directors Association, 4, 9–15. The content of this table is in the public domain.

might be related to pain, such as labored breathing, grimacing, moaning, groaning, and rigid, tense body posture. Other physiologic parameters such as heart rate or blood pressure can provide valuable information (Zwakhalen, Hamers, Abu-Saad, & Berger, 2006).

Principles of Pain Management for the Ambulatory Care Oncology Nurse

The nurse should integrate knowledge of the physiologic changes of aging that might affect the efficacy of pain medications (see Table 4-6). For patients with neuropathic pain, evaluate for the following (Fields, 1999; Galer, 1995; Jensen & Baron, 2003).

- Dysesthesia—unpleasant, abnormal sensations in response to unpainful stimuli
- Hyperalgesia—severe pain sensation in response to painful stimuli
- Hypoalgesia—reduced sensation to painful stimuli, such as a pin prick
- Allodynia—pain produced by a stimulus that usually does not produce pain, such as light touch

The World Health Organization (WHO, n.d.) pain ladder is a guideline for medication management of escalating pain. Three categories of drugs are includ-

Table 4-6. Common Physiologic Changes With Aging That Affect Analgesia	
Physiologic Parameter	**Changes With Aging**
Gastrointestinal absorption	Slowing of transit time may increase the incidence of constipation.
Transdermal absorption	Less subcutaneous fat in older patients may decrease absorption. Dosing of fentanyl patches may require adjustment.
Distribution	Increased ratio of fat to lean body weight may increase volume of distribution for fat-soluble drugs like fentanyl and may result in long drug half-life.
Liver metabolism	Metabolism is variable in elderly, which may result in prolonged half-life. Use acetaminophen cautiously.
Renal excretion	Glomerular filtration rate decreases with aging, resulting in decreased excretion and potentially increased toxicity. In patients with renal insufficiency, avoid morphine because of accumulation of metabolites, and avoid use of NSAIDs.

NSAIDs—nonsteroidal anti-inflammatory drugs

Note. Based on information from the American Geriatrics Society Panel on the Pharmacological Management of Persistent Pain in Older Persons, 2009; Lötsch, 2005; Pergolizzi et al., 2008.

ed in the WHO ladder and include nonopioids, opioids, and adjuvant analgesics. When pain occurs, oral administration of drugs should be given promptly in a stepwise manner. For mild pain, nonopioids (aspirin, acetaminophen, nonsteroidal anti-inflammatory drugs) should be used, as indicated on step 1 of the WHO ladder. For moderate to severe pain, a drug from step 2 or 3 of the WHO ladder should be used. For neuropathic pain, adjuvant drugs should be used. For chronic pain, opioids should be given around the clock rather than as needed. After initiation of opioid analgesics, patients should be closely monitored for drug efficacy and side effects, with careful dose titration for pain relief.

Adjuvant analgesics are medications not classified as analgesics but have been found to be helpful in certain pain syndromes and can be used at any stage of the pain ladder (WHO, n.d.). Some common adjuvant analgesics are
- Corticosteroids
- Antidepressants
- Anticonvulsants
- Topical therapy (e.g., lidocaine, capsaicin).

Side Effect Management

The most common and persistent side effect of opioid analgesics is constipation. A bowel regimen, such as a stimulant laxative, and a stool softener should be included as part of the pain management plan (see Constipation section). Other side effects include
- Nausea and vomiting
- Delayed gastric emptying
- Bladder dysfunction
- Pruritus
- Sexual dysfunction
- Sedation, impaired cognition, and delirium.

Respiratory depression, muscle rigidity, and myoclonus are seen with higher doses of opioids (Pergolizzi et al., 2008). Clinically significant respiratory depression is always seen with other signs of central nervous system depression, such as sedation and mental clouding. If present in the opioid-tolerant patient, other contributing factors usually are present. Fear of respiratory depression should not interfere with appropriate upward titration of opioid medications (American Pain Society, 2008).

Pharmacologic Interventions

Opioids are the mainstay of cancer pain treatment. When used as single agents, no ceiling effect appears to be present, meaning the dose can be increased until either adequate relief is reported or intolerable side effects occur (American Pain Society, 2008). Various long-acting preparations include oral extended and controlled release and transdermal routes of administration. Short-acting preparations include oral immediate release, transmucosal, and elixirs. The nurse should be aware of the available routes of administration for the ordered drug (e.g., oral, transdermal, transmucosal, subcutaneous, IV, epidural, intrathecal). When selecting a route of administration, the least invasive route should be used. Most patients can tolerate taking oral medications throughout the course of their disease; however, as the disease reaches late stages or after treatments (such as surgery) that make swallowing difficult, alternative routes can be employed to maintain comfort. See Figure 4-14 for principles of managing pain in the older adult with cancer.

For patients with severe, uncontrolled pain, the IV route is preferred. A portable pain pump can be used in the home setting for management of severe pain or severe pain with frequent episodes of breakthrough or incident-related pain. *Patient-controlled analgesia* is a method for the administration of IV or subcutaneous analgesia with the use of a small portable pump. Collaboration with homecare agencies, nurses, and pharmacists is needed. When

---

Figure 4-14. Principles of Pain Management in the Older Adult With Cancer

- Assess for cognitive, social, and psychological barriers in the older adult.
- Review physiologic parameters (e.g., renal and liver function, respiratory status) that may affect opioid dosing and effectiveness.
- Review past analgesic, opioid, and nonopioid drug use and response.
- Be informed of drug combinations that may potentiate side effects or preexisting co-morbidities.
- Plan for side effect management (e.g., bowel regimen, antiemetics).
- Educate the patient and caregivers about the pain management plan, potential side effects, and types of issues that should prompt a call to the doctor or nurse.
- Explain that the least invasive route of administration tolerated will be utilized, and the pain management plan will change with alterations in the patient's condition.
- Describe the rationale for around-the-clock dosing with long-acting opioids and rescue dosing with short-acting opioids for breakthrough pain.
- In opioid-naïve patients, administer short-acting opioids on an as-needed basis to determine opioid requirements, and then convert to a long-acting, around-the-clock preparation with as-needed short-acting opioids for breakthrough pain.
- When using combination drugs with acetaminophen, be aware that acetaminophen has a maximum daily ceiling dose.
- When using nonsteroidal anti-inflammatory drugs (NSAIDs), assess for gastrointestinal and renal toxicity, hypertension, and heart failure. Proton pump inhibitors or misoprostol can be administered for gastrointestinal protection when using NSAIDs on a consistent basis.
- Titrate short-acting opioids slowly, every two to three days if indicated, keeping in mind that they have no ceiling effect. Monitor for side effects and analgesic effect on a regular basis. After this titration phase, convert the patient to a long-acting preparation with a short-acting opioid to be given on an as-needed basis (rescue dose).
- Understand that effectiveness of the pain management plan will be influenced by cost and complexity. Advocate for simplicity in scheduling and cost-consciousness in selection of drugs.
- Frequently reassess for side effects and analgesic effect.

Note. Based on information from American Geriatrics Society Panel on the Pharmacological Management of Persistent Pain in Older Persons, 2009; American Pain Society, 2008.

all other routes of administration have failed to provide effective analgesia, interventions that may have effectiveness include anesthetic, neurosurgical, or neuroablative therapies, epidural, intrathecal administration of opioids and nonopioids, nerve blocks, radiofrequency ablation, and cryoablation (American Geriatrics Society Panel on the Pharmacological Management of Persistent Pain in Older Persons, 2009).

Nonpharmacologic Interventions

Nonpharmacologic interventions can be used alone or in combination with pharmacologic management. Integration of nonpharmacologic interventions into the pain management plan for all older adult patients should be considered (Brown & McCormack, 2006), including
- Physical exercise and physical therapy
- Progressive relaxation
- Music therapy
- Cognitive-behavioral therapy
- Biofeedback
- Acupuncture
- Transcutaneous electrical nerve stimulation
- Reflexology.

The ambulatory care oncology nurse should have an understanding of evidence-based supportive care for older adults with cancer, be familiar with pharmacologic and nonpharmacologic interventions, and be able to comprehensively integrate knowledge from these various domains to recognize barriers and improve the management of pain (Bourbonniere & Kagan, 2004). For further information on the assessment and management of cancer-related pain, see the Oncology Nursing Society Putting Evidence Into Practice resources (Aiello-Laws, Ameringer, Delzer, Peterson, & Reynolds, 2009; Eaton, 2009).

Sexuality

Overview

Loss of sexual activity and desire is not a part of the normal aging process. Sexual desire and activity continue well into later life, and age is not a deterrent to a happy and healthy sex life. Although a decrease in sexual activity occurs with age, sexual interest persists well into the senior years (Bancroft, 2007). Sexual interaction does not necessarily mean sexual intercourse. Sexuality encompasses partnership, activity, behavior, attitudes, and function (Lindau, Laumann, Levinson, & Waite, 2003). Sexual activity is associated with health, and illness may considerably interfere with sexual vigor (Lindau et al., 2007). The predominant influences on sexuality in later life include opportunities and attitudes, health and disability, and effective treatment for sexual problems (Stones & Stones, 2007).

Many people dealing with an illness find that being sexually active is not important for them in order to maintain a loving, intimate relationship or is not an important part of their relationship. Older adults often find that they can maintain loving, intimate relationships without being sexually active. However, for others, alterations manifested by a loss of libido or an inability to respond or perform sexually as they had in the past can be very distressing. Because cancer affects all aspects of life, including sexual feelings and the ways in which those feelings are expressed, the clinician should acknowledge that the older adult with cancer may have the same needs and desires as before the illness manifested and may have difficulty expressing those needs while coping with cancer and its treatment.

Cancer treatment can alter physical and physiologic function, resulting in pain with sexual intercourse, a loss of interest in sexual activity, and erectile dysfunction (Karakiewicz et al., 2008). The older adult may want to resume or continue sexual intimacy after a cancer has been diagnosed and treated or while undergoing treatment. This may require some adaptation of normal sexual patterns. The patient should express concerns with their partner and may also require specific information and guidance from the physician or nurse. Referral to a sexual counselor may assist the patient to overcome difficulties, reduce tensions, and improve communication. Intimacy does not require sexual intercourse and can be the balance for personal feelings, hopes, and closeness during cancer treatment.

Sexuality is a continuing human concern regardless of age. Even as normal and pathologic changes affect sexual health, older adults have an ongoing interest in sexual activity, which holds many benefits for them. Nurses have a role in assessing sexual health and assisting in developing plans for managing sexual problems. The ambulatory care oncology nurse can improve the care of older adults with cancer by careful consideration of intimacy and sexuality using standards of practice integrated with an understanding of the issues unique to older adults (Kagan, Holland, & Chalian, 2008).

Clinical Significance and Prevalence

Cancer and its treatment frequently affect intimacy and sexual functioning. Estimates of sexual dysfunction across cancer types range from 40% to 100% (Flynn et al., 2011). When an older adult is ill, maintaining sexual relations is not a priority during the course of the disease and treatment, much the same as with younger adults. Pain, discomfort, medications, or worry can overshadow sexual desire. For the older adult, the partner may be the caregiver, and sexual desire can become compromised by the stress of the caregiver role and concern for the loved one (Mayo Clinic, 2009). For older adults, having cancer is associated with reduced ability to perform many ADLs, with impact varying across cancer types. For example, patients with lung cancer experience significant increases in body pain and significant reductions in mental health scores (Goodwin & Stridhar, 2009).

The National Social Life, Health, and Aging Project, a nationally representative U.S. probability sample of 1,550 women and 1,455 men ages 57–85 at the time of interview, published results indicating that sexual problems among the elderly are not an inevitable consequence of aging, but instead are responses to the presence of stressors in multiple life domains. Moreover, this impact may partly be gender differentiated, with older women's sexual health being more sensitive to their physical health compared to men (Waite, Laumann, Das, & Schumm, 2009).

Interrelatedness to Aging and Etiology

Age-related, physical, physiologic, and psychological changes affect sexual fitness (Araujo, Mohr, & McKinlay, 2004). Additionally, older adults are more susceptible to a number of medical conditions that are associated with diminished sexual health and functioning (Gott, Hinchliff, & Galena, 2004). These include (a) cardiovascular disease, (b) Parkinson disease, (c) diabetes, (d) benign prostatic hypertrophy, and (e) cancer. Medications used among older adults, especially those used to treat common medical illnesses, also affect sexuality (Montejo, Llorca, Izquierdo, & Rico-Villademoros, 2001).

Interrelatedness to Treatment

Cancer and cancer treatment can cause changes in any phase of the sexual response. The sexual changes caused by cancer treatment may be long term or permanent. Decreased desire for sexual activity as well as decreased stamina is a common sexual problem for patients across the cancer continuum (Flynn et al., 2011). After cancer treatment, or just with aging, women may respond more slowly to sexual stimulation, produce less lubrication, and may feel that breast or genital caressing does not bring pleasure. Changes with arousal in men include not being able to attain or sustain an erection, having an erection that is not reliable, or not having erections as frequently as desired. Changes with orgasm may occur, such as taking longer to reach orgasm or being unable to achieve orgasm. Generally, sexual changes do not improve quickly. Finding the most helpful remedy may take time and patience because sexual changes can be caused by both psychological and physical factors, such as body image changes and organ loss (Flynn et al., 2011).

Assessment: The clinician should perform an assessment to determine the presence of physiologic changes through a health history, review of systems, and physical examination for changes that could affect sexual health (Wallace, 2008). The PLISSIT model (Annon, 1976) outlines an approach to sexual assessment and intervention and includes open-ended questions about sexuality. It has been used widely with older adults. The PLISSIT model begins by first seeking permission (P) to discuss sexuality with an older adult. The next step of the model affords an opportunity for the healthcare provider to share limited information (LI) with the patient. The third step guides the healthcare provider to provide specific suggestions (SS) to improve sexual health. The final part calls for intensive therapy (IT) when needed for clients whose sexual dysfunction goes beyond the scope of nursing management.

Intervention and Management

Communication and education are the first step. A discussion of age-, disease-, and treatment-related physiologic changes should be facilitated with the patient and his or her partner. The effects of medications and medical conditions on sexual functioning should be included. Ambulatory care oncology nurses may facilitate communication regarding sexual health with the following strategies.

- Open discussion of issues (see Figure 4-15 for examples for beginning dialogue)
- Safe sex practices
- Impact of current health on sexuality (e.g., fatigue, stamina, malaise)
- Strategies to compensate for alterations in sexual functioning, including
  - Water-based lubricants
  - Use of sildenafil citrate (Viagra®)
  - Use of centrally acting serotonin agonists
  - Vasodilating creams (Walsh & Berman, 2004)
  - Exploring sexual positions that place no weight on a scar or ostomy

Helping patients manage their sexual health is an important component of oncology care in all settings. Comprehensive pamphlets on sexuality and cancer for both men and women that provide illustrations and self-help information are available from organizations such as the American Cancer Society. Older adults experience normal and pathologic changes as they age, and many of these affect sexual health. Addressing older adults' sexuality can increase their self-esteem, promote companionship, restore function, inspire healing, and enhance energy.

Figure 4-15. Questions to Guide Sexuality Assessment Among Older Adults

- Can you share with me how you express your sexuality and sexual desires? Are there concerns or questions you have about how your ongoing sexual needs might be satisfied?
- How has the sexual rapport between you and your partner changed as you have aged or become ill?
- Would you be interested in learning about interventions or information that might help enrich your sexuality?

Note. Based on information from Wallace, 2000.

Conclusion

Numerous negative outcomes can result when care is inadequately attuned to the needs of older adults, particularly in an ambulatory care delivery system and when the disease is cancer. Older adults require time for listening, information gathering, medication review, examination, and counseling. In a system in which time is not a readily available commodity, the complexity of the older adult, the disease, and the treatment can easily result in inefficient and poorly coordinated care. Subsequently, vulnerable older adults' medical problems can go unrecognized or inadequately managed. Oncology nurses should understand that the physiologic diversity of aging makes designing standardized treatment and approaches to care especially challenging with older adult populations.

Care of the older adult with cancer bridges the domains of nursing, medicine, physical therapy, social work, occupational therapy, gerontology, and nutrition with the primary disease management team in a coordinated effort to treat the disease, readily recognize and respond to complications, and maintain pretreatment levels of performance and functional status. This chapter presented some significant symptoms associated with aging that the ambulatory care oncology nurse can influence during cancer treatment. It is hoped that knowledge of these significant symptoms and their interrelatedness to aging will enable the implementation of interventions to minimize severity, reduce distress, and improve QOL.

References

Aarsland, D., Londos, E., & Ballard, C. (2009). Parkinson's disease dementia and dementia with Lewy bodies: Different aspect of one entity. *International Psychogeriatrics, 21,* 216–219. doi:10.1017/S1041610208008612

Adams, L.A., Cunningham, R.S., Caruso, R.A., Norling, M.J., & Shepard, N. (2009). ONS PEP resource: Anorexia. In L.H. Eaton & J.M. Tipton (Eds.), *Putting evidence into practice: Improving oncology patient outcomes* (pp. 31–36). Pittsburgh, PA: Oncology Nursing Society.

Adams, L.A., Shepard, N., Caruso, R.A., Norling, M.J., Belansky, H., & Cunningham, R.S. (2009). Putting evidence into practice: Evidence-based interventions to prevent and manage anorexia. *Clinical Journal of Oncology Nursing, 13,* 95–102. doi:10.1188/09.CJON.95-102

Ahmed, T., & Haboubi, N. (2010). Assessment and management of nutrition in older people and its importance to health. *Clinical Interventions in Aging, 5,* 207–216. Retrieved from http://www.dovepress.com/articles.php?article_id=4939

Ahmedzai, S., & Brooks, D. (1997). Transdermal fentanyl versus sustained-release oral morphine in cancer pain: Preference, efficacy, and quality of life: The TTS fentanyl comparative trial group. *Journal of Pain and Symptom Management, 13,* 254–261.

Aiello-Laws, L.B., Ameringer, S.W., Delzer, N.A., Peterson, M.E., & Reynolds, J.K. (2009). ONS PEP resource: Pain. In L.H. Eaton & J.M. Tipton (Eds.), *Putting evidence into practice: Improving oncology patient outcomes* (pp. 223–234). Pittsburgh, PA: Oncology Nursing Society.

American Association of Neuroscience Nurses. (2007). *Neurologic assessment of the older adult a guide for nurses: AANN Clinical Practice Guideline Series.* Glenview, IL: Author.

American Geriatrics Society Panel on the Pharmacological Management of Persistent Pain in Older Persons. (2009). Pharmacological management of persistent pain in older persons. *Journal of the American Geriatrics Society, 57,* 1331–1346.

American Pain Society. (2008). *Principles of analgesic use in the treatment of acute pain and cancer pain* (6th ed.). Glenview, IL: Author.

Angevaren, M., Aufdemkampe, G., Verhaar, H.J., Aleman, A., & Vanhees, L. (2008). Physical activity and enhanced fitness to improve cognitive function in older people without known cognitive impairment. *Cochrane Database of Systematic Reviews* 2008, Issue 3. Art. No.: CD005381. doi:10.1002/14651858.CD005381.pub3

Annon, J. (1976). The PLISSIT model: A proposed conceptual scheme for behavioral treatment of sexual problems. *Journal of Sex Education and Therapy, 2*(2), 1–15.

Anthony, L. (2003). New strategies for the prevention and reduction of cancer treatment-induced diarrhea. *Seminars in Oncology Nursing, 19*(4), 17–21.

Araujo, A.B., Mohr, B.A., & McKinlay, J.B. (2004). Changes in sexual function in middle-aged and older men: Longitudinal data from the Massachusetts male aging study. *Journal of the American Geriatrics Society, 52*, 1502–1509. doi:10.1111/j.0002-8614.2004.52413.x

Arterburn, D.E., Crane, P.K., & Sullivan, S.D. (2004). The coming epidemic of obesity in elderly Americans. *Journal of the American Geriatrics Society, 52*, 1907–1912. doi:10.1111/j.1532-5415.2004.52517.x

Azarpazhooh, A., & Leake, J.L. (2006). Systematic review of the association between respiratory diseases and oral health. *Journal of Periodontology, 77*, 1465–1482. doi:10.1902/jop.2006.060010

Backonja, M.M. (2001). Painful neuropathies. In J.D. Loeser, S.H. Butler, C.R. Chapman, & D.C. Turk (Eds.), *Bonica's management of pain* (3rd ed., pp. 371–387). Baltimore, MD: Lippincott Williams & Wilkins.

Ballantyne, J.C. (2007). Opioid analgesia: Perspectives on right use and utility. *Pain Physician, 10*, 479–491.

Ballard, C., Corbett, A., Chitramohan, R., & Aarsland, D. (2009). Management of agitation and aggression associated with Alzheimer's disease: Controversies and possible solutions. *Current Opinion in Psychiatry, 22*, 532–540. doi:10.1097/YCO.0b013e32833111f9

Bancroft, J.H. (2007). Sex and aging. *New England Journal of Medicine, 357*, 820–822. doi:10.1056/NEJMe078137

Becker, G., Galandi, D., & Blum, H.E. (2007). Peripherally acting opioid antagonists in the treatment of opioid-related constipation: A systematic review. *Journal of Pain and Symptom Management, 34*, 547–565. doi:10.1016/j.jpainsymman.2006.12.018

Bennett, J.A., Thomas, V., & Riegel, B. (2004). Unrecognized chronic dehydration in older adults: Examining prevalence rates and risk factors. *Journal of Gerontological Nursing, 22*, 22–28.

Benson, A.B., III, Ajani, J.A., Catalano, R.B., Engelking, C., Kornblau, S.M., Martenson, J.A., Jr., ... Wadler, S. (2004). Recommended guidelines for the treatment of cancer treatment-induced diarrhea. *Journal of Clinical Oncology, 22*, 2919–2926. doi:10.1200/JCO.2004.04.132

Berg, D.T. (2006). The older adult with colorectal cancer. In D.G. Cope & A.M. Reb (Eds.), *An evidence-based approach to the treatment and care of the older adult with cancer* (pp. 135–165). Pittsburgh, PA: Oncology Nursing Society.

Berger, A.M., & Farr, L. (1999). The influence of daytime inactivity and nighttime restlessness on cancer-related fatigue. *Oncology Nursing Forum, 26*, 1663–1671.

Bisanz, A. (2005). Bowel management in patients with cancer. In J.A. Ajani, S.A. Curley, N.A. Janjan, & P.M. Lynch (Eds.), *Gastrointestinal cancer* (pp. 313–345). New York, NY: Springer Science+Business Media.

Bisanz, A.K., Woolery, M.J., Lyons, H.F., Gaido, L., Yenulevich, M., & Fulton, S. (2009). ONS PEP resource: Constipation. In L.H. Eaton & J.M. Tipton (Eds.), *Putting evidence into practice: Improving oncology patient outcomes* (pp. 93–104). Pittsburgh, PA: Oncology Nursing Society.

Bond, S.M. (2006). Symptom management of mucositis. In D. Cope & A. Reb (Eds.), *An evidence-based approach to the treatment and care of the older adult with cancer* (pp. 349–366). Pittsburgh, PA: Oncology Nursing Society.

Bosshard, W., Dreher, R., Schnegg, J.F., & Bula, C.J. (2004). The treatment of chronic constipation in elderly people: An update. *Drugs and Aging, 21,* 911–930.

Bouras, E.P., & Tangalos, E.G. (2009). Chronic constipation in the elderly. *Gastroenterology Clinics of North America, 38,* 463–480. doi:10.1016/j.gtc.2009.06.001

Bourbonniere, M., & Kagan, S.H. (2004). Nursing intervention and older adults who have cancer: Specific science and evidence based practice. *Nursing Clinics of North America, 39,* 529–543. doi:10.1016/j.cnur.2004.02.009

Braes, T., Milisen, K., & Foreman, M.D. (2008). Assessing cognitive function. In E. Capezuti, D. Zwicker, M. Mezey, & T. Fulmer (Eds.), *Evidence-based geriatric nursing protocols for best practice* (3rd ed., pp. 41–55). New York, NY: Springer.

Breitbart, W., Gibson, C., & Tremblay, A. (2002). The delirium experience: Delirium recall and delirium-related distress in hospitalized patients with cancer, their spouses/caregivers, and their nurses. *Psychosomatics, 43,* 183–194. Retrieved from http://psy.psychiatryonline.org/cgi/reprint/43/3/183

Brodaty, H., Breteler, M.M.B., DeKosky, S.T., Dorenlot, P., Fratiglioni, L., Hock, C., ... De Strooper, B. (2011). The world of dementia beyond 2020. *Journal of the American Geriatrics Society, 59,* 923–927. doi:10.1111/j.1532-5415.2011.03365.x

Broeckel, J.A., Jacobsen, P.B., Horton, J., Balducci, L., & Lyman, G.H. (1998). Characteristics and correlates of fatigue after adjuvant chemotherapy for breast cancer. *Journal of Clinical Oncology, 16,* 1689–1696.

Brown, D., & McCormack, B. (2006). Determining factors that have an impact upon effective evidence-based pain management with older people, following colorectal surgery: An ethnographic study. *Journal of Clinical Nursing, 15,* 1287–1298. doi:10.1111/j.1365-2702.2006.01553.x

Brown, J. (2002). A systematic review of the evidence on symptom management of cancer-related anorexia and cachexia. *Oncology Nursing Forum, 29,* 517–532. doi:10.1188/02.ONF.517-532

Byers, M., & Bonica, J.J. (2001). Peripheral pain mechanisms and nociceptor plasticity. In J.D. Loeser, S.H. Butler, C.R. Chapman, & D.C. Turk (Eds.), *Bonica's management of pain* (3rd ed., pp. 26–72). Baltimore, MD: Lippincott Williams & Wilkins.

Camilleri, M., & Bharucha, A.E. (2010). Behavioral and new treatments for constipation: Getting the balance right. *Gut, 59,* 1288–1296. doi:10.1136/gut.2009.199653

Camilleri, M., Lee, J.S., Viramontes, B., Bharucha, A.E., & Tangalos, E.G. (2000). Insights into the pathophysiology and mechanisms of constipation, irritable bowel syndrome, and diverticulosis in older people. *Journal of the American Geriatrics Society, 48,* 1142–1150.

Campbell, M.L., Templin, T., & Walch, J. (2010). A respiratory distress observation scale for patients unable to self-report dyspnea. *Journal of Palliative Medicine, 13,* 285–290. doi:10.1089/jpm.2009.0229

Campos, M.P.O., Hassan, B.J., Riechelmann, R., & Del-Giglio, A. (2011). Cancer-related fatigue: A review. *Revista da Associacao Medica Brasileira, 57,* 206–214.

Cancelli, I., Beltrame, M., Gigli, G.L., & Valente, M. (2009). Drugs with anticholinergic properties: Cognitive and neuropsychiatric side effects in elderly patients. *Neurological Sciences, 30,* 87–92. doi:10.1007/s10072-009-0033-y

Candy, B., Jones, L., Goodman, M.L., Drake, R., & Tookman, A. (2011). Laxatives or methylnaltrexone for the management of constipation in palliative care patients. *Cochrane Database of Systematic Reviews* 2011, Issue 1. Art. No.: CD003448. doi:10.1002/14651858.CD003448.pub3

Caraceni, A., Nanni, O., Maltoni, M., Piva, L., Indelli, M., Arnoldi, E., & De Conno, F. (2000). Impact of delirium on the short term prognosis of advanced cancer patients: Italian multicenter group on palliative care. *Cancer, 89,* 1145–1149.

Caraceni, A., & Simonetti, F. (2009). Palliating delirium in patients with cancer. *Lancet Oncology, 10,* 164–172. doi:10.1016/S1470-2045(09)70018-X

Carroll, J.K., Kohli, S., Mustian, K.M., Roscoe, J.A., & Morrow, G.R. (2007). Pharmacologic treatment of cancer-related fatigue. *Oncologist, 12*(Suppl. 1), 43–51. doi:10.1634/theoncologist.12-S1-43

Carroll, W.R., Locher, J.L., Canon, C.L., Bohannon, I.A., McColloch, N.L., & Magnuson, J.S., (2008). Pretreatment swallowing exercises improve swallow function after chemoradiation. *Laryngoscope, 118*, 39–44. doi:10.1097/MLG.0b013e31815659b0

Centeno, C., Sanz, A., & Bruera, E. (2004). Delirium in advanced cancer patients. *Palliative Medicine 18*, 184–194. doi:10.1191/0269216304pm879oa

Chapman, I. (2007). The anorexia of aging. *Clinics in Geriatric Medicine, 23*, 735–756. doi:10.1016/j.cger.2007.06.001

Chertkow, H. (2008). Diagnosis and treatment of dementia: Introduction. *Canadian Medical Association Journal, 178*, 316–321. doi:10.1503/cmaj.070795

Cheung, W.Y., & Zimmermann, C. (2010). Pharmacologic management of cancer-related pain, dyspnea, and nausea. *Seminars in Oncology, 38*, 450–459. doi:10.1053/j.seminoncol .2011.03.016

Clarkson, W.K., Pantano, M.M., Morley, J.E., Horowitz, M., Littlefield, J.M., & Burton, F.R. (1997). Evidence for the anorexia of aging: Gastrointestinal transit and hunger in healthy elderly vs. older adults. *American Journal of Physiology, 272*, R243–R248.

Cleeland, C.S. (1989). Measurement of pain by subjective report. In C.R. Chapman & J.D. Loeser (Eds.), *Advances in pain research and therapy, volume 12: Issues in pain management* (pp. 391–403). New York, NY: Raven.

Clemens, K.E., & Klaschik, E. (2010). Managing opioid-induced constipation in advanced illness: Focus on methylnaltrexone bromide. *Therapeutics and Clinical Risk Management, 6*, 77–82. doi:10.2147/TCRM.S4301

Coda, B.A., & Bonica, J.J. (2001). General considerations of acute pain. In J.D. Loeser, S.H. Butler, C.R. Chapman, & D.C. Turk (Eds.), *Bonica's management of pain* (3rd ed., pp. 222–240). Baltimore, MD: Lippincott Williams & Wilkins.

Cole, M.G. (2004). Delirium in elderly patients. *American Journal of Geriatric Psychiatry, 12*, 7–21.

Coleman, J. (2009). Diarrhea. In C.G. Brown (Ed.), *A guide to oncology symptom management* (pp. 173–198). Pittsburgh, PA: Oncology Nursing Society.

Cope, D. (2006). Fatigue. In D. Camp-Sorrell & R.A. Hawkins (Eds.), *Clinical manual for the oncology advanced practice nurse* (2nd ed., pp. 1127–1132). Pittsburgh, PA: Oncology Nursing Society.

Crum, R.M., Anthony, J.C., Bassett, S.S., & Folstein, M.F. (1993). Population-based norms for the mini-mental state examination by age and educational level. *JAMA, 269*, 2386–2391. doi:10.1001/jama.269.18.2386

Cummings, J.L., Mega, M., Gray, K., Rosenberg-Thompson, S., Carusi, D.A., & Gornbein, J. (1994). The neuropsychiatric inventory: Comprehensive assessment of psychopathology in dementia. *Neurology, 44*, 2308–2314.

Curt, G.A., Breitbart, W., Cella, D., Groopman, J.E., Horning, S.J., Itri, L.M., … Portenoy, R.K. (2000). Impact of cancer-related fatigue on the lives of patients: New findings from the fatigue coalition. *Oncologist, 5*, 252–360. doi:10.1634/theoncologist.5-5-353

Daniels, R. (2010). *Delmar's guide to laboratory and diagnostic tests* (2nd ed.). Clifton Park, NY: Delmar Cengage Learning.

Del Parigi, A., Panza, F., Capurso, C., & Solfrizzi, V. (2006). Nutritional factors, cognitive decline and dementia. *Brain Research Bulletin, 69*, 1–19. doi:10.1016/j.brainresbull .2005.09.020

Detsky, A.S., McLaughlin, J.R., Baker, J.P., Johnston, N., Whittacker, S., Mendelsohn, R.A., & Jeejeebhoy, K.N. (1987). What is subjective global assessment of nutritional status? *Journal of Parenteral and Enteral Nutrition, 11*, 8–13.

Dewys, W.D., Begg, C., Lavin, P.T., Band, P.R., Bennett, J.M., Bertino, J.R., … Tormey, D.C. (1980). Prognostic effect of weight loss prior to chemotherapy in cancer patients: Eastern Cooperative Oncology Group. *American Journal of Medicine, 69*, 491–497.

Dickerson, E.D., Benedetti, C., Davis, M.P., Grauer, P.A., Santa-Emma, P.H., & Zafirides, P. (2001). *Palliative care pocket consultant*. Dubuque, IA: Kendall-Hunt.

DiSalvo, W.M., Joyce, M.M., Culkin, A.E., Tyson, L.B., & Mackay, K. (2009). ONS PEP resource: Dyspnea. In L.H. Eaton & J.M. Tipton (Eds.), *Putting evidence into practice: Improving oncology patient outcomes* (pp. 93–104). Pittsburgh, PA: Oncology Nursing Society.

Donald, I.P., & Foy, C.A. (2004). A longitudinal study of joint pain in older people. *Rheumatology, 43,* 1256–1260. doi:10.1093/rheumatology/keh298

Donini, L.M., Saina, C., & Cannella, C. (2003). Eating habits and appetite control in the elderly: The anorexia of aging. *International Psychogeriatrics, 15,* 73–87.

Dworkin, R.H., Backonja, M., Rowbotham, M.C., Allen, R.R., Argoff, C.R., Bennett, G.J., ... Weinstein, S.M. (2003). Advances in neuropathic pain: Diagnosis, mechanisms, and treatment recommendations. *Archives of Neurology, 60,* 1524–1534. doi:10.1001/archneur.60.11.1524

Dworkin, R.H., O'Connor, A.B., Audette, J., Baron, R., Gourlay, G.K., Haanpää, M.L., ... Wells, C.D. (2010). Recommendations for the pharmacological management of neuropathic pain: An overview and literature update. *Mayo Clinic Proceedings, 85*(Suppl. 3), S3–S14. doi:10.4065/mcp.2009.0649

Dyspnea in cancer patients needs more attention. (2006). *Journal of Supportive Oncology, 4,* 62–64. Retrieved from http://www.supportiveoncology.net/jso/journal/articles/0402063.pdf

Eaton, L.H. (2009). Pain. In L.H. Eaton & J.M. Tipton (Eds.), *Putting evidence into practice: Improving oncology patient outcomes* (pp. 215–221). Pittsburgh, PA: Oncology Nursing Society.

Ekberg, O., Hamdy, S., Woisard, V., Wuttg-Hannig, A., & Ortega, P. (2002). Social and psychological burden of dysphagia: Its impact on diagnosis and treatment. *Dysphagia, 17,* 139–146. doi:10.1007/s00455-001-0113-5

Etters, L., Goodall, D., & Harrison, B.E. (2008). Caregiver burden among dementia patient caregivers: A review of the literature. *Journal of the American Academy of Nurse Practitioners, 20,* 423–428. doi:10.1111/j.1745-7599.2008.00342.x

Fields, H.L. (1999). Pain: An unpleasant topic. *Journal of the International Association for the Study of Pain, 82*(Suppl. 1), S61–S69.

Fillit, H.M., Butler, R.N., O'Connell, A.W., Albert, M.S., Birren, J.E., Cotman, C., ... Tully, T. (2002). Achieving and maintaining cognitive vitality with aging. *Mayo Clinical Practice, 77,* 681–696. doi:10.4065/77.7681

Fletcher, K. (2008). Dementia. In E. Capezuti, D. Zwicker, M. Mezey, T.T. Fulmer, D. Gray-Miceli, & M. Kluger (Eds.), *Evidence-based geriatric nursing protocols for best practice* (3rd ed., pp. 83–109). New York, NY: Springer.

Flynn, K.E., Jeffery, D.D., Keefe, F.J., Porter, L.S., Shelby, R.A., Fawzy, M.R., ... Weinfurt, K.P. (2011). Sexual functioning along the cancer continuum: Focus group results from the Patient Reported Outcomes Measurement Information System (PROMIS®). *Psycho-Oncology, 20,* 378–386. doi:10.1002/pon.1738

Foley, K.M. (2004). Acute and chronic pain syndromes. In D. Doyle, G.W. Hanks, N. Cherny, & K. Kalman (Eds.), *Oxford textbook of palliative medicine* (3rd ed., pp. 298–316). New York, NY: Oxford University Press.

Folstein, M.F., Folstein, S., & McHugh, P.R. (1975). Mini-mental state: A practical method for grading the cognitive state of patients for the clinician. *Journal of Psychiatric Research, 12,* 189–198. doi:10.1016/0022-3956(75)90026-6

Fong, T.G., Tulebaev, S.R., & Inouye, S.K. (2009). Delirium in elderly adults: Diagnosis, prevention and treatment. *Nature Reviews Neurology, 5,* 210–220. doi:10.1038/nrneurol.2009.24

Foreman, M.D., Mion, L.C., Trygstad, L., & Fletcher, K. (2003). Delirium: Strategies for assessing and treating. In M. Mezey, T. Fulmer, I. Abraham, & D.A. Zwicker (Eds.), *Geriatric nursing protocols for best practice* (2nd ed., pp. 116–140). New York, NY: Springer.

Foy, K., & Okpalugo, C. (2009). Usefulness of routine blood tests in dementia workup. *Psychiatrist, 33,* 481. doi:11.11921/pb.33.12.481

Friedman, J.D., & Dello Buono, F.A. (2001). Opioid antagonists in the treatment of opioid-induced constipation and pruritus. *Annals of Pharmacotherapy, 35,* 85–91. doi:10.1345/aph.10121

Fuhrman, M., Charney, P., & Mueller, C. (2004). Hepatic proteins and nutrition assessment. *Journal of American Dietetic Association, 104,* 1258–1264. doi:10.1016/j.jada.2004.05.213

Furman, E.F. (2006). Undernutrition in older adults across the continuum of care. *Journal of Gerontological Nursing, 32,* 22–27.

Galanakis, P., Bickel, H., Gradinger, R., von Gumppenberg, S., & Forstl, H. (2001). Acute confusional state in the elderly following hip surgery: Incidence, risk factors and complications. *International Journal of Geriatric Psychiatry, 16,* 349–355.

Galer, B.S. (1995). Neuropathic pain of peripheral origin: Advances in pharmacologic treatment. *Neurology, 45*(Suppl. 9), S517–S523.

Galer, B.S., Schwartz, L., & Allen, R.J. (2001). Complex regional pain syndromes-type 1: Reflex sympathetic dystrophy and type II causalgia. In J.D. Loeser, S.H. Butler, C.R. Chapman, & D.C. Turk (Eds.), *Bonica's management of pain* (3rd ed., pp. 388–411). Baltimore, MD: Lippincott Williams & Wilkins.

Gallagher, P., & O'Mahony, D. (2009). Constipation in old age. *Best Practice and Research Clinics of Gastroenterology, 23,* 875–887. doi:10.1016/j.bpg.2009.09.001

Gambert, S.R. (2005). Fatigue: Finding the cause of a common complaint. *Clinical Geriatrics, 13,* 6–8.

Gauthier, S., Reisberg, B., Zaudig, M., Petersen, R.C., Ritchie, K., Broich, K., ... Winblad, B. (2006). Mild cognitive impairment. *Lancet, 367,* 1262–1270. doi:10.1016/S0140-6736(06)68542-5

Gibson, S.J., & Helme, R.D. (2001). Age-related differences in pain perception and report. *Clinical Geriatric Medicine, 17,* 433–456.

Gielissen, M.F.M., Wiborg, J.F., Verhagen, C.A.H.H.V.M., Knoop, H., & Bleijenberg, G. (2011). Examining the role of physical activity in reducing post cancer fatigue. *Supportive Care in Cancer.* Advance online publication. doi:10.1007/s00520-011-1227-4

Gift, A.G. (1989). Validation of a vertical visual analogue scale as a measure of clinical dyspnea. *Rehabilitation Nursing, 14,* 323–325.

Gillman, P. (2009). Nutrition, hydration, electrolytes and acid base balance. In P. Gillman, P. Parker, & P. Tabloski (Eds.), *Gerontological nursing: ANCC nursing review and resource manual* (2nd ed., pp. 97–118). Silver Spring, MD: American Nurses Credentialing Center.

Given, B. (2008). Cancer-related fatigue: A brief overview of current nursing perspectives and experiences. *Clinical Journal of Oncology Nursing, 12*(Suppl. 5), 7–9. doi:10.1188/08.CJON.S2.7-9

Glaus, A. (1993). Assessment of fatigue in cancer and non-cancer patients and in healthy individuals. *Supportive Care in Cancer, 1,* 305–315.

Goodwin, P.J., & Stridhar, S.S. (2009). Health-related quality of life in cancer patients—More answers but many questions remain. *Journal of the National Cancer Institute, 101,* 838–839. doi:10.1093/jnci/djp140

Gott, M., Hinchliff, S., & Galena, E. (2004). General practitioner attitudes to discussing sexual health issues with older people. *Social Science and Medicine, 58,* 2093–2103. doi:10.1016/j.socscimed.2003.08.025

Grant, M., & Rivera, L. (1995). Anorexia, cachexia and dysphagia: The symptom experience. *Seminars in Oncology Nursing, 11,* 266–271.

Hall, G.R., & Buckwalter, K.C. (1987). Progressively lowered stress threshold: A conceptual model of care of adults with Alzheimer's disease. *Archives of Psychiatric Nursing, 1,* 399–406.

Hann, D.M., Jacobsen, P.B., Azzarello, L.M., Martin, S.C., Curran, S.L., Fields, K.K., ... Lyman, G. (1998). Measurement of fatigue in cancer patients: Development and validation of the Fatigue Symptom Inventory. *Quality of Life Research, 7,* 301–310.

Harrington, C.B., Hansen, J.A., Moskowitz, M., Todd, B.L., & Feuerstein, M. (2010). It's not over when it's over: Long-term symptoms in cancer survivors—A systematic review. *International Journal of Psychiatry in Medicine, 40,* 163–181.

Haugen, D.F., Hjermstad, M.J., Hagen, N., Caraceni, A., & Kaasa, S. (2010). Assessment and classification of cancer breakthrough pain: A systematic literature review. *Pain, 149,* 476–482.

Hebert, L.E., Scherr, P.A., Bienias, J.L., Bennett, D.A., & Evans, D.A. (2003). Alzheimer disease in the U.S. population: Prevalence estimates using the 2000 census. *Archives of Neurology, 60,* 1119–1122. doi:10.1001/archneur.60.8.1119

Herr, K., Titler, M., Fine, P., Sanders, S., Cavanaugh, J., Swegle, J., ... Tang, X. (2010). Assessing and treating pain in hospices: Current state of evidence-based practices. *Journal of Pain and Symptom Management, 39,* 803–819. doi:10.1016/j.jpainsymman.2009.09.025

Hodgkinson, B., Evans, D., & Wood, J. (2003). Maintaining oral hydration in older adults: A systematic review. *International Journal of Nursing Practice, 9*(3), S19–S21.

Holroyd-Leduc, J.M., Khandwala, F., & Sink, K.M. (2010). How can delirium best be prevented and managed in older patients in hospital? *Canadian Medical Association Journal, 182,* 465–469. doi:10.1503/cmaj.080519

Hooshiaran, A., van der Horst, F., Wesseling, G., Strik, J.J., Knottnerus, J.A., Gorgels, A., ... Muris, J.W. (2010). Quality of life in elderly dyspnea patients. In V.R. Preedy & R.R. Watson (Eds.), *Handbook of disease burdens and quality of life measures* (Pt. 3, pp. 2725–2744). New York, NY: Springer. doi:10.1007/978-0-387-78665-0_159

Hospice and Palliative Nurses Association. (1996). *Hospice and palliative care clinical practice protocol: Dyspnea.* Pittsburgh, PA: Author.

Howieson, D.B., Carlson, N.E., Moore, M.M., Wasserman, D., Abendroth, C.D., Payne-Murphy, J., & Kaye, J.A. (2008). Trajectory of mild cognitive impairment onset. *Journal of the International Neuropsychological Society, 14,* 192–198. doi:10.1017/S1355617708080375

Inouye, S.K. (2006). Current concepts: Delirium in older persons. *New England Journal of Medicine, 354,* 1157–1165.

International Cognition and Cancer Taskforce. (n.d.). ICCTF. Retrieved from http://www.icctf.com

Jansen, C.E., Miaskowski, C.A., Dodd, M.J., Dowling, G.A., & Kramer, J. (2005). Potential mechanisms for chemotherapy-induced impairments in cognitive function. *Oncology Nursing Forum, 32,* 1151–1163. doi:10.1188/05.ONF.1151-1163

Jensen, T.S., & Baron, R. (2003). Translation of symptoms and signs into mechanisms in neuropathic pain. *Pain, 102,* 1–8. doi:10.1016/s0304-3959(03)00006-x

Kagan, S.H., Holland, N., & Chalian, A.A. (2008). Sexual issues in special populations: Geriatric oncology—Sexuality and older adults. *Seminars in Oncology Nursing, 24,* 120–126. doi:10.1016/j.soncn.2008.02.005

Kale-Pradham, P.B., Jassal, H.K., & Wilhelm, S.M. (2010). Role of lactobacillus in the prevention of antibiotic associated diarrhea: A meta-analysis. *Pharmacotherapy, 30,* 119–126. doi:10.1592/phco.30.2.119

Kaleita, T.A., Wellisch, D.K., Cloughesy, T.F., Ford, J.M., Freeman, D., Belin, T.R., & Goldman, J. (2004). Prediction of neurocognitive outcome in adult brain tumor patients. *Journal of Neuro-Oncology, 67,* 245–253. doi:10.1023/B:NEON.0000021900.29176.58

Kalso, E., Edwards, J.E., Moore, R.A., & McQuay, H.J. (2004). Opioids in chronic non-cancer pain: Systematic review of efficacy safety. *Pain, 112,* 372–380. doi:10.1016/j.pain.2004.09.019

Karakiewicz, P.I., Bhojani, N., Neugut, A., Shariat, S.F., Jeldres, C., Graefen, M., ... Kattan, M.W. (2008). The effect of comorbidity and socioeconomic status on sexual and urinary function and on general health-related quality of life in men treated with radical prostatectomy for localized prostate cancer. *Journal of Sexual Medicine, 5,* 919–927. doi:10.1111/j.1743-6109.2007.00741.x

Kazanowski, M.K. (2003). Symptoms management in palliative care. In M.L. Mazo & D.W. Sherman (Eds.), *Palliative care nursing: Quality care to the end of life* (pp. 327–361). New York, NY: Springer.

Kohli, S., Fisher, S.G., Tra, Y., Wesnes, K., & Morrow, G.R. (2007). The cognitive effects of modafinil in breast cancer survivors: A randomized clinical trial [Abstract 9004]. *Journal of Clinical Oncology, 25*(Suppl. 18), 494s.

Kuhlbersh, B., Rosenthal, E., McGrew, B., Duncan, R., McCulloch, N., Carroll, W., & Magnuson, J. (2006). Pretreatment, preoperative swallowing exercises may improve dysphagia quality of life. *Laryngoscope, 116,* 883–887. doi:10.1097/01. mlg.0000217278.96901.fc

Kurz, A., & Sessler, D.I. (2003). Opioid-induced bowel dysfunction: Pathophysiology and potential new therapies. *Drugs, 63,* 649–671.

Lavizzo-Mourey, R., Johnson, J., & Stolley, P. (1988). Risk factors for dehydration among elderly nursing home residents. *Journal of the American Geriatrics Society, 36,* 213–218.

Lawlor, P.G. (2002). Delirium and dehydration: Some fluid for thought? *Supportive Care in Cancer, 10,* 445–454.

Lawrence, D.P., Kupelnick, B., Miller, K., Devine, D., & Lau, J. (2004). Evidence report on the occurrence, assessment, and treatment of fatigue in cancer patients. *Journal of the National Cancer Institute Monographs, 2004*(32), 40–50.

Leppert, W. (2010). The role of opioid receptor antagonists in the treatment of opioid-induced constipation: A review. *Advances in Therapy 27,* 714–730. doi:10.1007/s12325-010-0063-0

Levey, A., Lah, J., Goldstein, F., Steenland, K., & Bliwise, D. (2006). Mild cognitive impairment: An opportunity to identify patients at high risk for progression to Alzheimer's disease. *Clinical Therapeutics, 28,* 991–1001. doi:10.1016/j.clinthera.2006.07.006

Librach, S.L., Bouvette, M., De Angelis, C., Farley, J., Oneschuk, D., Pereira, J.L., & Sync, A. (2010). Consensus recommendations for the management of constipation in patients with advanced, progressive illness. *Journal of Pain and Symptom Management, 40,* 761–773. doi:10.1016/j.jpainsymman.2010.03.026

Lindau, S.T., Laumann, E.O., Levinson, W., & Waite, L.J. (2003). Synthesis of scientific disciplines in pursuit of health: The interactive biopsychosocial model. *Perspectives in Biology and Medicine, 46*(Suppl. 3), 74–86.

Lindau, S.T., Schumm, L.P., Laumann, E.O., Levinson, W., O'Muircheartaigh, C.A., & Waite, L.J. (2007). A study of sexuality and health among older adults in the United States. *New England Journal of Medicine, 357,* 762–774. doi:10.1056/NEJMoa067423

Lipowski, Z.J. (1989). Delirium in the elderly patient. *New England Journal of Medicine, 320,* 578–582. doi:10.1056/NEJM198903023200907

Litaker, D., Locala, J., Franco, K., Bronson, D.L., & Tannous, Z. (2001). Preoperative risk factors for postoperative delirium. *General Hospital Psychiatry, 23,* 84–89. doi:10.1016/S0163-8343(01)00117-7

Lonergan, E., Britton, A.M., & Luxenberg, J. (2007). Antipsychotics for delirium. *Cochrane Database of Systematic Reviews* 2007, Issue 2. Art. No.: CD005594. doi:10.1002/14651858. CD005594.pub2

Lötsch, J. (2005). Opioid metabolites. *Journal of Pain and Symptom Management, 29*(Suppl 5), S10–S24. Retrieved from http://www.jpsmjournal.com/article/S0885-3924(05)00030 -8/fulltext

Luckey, A.E., & Parsa, C.J. (2003). Fluid and electrolytes in the aged. *Archives of Surgery, 138,* 1055–1060. doi:10.1001/archsurg.138.10.1055

Luctkar-Flude, M.F., Groll, D.L., Tranmer, J.E., & Woodend, K. (2007). Fatigue and physical activity in older adult with cancer: A systematic review of the literature. *Cancer Nursing, 30,* E35–E45. doi:10.1097/01.NCC.0000290815.99323.75

Lynch, M.P. (2005). *Essentials of oncology care.* New York, NY: Professional Publishing Group.

Mahler, D.A., Selecky, P.A., Harrod, C.G., Benditt, J.O., Carrieri-Kohlman, V., Curtis, J.R., … Waller, A. (2010). American College of Chest Physicians consensus statement on the management of dyspnea in patients with advanced lung or heart disease. *Chest, 137,* 674–691. doi:10.1378/chest.09-1543

Manikantan, K., Khode, S., Sayad, S.I., Roe, J., Nutting, C., Rhys-Evans, P., … Kazi, R. (2009). Dysphagia in head and neck cancer. *Cancer Treatment Review, 35,* 724–732. doi:10.1016/j. ctrv.2009.08.008

Manning, C. (2004). Beyond memory: Neuropsychologic features in differential diagnosis of dementia. *Clinics in Geriatric Medicine, 20,* 93–119. doi:10.1016/j.cger.2003.10.002

Marcantonio, E.R., Simon, S.E., Bergmann, M.A., Jones, R.N., Murphy, K.M., & Morris, J.N. (2003). Delirium symptoms in post acute care: Prevalent, persistent and associated with poor functional recovery. *Journal of the American Geriatrics Society, 51,* 4–9. doi:10.1034/ j.1601-5215.2002.51002.x

Marik, P., & Kaplan, D. (2003). Aspiration pneumonia and dysphagia in the elderly. *Chest, 124,* 328–336. doi:10.1378/chest.124.1.328

Mayo Clinic. (2009, September 19). Sexual health and aging: Keep the passion alive. Retrieved from http://www.mayoclinic.com/health/sexual-health/HA00035

McAvay, G.J., Van Ness, P.H., Bogardus, S.T., Zhang, Y., Leslie, D.L., Leo-Summers, L.S., & Inouye, S.K. (2006). Older adults discharged from hospital with delirium: One year outcomes. *Journal of the American Geriatrics Society, 54,* 1245–1250.

McCrea, G.L., Miaskowski, C., Stotts, N.A., Macera, L., & Varma, M.G. (2008). Pathophysiology of constipation in the older adult. *World Journal of Gastroenterology, 14,* 2631–2638. doi:10.3748/wjg.14.2631

McCusker, J., Cole, M., Dendukuri, N., Belzile, E., & Primeau, F. (2001). Delirium in older medical inpatients and subsequent cognitive and functional status: A prospective study. *Canadian Medical Association Journal, 165,* 575–583.

McGee, S., Abernethy, W.B., III, & Simel, D.L. (1999). Is this patient hypovolemic? *JAMA, 281,* 1022–1029. doi:10.1001/jama.281.11.1022

McMillan, S.C., & Williams, F.A. (1989). Validity and reliability of the Constipation Assessment Scale. *Cancer Nursing, 1,* 183–188.

Mendoza, T.R., Wang, X.S., Cleeland, C.S., Morrissey, M., Johnson, B.A., Wendt, J.K., & Huber, S.L. (1999). The rapid assessment of fatigue severity in cancer patients: Use of the Brief Fatigue Inventory. *Cancer, 85,* 1186–1196.

Mentes, J. (2006). Oral hydration in older adults. *American Journal of Nursing, 106*(6), 40–49.

Mentes, J.C. (2008). Managing oral hydration. In E. Capezuti, D. Zwicker, M. Mezey, & T. Fulmer (Eds.), *Evidence-based geriatric nursing: Protocols for best practice* (pp. 369–390). New York, NY: Springer.

Mentes, J.C., Wakefield, B., & Culp, K. (2006). Use of a urine color chart to monitor hydration status in nursing home residents. *Biological Research for Nursing, 7,* 197–203. doi:10.1177/1099800405281607

Mercandante, S., Ferrera, P., & Casuccio, A. (2010). Effectiveness and tolerability of amidotrizoate for the treatment of constipation resistant to laxatives in advanced cancer patients. *Journal of Pain and Symptom Management.* Advance online publication. doi:10.1016/j. jpainsymman.2010.04.022

Metheny, N.M. (2000). *Fluid and electrolyte balance: Nursing considerations* (4th ed.). St. Louis, MO: Lippincott Williams & Wilkins.

Miaskowski, C. (2005). The next step to improving cancer pain management. *Pain Management Nursing, 6,* 1–2. doi:10.1016/j.pmn.2005.04.001

Miaskowski, C., Cleary, J., Burney, R., Coyne, P., Finley, R., Foster, R., ... Zahrbock, C. (2005). *Guidelines for the management of cancer pain in adults and children* (3rd ed.). Glenview, IL: American Pain Society.

Michaud, L., Büla, C., Berney, A., Camus, V., Voellinger, R., Stiefel, F., & Burnand, B. (2007). Delirium: Guidelines for general hospitals. *Journal of Psychosomatic Research, 62,* 371–383. doi:10.1016/j.jpsychores.2006.10.004

Milisen, K., Foreman, M.D., Abraham, I.L., DeGeest, S., Godderis, J., Vandermeulen, E., ... Broos, P.L. (2001). A nurse-led interdisciplinary intervention program for delirium in elderly hip-fracture patients. *Journal of the American Geriatrics Society, 49,* 523–532. doi:10.1046/j.1532-5415.2001.49109.x

Minton, O., Richardson, A., Sharpe, M., Hotopf, M., & Stone, P.A. (2008). A systematic review and meta-analysis of the pharmacological treatment of cancer-related fatigue. *Journal of the National Cancer Institute, 100,* 1155–1166. doi:10.1093/jnci/djn250

Mitchell, S.A., Beck, S.L., Hood, L.E., Moore, K., & Tanner, E.R. (2009). ONS PEP resource: Fatigue. In L.H. Eaton & J.M. Tipton (Eds.), *Putting evidence into practice:*

Improving oncology patient outcomes (pp. 155–174). Pittsburgh, PA: Oncology Nursing Society.

Mock, V., Abernethy, A.P., Atkinson, A., Barsevick, A., Berger, A.M., Cella, D., ... Wagner, L.I. (2007). Cancer-related fatigue. *Journal of the National Comprehensive Cancer Network, 5*, 1054–1078.

Mock, V., Atkinson, A., Barsevick, A., Cella, D., Cimprich, B., Cleeland, C., ... Stahl, C. (2000). NCCN practice guidelines for cancer-related fatigue. *Oncology, 14*(Suppl. 11A), 151–161.

Montejo, A.L., Llorca, G., Izquierdo, J.A., & Rico-Villademoros, F. (2001). Incidence of sexual dysfunction associated with antidepressant agents: A prospective multicenter study of 1,022 outpatients. Spanish Working Group for the Study of Psychotropic-Related Sexual Dysfunction. *Journal of Clinical Psychiatry, 62*(Suppl. 3), 10–21.

Morrow, G.R., Andrews, P.L., Hickok, J.T., Roscoe, J.A., & Matteson, S. (2002). Fatigue associated with cancer and its treatment. *Supportive Care in Cancer, 10*, 389–398. doi:10.1007/s005200100293

Muehlbauer, P., Thorpe, D., Davis, A.B., Drabot, R.C., Kiker, E.S., & Rawlings, B.L. (2009). ONS PEP resource: Diarrhea. In L.H. Eaton & J.M. Tipton (Eds.), *Putting evidence into practice: Improving oncology patient outcomes* (pp. 125–134). Pittsburgh, PA: Oncology Nursing Society.

Mukand, J., Cai, C., Zielinski, A., Danish, M., & Berman, J. (2003). The effects of dehydration on rehabilitation outcomes of elderly orthopedic patients. *Archives of Physical Medicine and Rehabilitation, 84*, 58–61. doi:10.1053/apmr.2003.50064

Müller-Lissner, S.A., Kamm, M.A., Scarpignato, C., & Wald, A. (2005). Myths and misconceptions about chronic constipation. *American Journal of Gastroenterology, 100*, 232–242. doi:10.1111/j.1572-0241.2005.40885.x

Mulrooney, T. (2010). Cognitive impairment. In C.G. Brown (Ed.), *A guide to oncology symptom management* (pp. 123–137). Pittsburgh, PA: Oncology Nursing Society.

Mungas, D. (1991). In-office mental status testing: A practical guide. *Geriatrics, 46*(7), 54–58, 63, 66.

Myers, J., Pierce, J., & Pazdernik, T. (2008). Neurotoxicity of chemotherapy in relation to cytokine release, the blood-brain barrier and cognitive impairment. *Oncology Nursing Forum, 35*, 916–920. doi:10.1188/08.ONF.916-920

National Cancer Institute. (2010). Gastrointestinal complications (PDQ®) [Health professional version]. Retrieved from http://www.cancer.gov/cancertopics/pdq/supportivecare/gastrointestinalcomplications/HealthProfessional

National Cancer Institute Cancer Therapy Evaluation Program. (2010, June 14). *Common terminology criteria for adverse events* [v.4.03]. Retrieved from http://evs.nci.nih.gov/ftp1/CTCAE/CTCAE_4.03_2010-06-14_QuickReference_5x7.pdf

National Comprehensive Cancer Network. (2011a). *NCCN Clinical Practice Guidelines in Oncology: Cancer-related fatigue* [v.1.2011]. Retrieved from http://www.nccn.org/professionals/physician_gls/pdf/fatigue.pdf

National Comprehensive Cancer Network. (2011b). *NCCN Clinical Practice Guidelines in Oncology: Palliative care* [v.2.2011]. Retrieved from http://www.nccn.org/professionals/physician_gls/pdf/palliative.pdf

Neef, D., & Walling, A.D. (2006). Dementia with Lewy bodies: An emerging disease. *American Family Physician, 73*, 1223–1229. Retrieved from http://www.aafp.org/afp/2006/0401/p1223.html

Neelemaata, F., Kruizengaa, H.M., de Vet, H.C.W., Seidell, J.C., Buttermand, M., & van Bokhorst-de van der Schuerena, M.A. (2008). Screening malnutrition in hospital outpatients: Can the SNAQ malnutrition screening tool also be applied to this population? *Clinical Nutrition, 27*, 439–446. doi:10.1016/j.clnu.2008.02.002

Ney, D., Weiss, J., Kind, A., & Robbins, J. (2009). Senescent swallowing: Impact strategies and interventions. *Nutrition in Clinical Practice, 24*, 395–413. doi:10.1177/0884533609332005

Nguyen, N.P., Frank, C., Moltz, C.C., Vos, P., Smith, H.J., Karlsson, U., ... Sallah, S. (2005). Impact of dysphagia on quality of life after treatment of head-and-neck cancer. *International Journal of Radiation Oncology, Biology, Physics, 61*, 772–778. doi:10.1016/j.ijrobp.2004.06.017

Oaklander, A.L. (2008). Mechanisms of pain and itch caused by herpes zoster (shingles). *Journal of Pain, 9*(1, Suppl. 1), 510–518. doi:10.1016/j.jpain.2007.10.003

O'Brien, J.T., Erkinjuntti, T., Reisberg, B., Roman, G., Sawada, T., Pantoni, L., ... DeKosky, S.T. (2003). Vascular cognitive impairment. *Lancet Neurology, 2,* 89–98. doi:10.1016/S1474-4422(03)00305-3

Orre, I.J., Fosså, S.D., Murison, R., Bremnes, R., Dahl, O., Klepp, O., ... Dahl, A.A.(2008). Chronic cancer-related fatigue in long-term survivors of testicular cancer. *Journal of Psychosomatic Research, 64,* 363–371. doi:10.1016/j.jpsychores.2008.01.002

Paik, N.-J. (2011). Dysphagia. Retrieved from http://emedicine.medscape.com/article/324096-overview#aw2aab6b3

Pan, C.X. (2003). Dyspnea. In R.S. Morrison & D.E. Meier (Eds.), *Geriatric palliative care* (pp. 232–255). New York, NY: Oxford University Press.

Panza, F., Capurso, C., D'Introno, A., Colacicco, M., Frisardi,V., Santamata, A., ... Solfrizzi, V. (2008). Vascular risk factors, alcohol intake, and cognitive decline. *Journal of Nutrition, Heath, and Aging, 12,* 376–381.

Pappagallo, M. (2001). Incidence, prevalence, and management of opioid bowel dysfunction. *American Journal of Surgery, 71,* 425–433.

Payne, R., & Gonzales, R.G. (2004). Pathophysiology of pain in cancer and other terminal diseases. In D. Doyle, G. Hanks, N. Cherny, & K. Calman (Eds.), *Oxford textbook of palliative medicine* (3rd ed., pp. 288–298). New York, NY: Oxford University Press.

Pergolizzi, J., Böger, R.H., Budd, K., Dahan, A., Erdine, S., Hans, G., ... Sacerdote, P. (2008). Opioids and the management of chronic severe pain in the elderly. *Pain Practice, 8,* 287–313. doi:10.1111/j.1533-2500.2008.00204.x

Peterson, R.C. (2011). Clinical practice: Mild cognitive impairment. *New England Journal of Medicine, 364,* 2227–2234. doi:10.1056/NEJMcp0910237

Pfeffer, R.I., Kurosaki, T.T., Harrah, C.H., Chance, J.M., & Filos, S. (1982). Measurement of functional activities of older adults in the community. *Journal of Gerontology, 37,* 323–329. doi:10.1093/geronj/37.3.323

Piquet, M.A., Ozsahin, I., Larpin, A., Zouhair, P., Coti, M., Monney, P., ... Roulet, M. (2002). Early nutritional intervention in oropharyngeal cancer patients undergoing radiotherapy. *Supportive Care in Cancer, 10,* 502–504. doi:10.1007/s00520-002-0364-1

Portenoy, R.K., Thomas, J., Boatwright, M.L.M., Tran, D., Galasso, F.L., Stambler, N., ... Israel, R.J. (2008). Subcutaneous methylnaltrexone for the treatment of opioid-induced constipation in patients with advanced illness: A double-blind, randomized, parallel group, dose-ranging study. *Journal of Pain and Symptom Management, 35,* 458–468. doi:10.1016/j.jpainsymman.2007.12.005

Potter, J. (2004). Fatigue experience in advanced cancer: A phenomenological approach. *International Journal of Palliative Nursing, 10,* 15–23.

Potter, J., Hami, F., Bryan, T., & Quigley, C. (2003). Symptoms in 400 patients referred to palliative care services: Prevalence and patterns. *Palliative Medicine, 17,* 310–314.

Price, K.A.R. (2010). Hydration in cancer patients. *Current Opinion in Supportive and Palliative Care, 4,* 276–280. doi:10.1097/SPC.0b013e32833e48d1

Prue, G., Rankin, J., Allen, J., Gracey, J., & Cramp, F. (2006). Cancer-related fatigue: A critical appraisal. *European Journal of Cancer, 42,* 846–863. doi:10.1016/j.ejca.2005.11.026

Quinten, C., Coens, C., Maver, M., Comte, S., Spranger, M., Cleeland, C., ... Bottomley, A. (2009). Baseline quality of life as a prognostic indicator of survival: A meta-analysis of individual patient data from EORTC clinical trials. *Lancet Oncology, 10,* 865–871. doi:10.1016/S1470-2045(09)70200-1

Radbruch, L., Sabatowski, R., Loick, G., Kulbe, C., Kasper, M., Grond, S., ... Lehmann, K.A. (2000). Constipation and the use of laxatives: A comparison between transdermal fentanyl and oral morphine. *Palliative Medicine, 14,* 111–119.

Raison, C.L., Capuron, L., & Miller, A.H. (2006). Cytokines sing the blues: Inflammation and the pathogenesis of depression. *Trends in Immunology, 27,* 24–31. doi:10.1016/j.it.2005.11.006

Rao, A.V., & Cohen, H.J. (2008). Fatigue in older cancer patients: Etiology, assessment, and treatment. *Seminars in Oncology, 35*, 633–642. doi:10.1053/j.seminoncol.2008.08.005

Rao, S.S., & Go, J.T. (2010). Update on the management of constipation in the elderly: New treatment options. *Clinical Interventions in Aging, 5*, 163–171. doi:10.1053/j.seminoncol.2008.08.005

Raschetti, R., Emiliano, A., Vanacore, N., & Maggini, M. (2007). Cholinesterase inhibitors in mild cognitive impairment: A systematic review of randomized trials. *PLoS Medicine, 4*(11), e338. doi:10.1371/journal.pmed.0040338

Rehwaldt, M., Wickham, R., Purl, S., Tariman, J., Blendowski, C., Shott, S., & Lappe, M. (2009). Self-care strategies to cope with taste changes after chemotherapy. *Oncology Nursing Forum, 36*, E47–E56. doi:10.1188/09.ONF.E47-E56

Ribaudo, J.M., Cella, D., Hahn, E.A., Lloyd, N.S., Tchekmedyian, J., VonRoenn, J., & Leslie, W.T. (2000). Re-validation and shortening of the Functional Assessment of Anorexia/Cachexia Therapy (FAACT) questionnaire. *Quality of Life Research, 9*, 1137–1146. doi:10.1023/A:1016670403148

Ricard, D., Taillia, H., & Renard, J. (2009). Brain damage from anticancer treatments in adults. *Current Opinion in Oncology, 21*, 559–565. doi:10.1097/CCO.0b013e328330c669

Robinson, S.B., & Rosher, R.B. (2002). Can a beverage cart help improve hydration? *Geriatric Nursing, 23*, 208–211. doi:10.1067/mgn.2002.126967

Rofes, L., Arreola, V., Almirall, J., Cabré, M., Campins, L., García-Peris, P., ... Clavé, P. (2011). Diagnosis and management of oropharyngeal dysphagia and its nutritional and respiratory complications in the elderly. *Gastroenterology Research and Practice.* Advance online publication. doi:10.1155/2011/818979

Román, G.C. (2008). The epidemiology of vascular dementia. *Handbook of Clinical Neurology, 89*, 639–658. doi:10.1016/S0072-9752(07)01259-6

Royall, D.R. (1996). Comments of the executive control of clock-drawing. *Journal of the American Geriatrics Society, 44*, 218–219.

Rubin, G.J., Cleare, A., & Hotopf, M. (2004). Psychological factors in postoperative fatigue. *Psychosomatic Medicine, 66*, 959–964.

Sawyer, P., Lillis, J.P., Bodner, E.U., & Allman, R.M. (2007). Substantial daily pain among nursing home residents. *Journal of the American Medical Directors Association, 8*, 158–165. doi:10.1016/j.jamda.2006.12.030

Schneck, M.J., & Janss, A. (2011, April 19). Radiation necrosis. Retrieved from http://emedicine.medscape.com/article/1157533-overview

Schols, J.M., De Groot, C.P., van der Cammen, T.J., & Rikkert, M.G.O. (2009). Preventing and treating dehydration in the elderly during periods of illness and warm weather. *Journal of Nutrition, Health, and Aging, 13*, 150–157.

Serlin, R.C., Mendoza, T.R., Nakamura, Y., Edwards, K.R., & Cleeland, C.S. (1995). When is cancer pain mild, moderate or severe? Grading pain severity by its interference with function. *Pain, 61*, 277–284. doi:10.1016/0304-3959(94)00178-H

Servaes, P., Verhagen, C., & Bleijenberg, G. (2002). Fatigue in cancer patients during and after treatment: Prevalence, correlates and interventions. *European Journal of Cancer, 38*, 27–43. doi:10.1016/S0959-8049(01)00332-X

Sjögren, P., Nilsson, E., Forsell, M., Johansson, O., & Hoogstraate, J. (2008). A systematic review of the preventive effect of oral hygiene on pneumonia and respiratory tract infection in elderly people in hospitals and nursing homes: Effect estimates and methodological quality of randomized controlled trials. *Journal of the American Geriatrics Society, 56*, 2124–2130. doi:10.1111/j.1532-5415.2008.01926.x

Solomon, R., & Cherny, N.I. (2006). Constipation and diarrhea in patients with cancer. *Cancer Journal, 12*, 355–364. doi:10.1097/00130404-200609000-00005

Stones, M., & Stones, L. (2007). Sexuality, sensuality and intimacy. In J.E. Berren (Ed.), *Encyclopedia of gerontology* (2nd ed., pp. 282–289). Boston, MA: Elsevier Academic Press.

Sultzer, D.L., Davis, S.M., Tariot, P.N., Dagerman, K.S., Lebowitz, B.D., Lyketsos, C.G., ... Schneider, L.S. (2008). Clinical symptom responses to atypical antipsychotic medications in Alzheimer's disease: Phase 1 outcomes from the CATIE-AD effectiveness trial. *American Journal of Psychiatry, 165,* 844–854. doi:10.1176/appi.ajp.2008.07111779

Sunderland, T., Hill, J.L., Mellow, A.M., Lawlor, B.A., Gundersheimer, J., & Newhouse, P.A. (1989). Clock drawing in Alzheimer's disease: A novel measure of dementia severity. *Journal of the American Geriatrics Society, 37,* 725–729.

Sykes, N.P. (2006). The pathogenesis of constipation. *Journal of Supportive Oncology, 4,* 213–218.

Tanaka, K., Akechi, T., Okuyama, T., Nishiwaki, Y., & Uchitomi, Y. (2000). Development and validation of the cancer dyspnea scale: A multidimensional, brief, self-rating scale. *British Journal of Cancer, 82,* 800–805.

Tannock, I.F., Ahles, T.A., Ganz, P.A., & van Dam, F.S. (2004). Cognitive impairment associated with chemotherapy for cancer: Report of a workshop. *Journal of Clinical Oncology, 22,* 2233–2239. doi:10.1200/JCO.2004.08.094

Tasker, R.R. (2001). Central pain states. In J.D. Loeser, S.H. Butler, C.R. Chapman, & D.C. Turk (Eds.), *Bonica's management of pain* (3rd ed., pp. 433–457). Baltimore, MD: Lippincott Williams & Wilkins.

Taylor, L.J., & Herr, K. (2003). Pain intensity assessment: A comparison of selected pain intensity scales for use in cognitively intact and cognitively impaired African American older adults. *Pain Management Nursing, 4,* 87–95. doi:10.1016/S1524-9042(02)54210-7

Thies, W., & Bleiler, L. (2011). 2011 Alzheimer's disease facts and figures. *Alzheimer's Dementia, 7,* 208–244. doi:10.1016/j.jalz.2011.02.004

Thomas, J. (2007). Cancer related constipation. *Current Oncology Reports, 9,* 278–284. doi:10.1007/s11912-007-0034-z

Timiras, P.S. (2007). Comparative aging, geriatric functional assessment, aging and disease. In P.S. Timiras (Ed.), *Physiological basis of aging and geriatrics* (4th ed., pp. 23–40). New York, NY: Informa HealthCare.

Tuma, R., & DeAngelis, L. (2000). Altered mental status in patients with cancer. *Archives of Neurology, 57,* 1727–1731.

Turk, D.C., & Okifuji, A. (2001). Pain terms and taxonomies of pain. In J.D. Loeser, S.H. Butler, C.R. Chapman, & D.C. Turk (Eds.), *Bonica's management of pain* (3rd ed., pp. 17–25). Baltimore, MD: Lippincott Williams & Wilkins.

Überall, M., & Müller-Schwege, G. (2006). Opioid-induced constipation—A frequent and distressing side effect in daily practice affecting oral and transdermal opioid applications. *European Journal of Pain, 10*(Suppl. 1), S172.

Urch, C.E. (2009). Pathophysiology of cancer pain. In T.D. Walsh, A.T. Caraceni, R. Fainsinger, K.M. Foley, P. Glare, C. Goh, ... L. Radbruch (Eds.), *Palliative medicine* (pp. 1378–1384). Philadelphia, PA: Elsevier Saunders.

U.S. Food and Drug Administration Psychopharmacologic Drugs Advisory Committee. (2008, June 16). Transcript for FDA media briefing on safety labeling changes for antipsychotic drugs. Retrieved from http://www.fda.gov/downloads/NewsEvents/Newsroom/Media Transcripts/UCM169331.pdf

Visvanathan, R., & Chapman, I.M. (2009). Undernutrition and anorexia in the older person. *Gastroenterology Clinics of North America, 38,* 393–409. doi:10.1016/j.gtc.2009.06.009

Vivanti, A., Harvey, K., Ash, S., & Battistutta, D. (2008). Clinical assessment of dehydration in older people admitted to hospital: What are the strongest indicators? *Archives of Gerontology and Geriatrics, 47,* 340–355. doi:10.1016/j.archger.2007.08.016

Volicer, L., & Hurley, A.C. (2003). Management of behavioral symptoms in progressive dementias. *Journals of Gerontology Series A: Biological Sciences and Medical Sciences, 58,* M837–M845.

Waite, L.J., Laumann, E.O., Das, A., & Schumm, L.P. (2009). Sexuality: Measures of partnerships, practices, attitudes, and problems in the National Social Life, Health and Aging Study. *Journals of Gerontology Series B: Psychological Sciences and Social Sciences, 64*(Suppl. 1), 156–166.

Wakefield, B., Mentes, J., Diggelmann, L., & Culp, K. (2002). Monitoring hydration status in elderly veterans. *Western Journal of Nursing Research, 24,* 132–142. doi:10.1177/01939450222045798

Wallace, M.A. (2000). Intimacy and sexuality. In A.G. Leuckenotte (Ed.), *Gerontologic nursing* (2nd ed., pp. 217–231). St. Louis, MO: Mosby.

Wallace, M.A. (2008). Assessment of sexual health in older adults. *American Journal of Nursing, 108*(7), 52–60. doi:10.1097/01.NAJ.0000325647.63678.b9

Walsh, K.E., & Berman, J.R. (2004). Sexual dysfunction in the older woman: An overview of the current understanding and management. *Drugs and Aging, 21,* 655–675. doi:10.2165/00002512-200421100-00004

Wang, X.S. (2008). Pathophysiology of cancer-related fatigue. *Clinical Journal of Oncology Nursing, 12*(Suppl. 5), 11–20. doi:10.1188/08.CJON.S2.11-20

Warden, V., Hurley, A.C., & Volicer, V. (2003). Development and psychometric evaluation of the Pain Assessment in Advanced Dementia (PAINAD) Scale. *Journal of the American Medical Directors Association, 4,* 9–15. doi:10.1016/S1525-8610(04)70258-3

White, G., O' Rourke, F., Ong, B., Cordato, D., & Chan, D. (2008). Dysphagia: Causes, assessment treatment and management. *Geriatrics, 63*(5), 15–20.

Wilson, M., Thomas, D., Rubenstein, L., Chibnall, J., Anderson, S., Baxi, A., ... Morley, J. (2005). Appetite assessment: Simple appetite questionnaire predicts weight loss in community-dwelling adults and nursing home residents. *American Journal of Clinical Nutrition, 82,* 1074–1081.

Winblad, B., Palmer, K., Kivipelto, M., Jelic, V., Fratiglioni, L., Wahlund, L.O., ... Petersen R.C. (2004). Mild cognitive impairment: Beyond controversies, towards a consensus—Report of the International Working Group on Mild Cognitive Impairment. *Journal of Internal Medicine, 256,* 240–246. doi:10.1111/j.1365-2796.2004.01380.x

Woolery, M., Bisanz, A., Lyons, H.F., Gaido, L., Yenulevich, M., Fulton, S., & McMillan, S.C. (2008). Putting evidence into practice: Evidence-based interventions for the prevention and management of constipation in patients with cancer. *Clinical Journal of Oncology Nursing, 12,* 317–337. doi:10.1188/08.CJON.317-337

World Health Organization. (n.d.). WHO pain relief ladder. Retrieved from http://www.who.int/cancer/palliative/painladder/en

Wynne, H. (2005). Drug metabolism and ageing. *Journal of the British Menopause Society, 11,* 51–56. doi:10.1258/136218005775544589

Xue, D., & Abernethy, A. (2010). Management of dyspnea in advanced lung cancer: Recent data and emerging concepts. *Current Opinion in Supportive and Palliative Care, 4,* 85–91. doi:10.1097/SPC.0b013e328339920d

Yancik, R., Ganz, P.A., Varricchio, C.G., & Conley, B. (2001). Perspectives on comorbidity and cancer in older patients: Approaches to expand the knowledge base. *Journal of Clinical Oncology, 19,* 1147–1151.

Yavuzsen, T., Davis, M., Walsh, D., Leggrans, S., & Lagman, R. (2005). Systematic review of the treatment of cancer associated anorexia and weight loss. *Journal of Clinical Oncology, 23,* 8500–8511. doi:10.1200/JCO.2005.01.8010

Yellen, S.B., Cella, D.F., Webster, K., Blendowski, C., & Kaplan, E. (1997). Measuring fatigue and other anemia-related symptoms with the Functional Assessment of Cancer Therapy (FACT) measurement system. *Journal of Pain and Symptom Management, 13,* 63–74. doi:10.1016/S0885-3924(96)00274-6

Yorke, J., Moosavi, S.H., Shuldham, C., & Jones, P.W. (2010). Quantification of dyspnoea using descriptors: Development and initial testing of Dyspnoea-12. *Thorax, 65,* 21–26. doi:10.1136/thx.2009.118521

Young, J., & Inouye, S.K. (2007). Delirium in older people. *BMJ, 334,* 842–846. doi:10.1136/bmj.39169.706574.AD

Zwakhalen, S.M., Hamers, J.P., Abu-Saad, H.H., & Berger, M.P. (2006). Pain in elderly people with severe dementia: A systematic review of behavioral pain assessment tools. *BMC Geriatrics, 6,* 3. doi:10.1186/1471-2318-6-3

CHAPTER 5

Hospice and Palliative Care

Nessa Coyle, PhD, ANP, ACHPN, FAAN, and Kathy Plakovic, FNP, ACHPN, AOCNP®

> What tormented Ivan Ilych was the lie, this lie that for some reason they all accepted, that he was only sick and not dying, and that if he would only remain calm and undergo treatment he could expect good results. Yet he knew that regardless of what was done, all he could expect was more agonizing suffering and death. And he was tortured by this lie, tortured by the fact that they refused to acknowledge what he and everyone knew . . . (Tolstoy, 2004, p. 103)

Introduction

Older individuals with cancer often live with multiple comorbid conditions. Long periods of physical decline and functional impairment may precede their death (O'Neill, Meier, & Morrison, 2009; Steel & Vitale, 2003). Ongoing discussions about goals of care and approaches to care are paramount. The progressive frailty commonly associated with aging makes older adults with cancer a particularly vulnerable population. The dependence on the professionals around them for knowledge, information, and care is similar to any patient with progressive disease (Freedman, 1993). Inadequate symptom control, undiagnosed depression and anxiety, and unaddressed existential distress, family distress, fatigue, burnout, and demoralization may all occur if goals of care are not clearly defined and the focus of care directed towards those goals (Irwin & von Gunten, 2010; Wright et al., 2008).

When the goal of care is to cure or prolong life, patients can benefit from palliative care that is integrated with their cancer treatment. When the goal of care changes to quality rather than quantity of life and life expectancy is six months or less, the patient may benefit from the hospice model of care. Although hospice care has long been accepted as the model of care for those close to death, palliative care is a relatively new and evolving discipline. Ambulatory care oncology nurses play a central role in introducing patients and their families to the concept of palliative care as an integral part of comprehensive cancer care. Later, if the disease progresses and the cancer is no longer amenable to treatment, the benefits of hospice care should be explored (Bakitas, Bishop, Caron, & Stephens, 2010; Beckstrand, Moore, Callister, & Bond, 2009; Ferrell, Virani, Malloy, & Kelly, 2010; Lawton, 2010; Zhou, Stolzfus, Houldin, Parks, & Swan, 2010).

The goal of this chapter is to familiarize the ambulatory care oncology nurse with the current practice of state-of-the-art palliative care and hospice care nursing. Another goal is to broaden the expertise of ambulatory care nurses so they can incorporate aspects of palliative care and hospice care into their current practice and make appropriate referrals. Key areas that will be covered include the special palliative care needs of older patients, the foundation of palliative care in hospice care and how one relates to the other, transitions in goals of care, and communication. A brief overview of procedures that may benefit patients with distressing symptoms at end of life is also given. Finally, ethical issues at end of life; specific needs of those within days to hours of death; loss, grief, and bereavement; and self-care for the staff are addressed.

What Are Palliative Care and Hospice Care, and How Do They Differ?

According to the World Health Organization (n.d.), palliative care is defined as "an approach that improves the quality of life of patients and their families facing the problem associated with life-threatening illness" (para. 1). Palliative care emphasizes the prevention and relief of suffering by early identification, skillful assessment, and treatment of pain and other problems: physical, psychosocial, and spiritual. While oncology treatment focuses on the disease, palliative care focuses on facilitating whole person care. In acknowledgment that oncology treatment with its disease focus and palliative care with its holistic focus are a natural fit, the National Comprehensive Cancer Network (NCCN, 2011) has clarified and highlighted key components of palliative care:

> Palliative care is both a philosophy of care and an organized, highly structured system for delivering care to persons with life threatening or debilitating illness. Palliative care is patient- and family-centered care that focuses on effective management of pain and other distressing symptoms while incorporating psychosocial and spiritual care according to patient/family needs, values, beliefs, and culture(s). The goal of palliative care is to prevent and relieve suffering and to support the best quality of life for patients and their families, regardless of the stage of their disease and need for other therapies. Palliative care

can be delivered concurrently with life-prolonging therapy or
as the main focus of care. (p. PAL-1)

The NCCN guidelines for palliative care, which are updated frequently, provide a useful framework for both identifying patients who would benefit from palliative care and delivering such care (NCCN, 2011).

An observant ambulatory care oncology nurse is often the one to identify patients who would benefit from integrating palliative care into their disease-focused treatment and later benefit from hospice care if goals of care change from life prolongation to quality of life and comfort.

This early identification of patients and families who would benefit from palliative care and later the hospice model of care is especially important when the individual has multiple distressing symptoms or has difficulty discussing goals of care or advance directives. To achieve this, the ambulatory care oncology nurse must have a clear understanding of the philosophy and goals of palliative care and hospice care and how palliative care and hospice care are both similar and different (Murphy-Ende, 2006; Panke & Coyne, 2006; Teno & Connor, 2009).

The key difference is that palliative care is provided at the same time the patient is receiving cancer therapy; closeness to death is not a criteria (World Health Organization, n.d.). The palliative care interdisciplinary team works alongside the disease management team. Hospice care, in contrast, is provided to patients with a life expectancy of six months or less, most of whom are no longer receiving active disease-focused therapy. Both palliative care and hospice care pay great attention to symptoms and suffering with the patient and family as the unit of care. Another way of understanding the differences between palliative care and hospice care is that palliative care is the care that provides attention to symptoms and suffering as well as the needs of the family during cancer treatment, whereas hospice care is the model of care in which palliative care is intensified at the end of life. The natural progression from cancer treatment and palliative care to hospice care when the focus of care changes from life prolongation to maintaining quality of life is illustrated in Figure 5-1. Palliative care is less available in the community than hospice programs, although most comprehensive cancer centers now have outpatient palliative care clinics (Teno & Connor, 2009).

As the cancer progresses despite therapy and disease-focused treatments become more burdensome than helpful, the benefits of hospice care should be discussed with the patient and family. Timing of these conversations is important so the patient and family know their various options (Steel & Vitale, 2003; Teno et al., 1997). A key concept of hospice is that physical, psychological, social, and spiritual aspects of suffering are often associated with dying (Clark, 1999; Ferrell & Coyle, 2008; Twycross & Lack, 1983). Because of the multidimensional level of care needed, hospice care is delivered by an interdisciplinary team. The patient and family is the unit of care. The same is true for specialized palliative care.

Only two criteria need to be met to initiate hospice care. First is that the patient is terminally ill, and second is that the patient has a life expectancy of six months or less. The Medicare hospice benefit was designed to address

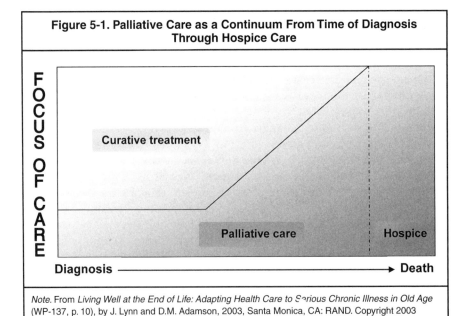

Figure 5-1. Palliative Care as a Continuum From Time of Diagnosis Through Hospice Care

Note. From *Living Well at the End of Life: Adapting Health Care to Serious Chronic Illness in Old Age* (WP-137, p. 10), by J. Lynn and D.M. Adamson, 2003, Santa Monica, CA: RAND. Copyright 2003 by RAND. Retrieved from http://www.rand.org/pubs/white_papers/2005/WP137.pdf. Adapted with permission.

the variations in care intensity that is required to meet the patient and family needs at end of life. The four levels of care are (a) routine home care, provided wherever the patient resides (e.g., home, nursing home, residential care setting), (b) continuous home care provided during a brief period of crisis that enables the patient to remain at home, (c) general inpatient care where a patient is admitted to the hospital for symptom control that cannot be managed at home, and (d) inpatient respite care on a short-term basis where the patient is admitted to the hospital to allow the family respite from the care of the patient at home (Connor, 2009).

Why Do Patients Need Access to Both Palliative and Hospice Care?

With advances in science, technology, and medical care in the United States, the trajectory of dying has changed. Today, the mean age at death is older than 77 years, and chronic diseases such as heart disease, cancer, and stroke are the leading causes of death (Steel & Vitale, 2003). Through screening, early detection, and the variety of therapeutic options available, cancer has become a chronic disease for many. For the older adult, however, living with cancer and the associated symptoms of the disease or treatment is often not the only health issue. Many older adults with cancer have a number of chronic and sometimes debilitating conditions, such as arthritis, diabetes, congestive heart failure, and hypertension. Cancer, for some, is a comorbid condition.

A review of Medicare data identified a typical trajectory for advanced cancer toward death. The course is most often marked by a slow decline over months, followed by a rapid decline in the last two months of life (Lunney, Lynn, Foley, Lipson, & Guralnik, 2003). The combination of advanced cancer and comorbid conditions can result in the individual experiencing multiple interacting and distressing symptoms, which may manifest as physical, social, psychological, spiritual, or existential difficulties. These distressing symptoms interfere with quality of life and well-being. Increasing frailty, dependence on others, multiple and accumulated losses, and worry about being unable to stay in familiar surroundings or having to die among strangers adds to the distress. Dame Cecily Saunders, the founder of the modern hospice movement, captures the essence of this suffering in her concept of "total pain" (Clark, 1999). "Total pain" is described as suffering that is more than physical pain and related symptoms but also includes impairments and disabilities; psychological distress with grief over loss and change; social disruption with financial, residential, family, and roles strains; and spiritual and existential distress. "Total pain" can occur when the patient is receiving active cancer treatment, which further supports the importance of incorporating the principles of palliative care into ambulatory care nursing practice (Saunders, 2010).

Literature indicates that during the last few months to weeks of life, whether the older adult is being cared for at home or in a nursing home, the prevalence of poorly managed symptoms, psychosocial distress, caregiver burden, and financial distress is high (Steel & Vitale, 2003). Families can feel overwhelmed, burdened, and guilty, especially if their relative is no longer able to be cared for at home. Complicating choices and decisions are the technologic advances that have made it possible to prolong life even when health-related quality of life is no longer present. Without advance care planning, many deaths can become protracted, and families are put in the position of having to make decisions about the implementation or discontinuation of life-prolonging technologies. Feeding tubes, ventilators, and IV fluids are examples. Advance care planning can decrease the burden on family members regarding these decisions. The ambulatory care oncology nurse can determine if advance care planning has been addressed or facilitate these conversations through education, the provision of educational materials, or appropriate referrals.

What makes palliative care different in the older adult with cancer from patients who are younger are the multiple comorbidities and associated frailty that develop over time. Symptom distress is multifactorial, and meticulous attention to assessment and management is an important aspect of ambulatory care. The high prevalence of long-term functional and cognitive impairments in this age group leads to significant and chronic family caregiver burden. Ongoing support for family caregivers is critical (Andersson, Ekwall, Hallberg, & Edberg, 2010; Davis & Steele, 2010; Kissane, Lichtenthal, & Zaider, 2007–2008; Levine, 2003; Zaider & Kissane, 2009). Older adults benefit from palliative care that is introduced early in the cancer disease treatment process. This facilitates the provision of additional services, such as physical, psychological, social, and spiritual support to patients and their families, as well as the opportunity to rapidly address symptoms as they occur. When educating the patient and family about palliative care as an important addition to the treatment plan of care, the ambulatory care oncology nurse may need to reinforce that palliative care does not mean end-of-life care, giving up on treatment, or that their oncologist will no longer be directing their care. The ambulatory care oncology nurse may need to reinforce that hospice care and palliative care are not the same and that palliative care is delivered concurrently with cancer therapy, whereas hospice care is provided to individuals who are no longer benefiting from cancer therapy and are coming toward the end of their lives.

AARP conducted a survey regarding hospice care and found that more than 90% of respondents had heard of hospice, but fewer than 4 in 10 of those surveyed knew that it was a Medicare benefit. Three-quarters of those who knew about hospice care said they would want it if they knew that they were dying (Connor, 2009; Guengerich, 2009). Comparing the AARP statistics with the national statistics, a large gap exists between what people say they would want if they knew that they were dying and how they are actually cared for at the end of life. The National Hospice and Palliative Care Organization (2010) estimated that approximately 41.6% of all deaths in the United States were under the care of a hospice program, and half received care for less than three weeks. It is not known how many of these people were receiving palliative care outside of hospice care. Oncology nurses have a role in ensuring that their patients are aware of the care options available to them throughout the trajectory of disease.

Transitions in Goals of Care and Communication

An abundance of literature addresses the importance of communication in advanced disease about transitions in care goals from cure and life-prolongation to comfort (Coyle & Sculco, 2003; Hallenbeck & Arnold, 2007; Pantilat, 2009; Quill, Arnold, & Back, 2009). Unfortunately, patients can receive ambiguous or conflicting information from their care providers. This increases uncertainty and erodes the confidence of the patient and family on how best to proceed. Patients need accurate information to plan ahead for themselves and their families. Care goals and personal values will then drive the therapy rather than the other way around. Many people fear the process of dying, and open conversations about death and dying can be helpful in demystifying what to expect. Addressing specific fears, correcting myths, and giving helpful medical information about symptoms that may occur and how they will be managed can all help restore a sense of control and decrease uncertainty. Knowledge that the patient and family will not have to go through this alone but will be well supported is also reassuring. The ambulatory care oncology nurse may be the first one to hear these concerns and can provide reassurance that the care team will discuss and address these issues. A family meeting can be convened involving key individuals of the multidisciplinary care team, such as the social worker, case manager, physician, nurse, and chaplain (Coyle & Kissane, 2010). The clinical environment and available resources will determine the format used.

A typical trajectory for advanced cancer is slow decline over months, followed by a more rapid decline, leading to death, in the last two months (Lunney et al., 2003). This is important information for the ambulatory care oncology nurse, as it helps to identify the appropriate timing to revisit goals of care and review options to achieve those goals. Unless open and honest communication with the patient and family has occurred throughout this trajectory, they may be subjected to ineffective treatment and deprived of the information needed to make important quality-of-life decisions. The opportunity to integrate this phase of life into their whole life's story may be lost, and the person and family may be left with a feeling of abandonment or betrayal. Studies have found that end-of-life discussions are associated with less-aggressive medical care near death and earlier hospice referrals (Trice & Prigerson, 2009; Wright et al., 2008). This is an important finding because aggressive, disease-focused medical care at the end of life has been associated with worse quality of life (Mack et al., 2009).

The ambulatory care oncology nurse often develops close relationships with patients and their families and is often the one who hears their deepest worries and concerns. The patient and family may tell the nurse many things that they do not share with each other or the physician. As the nurse hears the story of a life interrupted, the hopes that had been held for treatment, the quality of the patient's and family's life, and whether continued treatment is worthwhile for them, the nurse has an opportunity to open or continue the discussion on advance care planning. Hoping for the best but preparing for the worst is a concept that normalizes advance care planning and gives individuals the opportunity to articulate what they would want at end of life. Their wishes can then be formalized in advance directives.

The ability to communicate compassionately and effectively with patients facing a life-threatening illness is an essential skill for ambulatory care oncology nurses. It sometimes comes naturally but is a skill that can be taught. For patients to have autonomy and make informed choices, they have to understand the information given to them and the consequences of each decision. The functions of information are to decrease uncertainty and produce a basis for action in order to make decisions. The way information is presented can decrease uncertainty and improve the clinician/patient/family relationship, or it can create uncertainty, paralyze action, and destroy the relationship (Coyle & Sculco, 2003; Pantilat, 2009). Not all nurses and oncologists are good communicators, especially concerning end-of-life issues. Significant barriers include lack of experience in holding these conversations, fear of mortality, fear of not knowing how to respond to a patient's or family's emotions, lack of mentors, greater comfort in talking about interventions, and a sense of guilt at not being able to achieve a cure (Maguire & Weiner, 2009). Facilitating these difficult conversations is a skill that can be learned, and training programs are available in some academic medical centers in the United States and elsewhere (Kissane, Bultz, Butow, & Finlay, 2010). Guidelines have been developed for holding difficult conversations, especially regarding transitions in goals of care. A sequence of steps is suggested, always initially exploring what the patient knows about their situation and proceeding from there (Kaplan, 2010).

Because terminal illness is a family experience, holding periodic family meetings is an important opportunity for communication, especially with a change in care goals or the approach to care (Coyle & Kissane, 2010). Family meetings include the patient and family members and friends who are important in the patient's life whenever possible and the interdisciplinary team members involved in the patient's care. Family meetings are undertaken for multiple purposes and provide an ideal avenue to inform, deliberate, clarify and establish care goals, and discuss advance care planning.

Ethical Issues

In tertiary cancer settings where advanced technology is so abundant, decisions are made on a daily basis about life-sustaining and life-limiting interventions (Cassell & Rich, 2010; Mahon, 2010; Olsen, Swetz, & Mueller, 2010; Pellegrino & Sulmasy, 2009; Schwarz & Tarzian, 2010). Conflicts and ethical issues can arise regarding what is an appropriate level of care for an individual. Specific to the ambulatory care setting, conflicts are sometimes seen at the time of transition from disease-focused treatment to end-of-life and hospice care. This shift in the care focus may be difficult for patients and families to initially accept, particularly if palliative care has not been integrated with the oncology treatment. Frequent blood work, transfusions, supportive hydration, and trips to the emergency department for complications may have been the patient's and family's routine, giving them a sense of safety and security. When the focus of care transitions to end-of-life care, this routine is changed. Symptoms are managed at home by the hospice team and family caregivers, not through trips to the emergency department. Blood work is infrequent if at all, artificial hydration or nutrition is uncommon, and quality of life, rather than prolonging life, is the focus. The ambulatory care oncology nurse plays a key role during this period of change by providing support and remaining available to the patient and family, maintaining contact with the hospice providers, and supporting the transition of care to the hospice team.

As norms of society change around options and choices at end of life, it is essential that nurses know the law regarding certain end-of-life options, as well as their own professional code of ethics. For example, Oregon, Washington, and Montana permit physician-assisted suicide (also known as physician-assisted death or aid in dying) when strict guidelines are followed. In all other states, physician-assisted suicide is illegal. Euthanasia is not permitted anywhere in the United States. Withdrawal of all and any life-prolonging treatment, including ventilator support, is permitted in all states based on the federally mandated Patient Self-Determination Act (Teno et al., 1997). Treatment of pain at the end of life is also an essential component of end-of-life care that the American Nurses Association (2010) includes in their position statement *Registered Nurses' Roles and Responsibilities in Providing Expert Care and Counseling at End of Life.*

Symptom Assessment and Management

Patients and their families are our teachers regarding what is important to them during their disease course and at the end of life. Studies have shown consistent themes emerge as important to patients and families: freedom from pain, attaining peace with God, having the presence of family, being mentally aware, having their treatment choices followed, having their finances in order, feeling their life was meaningful, and resolving conflicts (Steinhauser et al., 2000). These findings reflect that patients desire a system of care that will provide skilled, compassionate, and personalized attention during the last phase of their life. Steinhauser and colleagues (2000) identified that the components of such care are (a) vigorous treatment of pain and other symptoms, (b) relief from worry, anxiety, and depression, (c) communication about care over time, (d) coordinated care throughout the course of illness, (e) support for family caregivers and practical support, and (f) a sense of safety in the healthcare system.

The interdisciplinary team approach embedded in both palliative care and the hospice care model was specifically designed to meet these patient and family needs: the palliative care model while the patient is still being treated actively for their disease and the hospice model when the focus of care is quality of life and when the patient has a life expectancy of six months or less. Some specific palliative care procedures to alleviate specific symptoms are outlined in the next section. These can be performed for patients who are in active treatment as well as for patients who are no longer in active treatment and prior to being transitioned to hospice care.

Examples of Palliative Care Symptom Management Procedures

Percutaneous endoscopic gastrostomy for decompression may be useful to alleviate nausea and vomiting in patients with malignant obstruction. The rate of minor complications is 9%–25%, and major complications occur in less than 9% of cases (McClave & Ritchie, 2006; Pothuri et al., 2005). Most patients achieve symptom relief in seven days and are able to eat soft foods and liquids after the procedure (Pothuri et al., 2005).

Palliative radiation may be offered to treat painful bone metastases. Janjan and colleagues (2009) reported that 70% of patients had pain relief that lasted for up to three months. Response to therapy, however, can take up to 12 weeks, so it is important to carefully consider prognosis and offer single-dose radiation fractions when possible (Gripp, Mjartan, Boelke, & Willers, 2010). Single fraction radiation has similar response rates to multiple fraction radiation with lower rates of toxicity (Janjan et al., 2009).

Refractory ascites can occur with gastrointestinal and gynecologic malignancies and may cause dyspnea, nausea, and pain. Patients often have relief of these symptoms with palliative paracentesis. Despite this treatment, rapid re-accumulation may require frequent office visits to repeat the procedure. One option is placement of a tunneled catheter for periodic drainage of malignant ascites. The procedure can be done in the outpatient setting, and infection rates are relatively low (Fleming, Alvarez-Secord, Von Grueningen, Miller, & Abernathy, 2009).

Malignant pleural effusions caused by breast, lung, and ovarian cancers have a deleterious impact on quality of life. Dyspnea due to effusions can cause anxiety for patients and families. A chronic indwelling catheter, such as a PleurX® catheter, can allow patients to manage their symptoms at home. The procedure has a complication rate of 12% and has been shown to be effective in managing dyspnea, pain, and cough in 86% of patients (Bazerbashi et al., 2009).

Careful assessment on the benefit and burden of each intervention and associated morbidity, especially in the older adult, is a critical part of ethical care. The ambulatory care oncology nurse can assist the family in weighing the benefits and risks.

Last Days to Hours of Living

Basic knowledge about prognostication and the dying process is important for the nurse to acquire so that a level of comfort is present when responding to patients' questions or referring them to an appropriate resource such as a palliative care team member or a social worker. As previously reviewed, most deaths in the older adult will occur in the setting of multiple comorbidities with associated frailty and dependency on others.

Despite this common experience among friends and family, many people have little experience with the actual dying process. In addition, although increasing attention has been given to prognostication, this remains an imprecise science, especially in older adults with cancer and multiple comorbid conditions. Often multiple determinants must be considered (Glare et al., 2008; Glare & Sinclair, 2008; Parker et al., 2007).

The benefits of prognostication include the ability to make informed decisions, an opportunity for reconciliation and to say goodbye, alleviation of the stress that not knowing creates, and less reluctance of families to discuss options. A variety of prognostic tools that help with prognostication are available in addition to the subjective assessment. For example, functional status can be measured using the Eastern Cooperative Group Performance Scale (Oken et al., 1982), the Karnofsky Performance Status (Crooks, Waller, Smith, & Hahn, 1991), or the Palliative Performance Scale (Anderson, Downing, Hill, Casorso, & Lerch, 1996). Disease-specific markers of poor prognosis are also available (Thomas, 2010). Asking the question "Would you be surprised if this person died within six months, three months, or days?" can redirect care goals and foster education of the patient and family to the reality of the situation (Lynn, Harrell, Cohn, Wagner, & Conners, 1997). The ambulatory care oncology nurse may be in the position to suggest this redirection to the disease management team.

What to Expect at the End of Life

Families, and sometimes patients, may ask the ambulatory care oncology nurse what to expect as life draws to a close. These conversations most commonly occur when the goals of care are in transition from life-prolonging therapy to comfort. Included are questions about the physiologic changes that occur and how any distressing symptoms will be managed. Although death may appear to be imminent, the actual time for a particular patient in terms of hours or days can be unpredictable. This uncertainty can be distressing for families as they wait for the inevitable and find the waiting to be emotionally exhausting.

Physiologic changes that occur during the dying process include increasing weakness and extreme fatigue. This places the patient at a higher risk for pressure ulcers and requires increased care such as turning, positioning, and massage. Decreased appetite and food intake is natural as the body slows down but may be distressing to the family as they associate lack of food with starvation. Helping the family to understand the natural dying process, the risk of aspiration if food is forced, that hunger is rarely felt, and other ways to care are all part of care of the family at this time. Diminished fluid intake can cause family and caregivers distress about dehydration and thirst. Families who have a close relationship with the ambulatory care oncology nurse may turn to that nurse for advice. It is important to make the family and caregivers aware that parenteral fluids can cause fluid overload, breathlessness, cough, and increased secretions. The family and caregivers can at the same time be reassured that there is no evidence that dehydration causes distress and that if any signs of distress do occur they will be promptly managed.

Cardiac and renal dysfunction can be evidenced by tachycardia and hypotension. The patient may experience peripheral cooling, mottling of the skin, and cyanosis. Urine output will be diminished. The family should be coached and reassured each step of the normal process of dying. Although the hospice team will work with the family throughout this process, the family may reach out to the ambulatory care oncology nurse for reassurance about what is happening. Neurologic dysfunction is evidenced by decreasing levels of consciousness, decreased or absent communication, confusion or delirium, loss of ability to swallow, and loss of sphincter control. Loss of the gag reflex can result in the buildup of saliva and secretions, which results in what is known as the "death rattle." This can usually be managed by the use of anticholinergics (scopolamine patches, atropine drops, or glycopyrrolate subcutaneously or intravenously). Suctioning is rarely helpful. Moaning or "phonation" sometimes occurs as the muscles relax and lose their tone. This can be extremely distressing for families and caregivers as they equate this as indicative of pain. Changing the patient's position can sometimes help. The respiratory pattern may change with increasing periods of apnea, Cheyne-Stokes respirations, increased use of accessory muscles, and last reflex breaths. The last reflex breaths can be frightening to families unless they have been prepared. Sometimes patients lose the ability to close their eyes fully. This is associated with the loss of the retro-orbital fat pad. Attention to the conjunctiva is important because of the risk of increased dryness and irritation.

Families are frequently uncertain about what to do as they stand at the foot of the bed, watching the dying process unfold. Explaining to them what is happening in a language that is understandable can be extremely reassuring. Teaching them the importance of presence, touch, and talking to the patients and assuring them that they are safe, they are not alone, they will not be forgotten, the family will miss them but will continue forward, and they can sleep in peace now are long-held hospice concepts in aiding patients' transition through the dying process.

New symptoms that may occur or old symptoms that may escalate in intensity can usually be anticipated for a particular person. Pain, terminal delirium, dyspnea, and difficulty clearing secretions are a symptom cluster frequently seen at end of life. Tools to manage these symptoms should be readily available in the home, including 20 mg/ml morphine sulfate, 2 mg/ml lorazepam intensol, 2 mg/ml high-potency haloperidol, scopolamine patches, and atropine drops. Hospice programs frequently provide a comfort pack with such medications and instruct the family in their use as the need arises. The ambulatory care nurse can be very helpful in reassuring the family that the hospice team's expertise is in this area. In the few instances where symptoms cannot be controlled at end of life and the person remains awake and alert, palliative sedation is an option. Comfort rather than level of alertness becomes the primary goal of care for the patient.

Loss, Grief, and Bereavement

Cumulative losses over time are a common experience for the patient with cancer. Because these losses, some actual and some anticipated, escalate in the setting of advanced disease, it is important for the ambulatory care oncology nurse to recognize their impact and to initiate appropriate referrals. The ambulatory care oncology nurse needs a basic understanding of grief and loss. People grieve their losses in different ways that personal, cultural, and spiritual factors influence. Grief work includes acknowledging the loss, expressing the associated emotions, adjusting to a changed life, and approaching death (Corless, 2010). A search for meaning is common at this time, and a variety of interventions have been designed specifically to facilitate this exploration (Breitbart et al., 2010). Ongoing support for patients and their families experiencing grief and bereavement is an integral component of palliative and hospice care. In addition, nurses need to acknowledge their own feelings of grief and loss when a patient is no longer responding to treatment and is transitioned to hospice care. Unacknowledged grief and loss can contribute to burnout and compassion fatigue on the part of staff.

Burnout and Compassion Fatigue

Ambulatory care oncology nurses and others caring for patients with progressive disease are subject to multiple stressors. These may lead to burnout and compassion fatigue. Burnout results from the clinician's interaction with the work environment, whereas compassion fatigue evolves specifically from the relationship between the clinician and the patient. Dimensions of burnout include persistent exhaustion, constant frustration, cynicism, depersonalization or detachment from the job, a sense of ineffectiveness, and a lack of personal accomplishment (Vachon & Huggard, 2010). The source of the stress is the context in which one works, as opposed to the content of one's work. Burnout is grounded in our reaction to our environment, whereas compassion fatigue is grounded in the clinical work and our reaction to it. Symptoms of compassion fatigue include disturbed sleep; irritability; reduced frustration tolerance and increased outbursts of anger; hypervigilance; the desire to avoid thoughts, feelings, and conversations about the patient's pain and suffering; transference and countertransference; and psychological or physiologic distress in response to reminders of work with people who are dying (Vachon & Huggard, 2010). Compassion fatigue can lead to burnout (Potter et al., 2010).

Personal factors that have been found to mitigate burnout are the personality characteristics of hardiness, including a sense of commitment, control, and challenge (Grafton, Gillepsie, & Henderson, 2010; Perry, 2008; Vachon & Huggard, 2010). Exquisite empathy is the ability to be highly present and sensitively attuned, as well as to have well-defined boundaries and to exhibit heartfelt engagement. Exquisite empathy can invigorate professional connections and safeguard against compassion fatigue and burnout (Vachon & Huggard, 2010). Meaningful and rewarding involvement in one's work is the opposite of burnout. It involves a sustainable workload, feelings of choice and control, appropriate recognition and reward, a supportive work community, fairness and justice, and meaningful and valued work (Aycock & Boyle, 2009).

The importance of self-care to manage the stress related to caring for patients with advanced cancer cannot be overemphasized. Oncology nurses, however, often do not take the time to grieve the losses they encounter (Boyle, 2000). Ferrell and Coyle (2008) stated that "providing care for others without caring for oneself is unsustainable" (p. 20). Unfortunately, self-care does not come naturally for many nurses, but positive coping behaviors can be taught. It is important to create an approach for dealing with the emotions that are common when providing care to patients with advanced cancer. One key step is seeking out a colleague to discuss difficult cases (Meier, Back, & Morrison, 2001). Kutner and Kilbourn (2009) found this technique obvious but often forgotten. Acknowledging the emotions inherent in caring for patients with cancer helps to promote healthy coping. Medland, Howard-Ruben, and Whitaker (2004) found that implementing a CARES program promoted psychosocial wellness for staff members. This included

• Creation of a community of care and awareness of the signs and symptoms of stress and burnout
• Reinforcement of the importance of relaxation and rejuvenation
• Emphasis on regular aerobic exercise and healthy eating
• Spiritual awareness and reconnection to whatever is personally meaningful.

These skills are essential in helping to reduce the psychological impact of caring for the patient with advanced disease.

Conclusion

The differences between palliative care needs in the older adult with cancer and palliative care for younger patients are the multiple comorbidities, losses, and associated frailty. Significant and chronic family caregiver burden is often present. Special education and training are needed foundations for palliative nursing care and end-of-life care, especially for clinicians who serve the older adult population. Ambulatory care oncology nurses would benefit from having such knowledge and training available to them, as palliative care is an integral part of comprehensive cancer care.

References

American Nurses Association. (2010, June 14). Position statement: Registered nurses' roles and responsibilities in providing expert care and counseling at the end of life. Retrieved from http://www.nursingworld.org/MainMenuCategories/EthicsStandards/Ethics -Position-Statements/etpain14426.aspx

Anderson, F., Downing, G.M., Hill, J., Casorso, L., & Lerch, N. (1996). Palliative Performance Scale (PPS): A new tool. *Journal of Palliative Care, 12,* 5–11.

Andersson, M., Ekwall, A.K., Hallberg, I.R., & Edberg, A.K. (2010). The experience of being next of kin to an older person in the last phase of life. *Palliative Supportive Care, 8,* 17–26. doi:10.1017/S1478951509990666

Aycock, N., & Boyle, D. (2009). Interventions to manage compassion fatigue in oncology nursing. *Clinical Journal of Oncology Nursing, 13,* 183–191. doi:10.1188/09.CJON.183-191

Bakitas, M., Bishop, M.F., Caron, P., & Stephens, L. (2010). Developing successful models of cancer palliative care services. *Seminars in Oncology Nursing, 26,* 266–284. doi:10.1016/j.soncn.2010.08.006

Bazerbashi, S., Villaquiran, J., Awan, M.Y., Unsworth-White, M.J., Rahamim, J., & Marchbank, A. (2009). Ambulatory intercostal drainage for the management of malignant pleural effusion: A single center experience. *Annals of Surgical Oncology, 16,* 3482–3487. doi:10.1245/s10434-009-0691-2

Beckstrand, R.L., Moore, J., Callister, L., & Bond, A.E. (2009). Oncology nurses' perceptions of obstacles and supportive behaviors at the end of life. *Oncology Nursing Forum, 36,* 446–453. doi:10.1188/09.ONF.446-453

Boyle, D. (2000). Pathos in practice: Exploring the affective domain of oncology nursing. *Oncology Nursing Forum, 27,* 915–919.

Breitbart, W., Rosenfeld, B., Gibson, C., Pessin, H., Poppito, S., Nelson, C., ... Olden, M. (2010). Meaning-centered group psychotherapy for patients with advanced cancer: A pilot randomized controlled trial. *Psycho-Oncology, 19,* 21–28. doi:10.1002/pon.1556

Cassell, E.J., & Rich, B.A. (2010). Intractable end-of-life suffering and the ethics of palliative sedation. *Pain Medicine, 11,* 435–438. doi:10.1111/j.1526-4637.2009.00786.x

Clark, D. (1999). "Total pain," disciplinary power and the body of work of Cicely Saunders, 1958–1967. *Social Science and Medicine, 49,* 727–736. doi:10.1016/S0277-9536(99)00098-2

Connor, S.R. (2009). *Hospice and palliative care: The essential guide* (2nd ed.). New York, NY: Taylor & Francis.

Corless, I.B. (2010). Bereavement. In B.R. Ferrell & N. Coyle (Eds.), *Oxford textbook of palliative nursing* (3rd ed., pp. 597–627). New York, NY: Oxford University Press.

Coyle, N., & Kissane, D.W. (2010). Conducting a family meeting. In D.W. Kissane, B.D. Bultz, P.M. Butow, & I.G. Finlay (Eds.), *Handbook of communication in oncology and palliative care* (pp. 165–175). New York, NY: Oxford University Press.

Coyle, N., & Sculco, L. (2003). Communication and the patient/physician relationship: A phenomenological inquiry. *Journal of Supportive Oncology, 1,* 206–215.

Crooks, V., Waller, S., Smith, T., & Hahn, T.J. (1991). The use of the Karnofsky Performance Scale in determining outcomes and risk in geriatric outpatients. *Journal of Gerontology, 46,* M139–M144. doi:10.1093/geronj/46.4.M139

Davis, B., & Steele, R. (2010). Supporting families in palliative care. In B.R. Ferrell & N. Coyle (Eds.), *Oxford textbook of palliative nursing* (3rd ed., pp. 613–628). New York, NY: Oxford University Press.

Ferrell, B.R., & Coyle, N. (2008). The nature of suffering and the goals of nursing. *Oncology Nursing Forum, 35,* 241–247. doi:10.1188/08.ONF.241-247

Ferrell, B., Virani, R., Malloy, P., & Kelly, K. (2010). The preparation of oncology nurses in palliative care. *Seminars in Oncology Nursing, 26,* 259–265.

Fleming, N.D., Alvarez-Secord, A., Von Grueningen, V., Miller, M.J., & Abernathy, A.P. (2009). Indwelling catheters for the management of refractory malignant ascites: A systematic literature overview and retrospective chart review. *Journal of Pain and Symptom Management, 38,* 342–349. doi:10.1016/j.jpainsymman.2008.09.008

Freedman, B. (1993). Offering truth: One ethical approach to the uninformed cancer patient. *Archives of Internal Medicine, 153,* 572–576.

Glare, P., Sinclair, C., Downing, M., Stone, P., Maltoni, M., & Vigano, A. (2008). Predicting survival in patients with advanced disease. *European Journal of Cancer, 44,* 1146–1156. doi:10.1016/j.ejca.2008.02.030

Glare, P., & Sinclair, C.T. (2008). Palliative medicine review: Prognostication. *Journal of Palliative Medicine, 11,* 84–103. doi:10.1089/jpm.2008.9992

Grafton, E., Gillespie, B., & Henderson, S. (2010). Resilience: The power within. *Oncology Nursing Forum, 37,* 698–705. doi:10.1188/10.ONF.698-705

Gripp, S., Mjartan, S., Boelke, E., & Willers, R. (2010). Palliative radiotherapy tailored to life expectancy in end-stage cancer patients: Reality or myth? *Cancer, 116,* 3251–3256. doi:10.1002/cncr.25112

Guengerich, T. (2009, February). Caregiving and end of life issues: A survey of AARP members in Florida. Retrieved from http://www.aarp.org/relationships/grief-loss/info-02-2009/fl_eol_08.html

Hallenbeck, J., & Arnold, R. (2007). A request for nondisclosure: Don't tell Mother. *Journal of Clinical Oncology, 25,* 5030–5034. doi:10.1200/JCO.2007.11.8802

Irwin, S.A., & von Gunten, C.F. (2010). The role of palliative care in cancer care transitions. In J.C. Holland, P.B. Jacobsen, & R. McCorkle (Eds.), *Psycho-oncology* (2nd ed., pp. 277–283). New York, NY: Oxford University Press.

Janjan, N., Lutz, S.T., Bedwinek, J.M., Hartsell, W.F., Ng, A., Pieters, R.S., … Rettenmaier, A. (2009). Therapeutic guidelines for the treatment of bone metastasis: A report from the American College of Radiology appropriateness criteria expert panel on radiation oncology. *Journal of Palliative Medicine, 12,* 417–426. doi:10.1089/jpm.2009.9633

Kaplan, M. (2010). SPIKES: A framework for breaking bad news to patients with cancer. *Clinical Journal of Oncology Nursing, 14,* 514–516. doi:10.1188/10.CJON.514-516

Kissane, D., Lichtenthal, W.G., & Zaider, T. (2007–2008). Family care before and after bereavement. *Omega, 56,* 21–32.

Kissane, D.R., Bultz, B.D., Butow, P., & Finlay, I. (Eds.). (2010). *Handbook of communication in oncology and palliative care.* New York, NY: Oxford University Press.

Kutner, J.S., & Kilbourn, K.M. (2009). Bereavement: Addressing challenges faced by advanced cancer patients, their caregivers, and their physicians. *Primary Care, 36,* 825–844. doi:10.1016/j.pop.2009.07.004

Lawton, C. (2010). Developing a nurse led hospice outpatient clinic to improve palliative care services. *Nursing Times, 106*(34), 18–20.

Levine, C. (2003). Family caregivers: Burdens and opportunities. In R.S. Morrison, D.E. Meier, & C. Capello (Eds.), *Geriatric palliative care* (pp. 376–385). New York, NY: Oxford University Press.

Lunney, J.R., Lynn, J., Foley, K.M., Lipson, S., & Guralnik, J.M. (2003). Patterns of functional decline at the end of life. *JAMA, 289,* 2387–2392. doi:10.1001/jama.289.18.2387

Lynn J., Harrell, F., Cohn, F., Wagner, D., & Conners, A.F., Jr. (1997). Prognoses of seriously ill hospitalized patients on the days before death: Implications for patient care and public policy. *New Horizon, 5,* 56–61.

Mack, J.W., Block, S.D., Nilsson, B.S., Wright, A., Trice, E., Friedlander, R., … Prigerson, H.G. (2009). Measuring therapeutic alliance between oncologists and patients with advanced cancer: The human connection scale. *Cancer, 115,* 3302–3311. doi:10.1002/cncr.24360

Maguire, P., & Weiner, J.S. (2009). Communication with terminally ill patients and their families. In H.M. Chochinov & W. Breitbart (Eds.), *Handbook of psychiatry in palliative medicine* (2nd ed., pp. 157–171). New York, NY: Oxford University Press.

Mahon, M.M. (2010). Clinical decision making in palliative care and end of life care. *Nursing Clinics of North America, 45,* 345–362. doi:10.1016/j.cnur.2010.03.002

McClave, S.A., & Ritchie, C.S. (2006). The role of endoscopically placed feeding or decompression tubes. *Gastroenterology Clinics of North America, 35,* 83–100. doi:10.1016/j.gtc.2005.12.003

Medland, J., Howard-Ruben, J., & Whitaker, E. (2004). Fostering psychosocial wellness in oncology nurses: Addressing burnout and social support in the workplace. *Oncology Nursing Forum, 31,* 47–54. doi:10.1188/04.ONF.47–54

Meier, D.E., Back, A.L., & Morrison, R.S. (2001). The inner life of physicians and care of the seriously ill. *JAMA, 286,* 3007–3014. doi:10.1001/jama.286.23.3007

Murphy-Ende, K. (2006). Palliative care of the older adult with cancer. In D.G. Cope & A. Reb (Eds.), *An evidence-based approach to the treatment and care of the older adult with cancer* (pp. 465–466). Pittsburgh, PA: Oncology Nursing Society.

National Comprehensive Cancer Network. (2011). *NCCN Clinical Practice Guidelines in Oncology: Palliative care* [v.2.2011]. Retrieved from http://www.nccn.org/professionals/physician_gls/PDF/palliative.pdf

National Hospice and Palliative Care Organization. (2010, October). NHPCO facts and figures: Hospice care in America. Retrieved from http://www.nhpco.org/files/public/Statistics_Research/Hospice_Facts_Figures_Oct-2010.pdf

Oken, M.M., Creech, R.H., Tormey, D.C., Horton, J., Davis, T.E., McFadden, E.T., & Carbone, P.P. (1982). Toxicity and response criteria of the Eastern Cooperative Oncology Group. *American Journal of Clinical Oncology, 5,* 649–655.

Olsen, M.L., Swetz, K.M., & Mueller, P.S. (2010). Ethical decision making with end-of-life care: Palliative sedation and withholding or withdrawing life-sustaining treatments. *Mayo Clinic Proceedings, 85,* 949–954. doi:10.4065/mcp.2010.0201

O'Neill, L.B., Meier, D.E., & Morrison, R.S. (2009). Special considerations for the seriously ill older adult. In H.M. Chochinov & W. Breitbart (Eds.), *Handbook of psychiatric palliative medicine* (2nd ed., pp. 544–552). New York, NY: Oxford University Press.

Panke, J.T., & Coyne, P. (2006). *Conversations in palliative care* (2nd ed.). Pittsburgh, PA: Hospice and Palliative Nurses Association.

Pantilat, S.Z. (2009). Communicating with seriously ill patients: Better words to say. *JAMA, 301,* 1279–1281. doi:10.1001/jama.2009.396

Parker, S.M., Clayton, J.M., Hancock, K., Walder, S., Butow, P.N., Currow, D., ... Tattersall, M.H. (2007). A systematic review of prognostic/end-of-life communication with adults in the advanced stages of a life limiting illness: Patient/caregiver preferences for the content, style, and timing of information. *Journal of Pain and Symptom Management, 34,* 81–93. doi:10.1016/j.jpainsymman.2006.09.035

Pellegrino, E.D., & Sulmasy, D.P. (2009). Ethical issues in palliative care. In H.M. Chochinov & W. Breitbart (Eds.), *Handbook of psychiatry in palliative medicine* (2nd ed., pp. 267–280). New York, NY: Oxford University Press.

Perry, B. (2008). Why exemplary oncology nurses seem to avoid compassion fatigue. *Canadian Oncology Nursing Journal, 18,* 87–99.

Pothuri, B. Montmanrano, M., Gerardi, M., Shike, M., Ben-Porat, L., Sabbatini, P., & Barakat, R.R. (2005). Percutaneous endoscopic gastrostomy tube placement in patients with malignant bowel obstruction due to ovarian cancer. *Gynecologic Oncology, 96,* 330–334. doi:10.1016/j.ygyno.2004.09.058

Potter, P., Deshields, T., Divanbeigi, J., Berger, J., Cipriano, D., Norris, L., & Olsen, S. (2010). Compassion fatigue and burnout: Prevalence among oncology nurses [Online exclusive]. *Clinical Journal of Oncology Nursing, 14,* E56–E62. doi:10.1188/10.CJON.E56-E62

Quill, T.E., Arnold, R., & Back, A.L. (2009). Discussing treatment preferences with patients who want "everything." *Annals of Internal Medicine, 151,* 345–349.

Saunders, C. (2010). Foreword. In B.R. Ferrell & N. Coyle (Eds.), *Oxford textbook of palliative nursing* (3rd ed., pp. v–vi). New York, NY: Oxford University Press.

Schwarz, J.K., & Tarzian, A.J. (2010). Ethical aspects of palliative care. In M.L. Matzo & D.W. Sherman (Eds.), *Palliative care nursing: Quality care to the end of life* (3rd ed., pp. 119–141). New York, NY: Springer.

Steel, K., & Vitale, C. (2003). Home care for frail, older adults. In R.S. Morrison, D.E. Meier, & C. Capello (Eds.), *Geriatric palliative care* (pp. 386–401). New York, NY: Oxford University Press.

Steinhauser, K.E., Christakis, N.A., Clipp, E.C., McNeilly, M., McIntyre, L., & Tulsky, J.A. (2000). Factors considered important at the end of life by patients, family, physicians, and other care providers. *JAMA, 284,* 2476–2482. doi:10.1001/jama.284.19.2476

Teno, J.M., & Connor, S.R. (2009). Referring a patient and family to high quality palliative care at the close of life: "We met a new personality ... with this level of compassion and empathy." *JAMA, 301,* 651–659. doi:10.1001/jama.2009.109

Teno, J., Lynn, J., Wenger, N., Phillips, R.S., Murphy, D.P., Connors, A.F., Jr., ... Knaus, W.A. (1997). Advance directives for seriously ill hospitalized patients: Effectiveness with the

Patient Self-Determination Act and the SUPPORT intervention. *Journal of the American Geriatrics Society, 45,* 500–507.

Thomas, K. (2010). The Gold Standards Framework: The GSF Prognostic Indicator Guidance. *End of Life Care, 4,* 62–64. Retrieved from http://www.goldstandardsframework. nhs.uk/OneStopCMS/Core/CrawlerResourceServer.aspx?resource=68FE53BA-A79B -4DBD-A32A-E76B40BC7828&mode=link&guid=9d9423c7b38d49c9b74c02cdc95f1aa2

Tolstoy, L. (2004). *The death of Ivan Ilych and other stories.* New York, NY: Barnes and Noble.

Trice, E.D., & Prigerson, H.G. (2009). Communication in end-stage cancer: Review of the literature and future research. *Journal of Health Communication, 14,* 95–108. 10.1080/10810730902806786

Twycross, R.G., & Lack, S.A. (1983). Pain—A broader concept. In R.G. Twycross & S.A. Lack (Eds.), *Symptom control in far advanced cancer* (pp. 43–55). London, England: Pitman Books.

Vachon, M., & Huggard, J. (2010). Experiences of the nurse in end-of-life care in the 21st century. In B.R. Ferrell & N. Coyle (Eds.), *Oxford textbook of palliative nursing* (3rd ed., pp. 1137–1155). New York, NY: Oxford University Press.

World Health Organization. (n.d.). WHO definition of palliative care. Retrieved from http://www.who.int/cancer/palliative/definition

Wright, A.A., Zhang, B., Ray, A., Mack, J.W., Trice, E., Balboni, T., … Prigerson, H.G. (2008). Associations between end-of-life discussions, patient mental health, medical care near death, and caregiver bereavement adjustment. *JAMA, 300,* 1665–1673. doi:10.1001/ jama.300.14.1665

Zaider, T., & Kissane, D. (2009). The assessment and management of family distress during palliative care. *Current Opinion in Supportive Palliative Care, 3,* 67–71. doi:10.1097/ SPC.0b013e328325a5ab

Zhou, G., Stoltzfus, J.C., Houldin, A.D., Parks, S.M., & Swan, B.A. (2010). Knowledge, attitudes, and practice behaviors of oncology advanced practice nurses regarding advanced care planning for patients with cancer [Online exclusive]. *Oncology Nursing Forum, 37,* E400–E410. doi:10.1188/10.ONF.E400-E410

CHAPTER 6

Survivorship Issues

Kimberly A. Christopher, PhD, RN, OCN®

Introduction

Cancer incidence rates are projected to increase significantly over the next few decades in people who are 65 years old or older. By 2030, the older adult population is expected to have a 67% increase in cancer incidence (Smith, Smith, Hurria, Hortobagyi, & Buchholz, 2009). This increase is in part due to the aging Baby Boomers and the overall growth in the older adult population. Despite the increase in cancer incidence, mortality rates overall have declined as a result of ongoing advances in oncologic treatment (Shulman et al., 2009; Smith et al., 2009). According to the American Cancer Society (ACS), at least 12 million cancer survivors live in the United States, of which approximately 60% are 65 years old or older, and these numbers continue to increase each year (ACS, 2010). Cancer survivorship can be stressful, and patients must face many physical and psychosocial challenges following diagnosis and treatment. Ambulatory care oncology nurses have a unique opportunity to assess patients and plan for individualized post-treatment care. This chapter will address older adult demographic characteristics and survivorship issues, development of the survivorship care plan, long-term and late effects of cancer and cancer treatment, and recommendations for a holistic approach to assessing older adult cancer survivors.

Demographics of the Older Adult Population

Awareness of demographic characteristics of the current older adult population will assist ambulatory care oncology nurses when planning survivorship care. The Department of Health and Human Services Administration on Aging (AoA) *Profile of Older Americans* (AoA, 2009) provides a resource for complete data about this population. Chapter 1 of this report presents general data about older adults in the United States. Specific characteristics that potentially affect survivorship care, including life expectancy, marital status, living arrangement, income, and geographic distribution, will be presented here.

The average life expectancy of a person reaching 65 years is an additional 18.6 years (AoA, 2009). Older women (22.4 million) outnumber older men (16.5 million). Older men (72%) are more likely to be married than older women (42%). Therefore, older women are more likely to live alone, and of women 75 years old and older, an estimated 50% live alone (AoA, 2009). In 2008, households headed by people 65 years old or older reported a median income of $44,188. However, for that year, individual median income was $25,503 for males and $14,559 for females, almost 50% less than men. Thirty-five percent of all Social Security beneficiaries reported that Social Security constituted 90% or more of their income (AoA, 2009).

The first of the Baby Boomer generation began reaching 65 years of age on January 1, 2011. The 65 and older population, estimated at 40 million in 2010, is expected to increase to 55 million in 2020, a 36% increase over the decade. The number of adults 85 years and older, estimated at 5.7 million in 2010, is expected to increase to 6.6 million in 2020, a 15% increase over the decade. In addition, the United States is experiencing and will continue to experience increases in minority older adult populations. Projections estimate that the number of minorities 65 and older will increase by 172% between 2008 and 2030, whereas the older White population is estimated to increase by 64% (AoA, 2009). This increasing older adult population is at risk for cancer and will require increased healthcare services (Rose, O'Toole, Koroukian, & Berger, 2009; Rowland & Bellizzi, 2008).

The geographic distribution of the older adult population varies across the United States, resulting in some states having much higher populations of older adults (AoA, 2009). According to data from 2008, 51% of adults 65 and older lived in nine states: California (4.1 million), Florida (3.2 million), New York (2.6 million), Texas (2.5 million), Pennsylvania (1.9 million) and Illinois, Ohio, Michigan, and New Jersey (more than 1 million each) (AoA, 2009). Approximately 81% of the older adult population resided in metropolitan areas; the remaining lived in nonmetropolitan areas. Of those in metropolitan areas, about 35% lived in the principal cities and 65% outside of the cities (AoA, 2009). In addition, the data indicate that older adults are not likely to change residence. Between 2007 and 2008, 3.7% of older adults moved compared to about 13% of individuals who are younger than 65 years old (AoA, 2009). Of the older adults who did move, only about 20% changed state residence (AoA, 2009).

Ambulatory care oncology nurses' assessment and care planning for older adult cancer survivors must take into consideration these demographic trends in order to provide high quality care. These trends indicate that older women and older men have different resources, and this will potentially affect their survivorship experience. Older women are likely to be unpartnered and have less income in comparison to older men. Therefore, older women's resources such as social support, caregiver assistance, and financial capacity should be carefully assessed when planning survivorship care. Although all oncology nurses need knowledge and clinical expertise in the care of older adults, competency in caring for older adults should be a high priority for those nurses working in states with high concentrations of this population. In addition, as older adult minority populations increase, oncology nursing competency in minority health issues will be increasingly necessary.

Transitioning to Survivorship Care

The 2005 Institute of Medicine (IOM) report *From Cancer Patient to Cancer Survivor: Lost in Transition* (Hewitt, Greenfield, & Stovall, 2006) identifies cancer survivorship as a distinct phase of cancer care. The report stressed that successfully transitioning patients from primary treatment to the post-treatment survivorship phase of the cancer care trajectory requires a comprehensive and coordinated plan designed to assist patients in the next phase of their life (Hewitt et al., 2006). Although there is currently no agreement on whether cancer survivors should be followed post-treatment by the oncology, primary care, or multidisciplinary healthcare team (Cheung, Neville, Cameron, Cook, & Earle, 2009; Grunfeld, 2009; Hewitt et al., 2006; Horning, 2008; Jacobs et al., 2009; Morgan, 2009; Rose et al., 2009; Shulman et al., 2009), ambulatory care oncology nurses are well-positioned to advocate for quality survivorship care. Whether oncology nurses are directly caring for survivors or transitioning patients to primary care clinicians, nurses have a role in ensuring good communication and education about the patient's treatment history and the next phase of their cancer care—survivorship (Haylock, Mitchell, Cox, Temple, & Curtiss, 2007).

Moving from the primary treatment to survivorship phase of care is a potentially stressful time for patients with cancer. Research findings identify that patients report mixed emotions at this transition time, including grief, anxiety, and uncertainty (Holland & Weiss, 2008; Mellon, 2002; Morgan, 2009; Reuben, 2004; Rowland, 2008b; Wonghongkul, Moore, Musil, Schneider, & Deimling, 2000). Completing treatment represents meeting goals associated with "getting through" therapies designed to cure or arrest the disease. Completing treatment is also associated with a new plan for follow-up, less regular contact with oncology clinicians, and potentially a transfer of follow-up care to a primary care physician (Rose et al., 2009). Recognizing patients' potential distress, ambulatory care oncology nurses need to assess patients in a holistic manner in order to determine, coordinate, and communicate an appropriate plan of care. Research suggests that some patients believe that communication among clinicians and with patients can influence cancer outcomes, further emphasizing the need for good communication (Thorne, Hislop, Armstrong, & Oglov, 2007).

The Survivorship Care Plan: Facilitating Quality Care

The IOM report strongly recommended that every patient receive a "comprehensive care summary and follow-up plan" (Hewitt et al., 2006, p.4) upon completion of primary treatment. The survivorship care plan (SCP) expanded previous follow-up guidelines focusing primarily on surveillance for disease recurrence to address a broad range of areas designed to ensure that survivors receive coordinated, high-quality, holistic care (Earle, 2006; Hoffman & Stovall, 2006; Morgan, 2009). Since the 2005 IOM recommendation for SCPs, numerous oncology institutions and organizations have developed SCPs, and evaluation by patients, oncology professionals, and primary care clinicians—which has been positive to date—is ongoing (Baravelli et al., 2009; Hill-Kayser, Vachani, Hampshire, Jacobs, & Metz, 2009; Miller, 2008).

Although SCP templates vary somewhat by institution and organization (Figure 6-1), there is agreement that the core elements identified in the IOM report (Hewitt et al., 2006) are essential to ensure good communication with the patient and the patient's healthcare providers (Baravelli et al., 2009; Earle, 2006; Ganz, Casillas, & Hahn, 2008). The SCP provides patients with key educational information that will assist them as they advocate for their own best survivorship care (Ganz et al., 2008; Hoffman & Stovall, 2006). The core elements include cancer treatment history, potential long-term and late effects of therapy, recommendations for surveillance for long-term and late effects of therapy, surveillance for new cancers, time intervals for follow-up care, and specific identification of the appropriate clinician for follow-up care (Hewitt et al., 2006). The individual patient's responses to therapy should be accurately described within the core elements; for example, side effects and toxicities associated with the patient's therapy should be identified (Miller, 2008).

Research findings support anecdotal experiences that cancer survivors have a broad range of physical and emotional needs (Wolf et al., 2005). Therefore, the SCP should include information on the psychosocial impact of cancer, health promotion activities, cancer-related resources, and comorbidities (Ganz et al., 2008; Hewitt et al., 2006; Jacobsen, 2009). Patients need

---

Figure 6-1. Online Resources for Survivorship Care Plans

- American Society of Clinical Oncology
  www.cancer.net/patient/survivorship/ASCO+Cancer+Treatment+Summaries
- Journey Forward, a collaboration of National Coalition for Cancer Survivorship, Oncology Nursing Society, UCLA Cancer Survivorship Center, WellPoint, Inc., and Genentech
  http://journeyforward.org
- LIVESTRONG Care Plan
  www.livestrongcareplan.org
- National Comprehensive Cancer Network treatment summaries
  www.nccn.com/treatment-summaries.html
- A Prescription for Living Care Plan
  www.nursingcenter.com/library/static.asp?pageid=721732

information on how cancer and treatment may impact marriage/partner relationships, sexual functioning, mood state, and role responsibilities such as parenting and work (Holland & Weiss, 2008; Jacobsen, 2009). Referrals to clinicians and support groups to address psychosocial needs should be provided, as needed, in the SCP. In addition, lifestyle adjustments will potentially improve overall quality of life (QOL) and comorbid conditions (Rowland, 2008a, 2008b). Information on health-promoting activities appropriate for individual patient needs (e.g., stress management, exercise, weight control, smoking cessation, osteoporosis prevention) should be included in the SCP as appropriate (Ganz et al., 2008; Miller, 2008). In addition to the medical and psychosocial information, the SCP should include information on how cancer potentially affects employment, insurance, and financial aspects of patients' lives (Earle, 2006; Haylock et al., 2007; Hewitt et al., 2006; Miller, 2008). Unfortunately, the Americans with Disabilities Act does not prevent some cancer survivors from experiencing job loss, discrimination in hiring, limited employment benefits, and insurance issues (Earle, 2006). Therefore, information on employment and health insurance should be provided as part of survivorship care.

Monitoring for Long-Term and Late Effects of Cancer and Cancer Therapy

Continuing advances in cancer care (e.g., early detection, improved treatment modalities, increased treatment options) have resulted in more people surviving cancer for longer periods of time (American Society of Clinical Oncology [ASCO], 2010a; Meneses & Benz, 2010). For increasing numbers of patients, cancer is curable, and for many others cancer is a chronic disease (Rowland, 2008b). Improving cancer survivors' QOL along with length of life is a primary goal of survivorship care, and clinicians and other health professionals must be committed to assisting survivors to manage the negative effects of surviving cancer (Rowland, 2008b). Adopting a health promotion and disease prevention focus as a framework for survivorship care will help to decrease morbidity and mortality and optimize health (Haylock et al., 2007; Lewis, 2006; Rowland, 2008a, 2008b).

Ambulatory care oncology nurses are positioned to educate cancer survivors about potential or actual long-term and late effects of cancer therapy while providing care during the cancer treatment phase. Because research findings suggest that health professionals are not all knowledgeable about key survivorship areas (Uijtdehaage et al., 2009), defining *long-term* and *late effects* is a first step. Long-term effects, also referred to as *persistent effects*, are the adverse effects or complications of treatment. Long-term effects begin during treatment and persist after treatment is completed (Haylock et al., 2007). Late effects are side effects of cancer and cancer treatment manifested after treatment is completed (Haylock et al., 2007). Some definitions describe late effects as those side effects that occur more than five years after a diagnosis of cancer (ASCO, 2010b). Late effects are the result of treatments such as chemotherapy, radiation therapy, or surgery (ASCO, 2010b; Haylock et al., 2007).

Survivors are a heterogeneous group. Their response to treatment and their experience with long-term and late effects will vary from individual to individual depending on the type of disease, which treatment they received, when treatment was delivered, and the length of time since treatment (ASCO, 2010b; Earle, 2007; Rowland & Bellizzi, 2008). Although some survivors will experience few effects and others will experience multiple (Miller & Triano, 2008; Rowland, 2008b; Rowland & Bellizzi, 2008), about 75% of survivors will experience some adverse response to treatment (Aziz & Rowland, 2003). Long-term and late effects can affect survivors of all ages. However, for older adult cancer survivors, distinguishing adverse effects from other comorbidities may be challenging (Earle, 2007; Rowland & Yancik, 2006). In addition, some late effects take many years to manifest, requiring diligent ongoing assessment (Earle, 2006). Long-term and late effects of cancer further increase survivors', families', and societies' illness burden (Rowland, 2008b; Rowland & Bellizzi, 2008; Yabroff, Lawrence, Clauser, Davis, & Brown, 2004). Unfortunately, predicting which survivors are at risk is difficult.

Assessing older adults for long-term and late effects of cancer therapy is challenging. To date, evidence-based recommendations and consensus guidelines are not available (Earle, 2007; Rowland & Bellizi, 2008). Planning care based on extrapolations from younger population experiences should be done with an abundance of caution, if at all, because older adults are physiologically, psychologically, and socially different (Earle, 2007; Rowland & Bellizzi, 2008). Comorbid conditions such as heart disease, arthritis, diabetes, and geriatric syndromes affect patients' treatment options, responses to treatment, QOL, and symptom burden after treatment (Burkett & Cleeland, 2007; Rowland & Bellizzi, 2008). When compared to the general population, older adults with cancer tend to have poorer health, two or more chronic medical problems, more functional limitations, and more limitations with activities of daily living, especially instrumental activities of daily living (Hewitt, Rowland, & Yancik, 2003).

Although the research evidence for long-term and late effects of cancer and cancer therapy continues to be explored in adults of all ages, research findings suggest that adverse outcomes are more prevalent than expected (Houldin, Curtiss, & Haylock, 2006). As survivors live longer and grow older, manifestations of long-term and late effects will likely change. Therefore, oncology nurses and other healthcare professionals continually need to update their knowledge and clinical expertise in this area. Patient educational resources on ASCO's Cancer.net Web site provide an explanation of late effects written for consumers. Miller and Triano (2008) provide clinicians with a detailed review of medical issues and the many possible sequelae of cancer treatment. Figure 6-2 lists some of the more common effects of treatment. Whether as a result of treatment itself or the additional burden of comorbidities, older adults are at risk for cardiac, pulmonary, and renal toxicities (Ganz et al., 2008). Some of the toxicities, which first manifest during treatment and then persist as long-term effects, include fatigue, pain, lymphedema, changes in memory and concentration, sexual dysfunction, and fear of recurrence (Rowland, 2008b; Rowland & Yancik, 2006). Problems that manifest months or years after therapy include cardiac dysfunction, osteoporosis, pulmonary fibrosis, mood disturbances, and secondary malignancies (Rowland, 2008b; Rowland & Yancik, 2006). Ambulatory care oncology nurses should continually assess survivors for surgical, radiation, and chemotherapy treatment effects. For example, surgery results in cosmetic changes and functional impairment (Haylock et al., 2007). Radiation therapy, depending on the dose, damages healthy tissue and organs in surrounding areas. For example, radiation to the head and neck can result in damage to the oral cavity with diminished salivary gland production and dental decay. Changes in oral health can potentially affect nutritional status (Haylock et al., 2007). Radiation to the chest for breast cancer, lung cancer, or lymphoma often results in cardiac and pulmonary damage (Haylock et al., 2007). Chemotherapy is also associated with risks. For example, alkylating agents are neurotoxic and nephrotoxic; antimetabolites can cause persistent gastrointestinal changes; antitumor antibiotics are myelosuppressive and associated with cardiac and pulmonary toxicities; and hormonal therapy is associated with osteoporosis, stroke, and clotting abnormalities (Haylock et al., 2007).

Figure 6-2. Common Long-Term Sequelae of Cancer Treatment

Cardiovascular
- Cardiomyopathy
- Valvular heart disease
- Coronary artery disease

Pulmonary
- Pulmonary fibrosis
- Interstitial lung disease
- Stricture/obstruction

Gastrointestinal
- Malabsorption
- Second malignancies
- Post-chemotherapy rheumatism

Rheumatologic
- Osteopenia/osteoporosis
- Osteonecrosis
- Lymphedema
- Panhypopituitarism

Endocrine
- Hypothyroidism
- Adrenal insufficiency
- Diabetes mellitus

Renal
- Chronic kidney disease

Sensory/Neurologic
- Hearing loss
- Visual changes
- Neuropathy

Note. From "Medical Issues in Cancer Survivors—A Review," by K. Miller and L. Triano, 2008, *The Cancer Journal, 14,* p. 376. doi:10.1097/PPO.0b013e31818ee3dc. Copyright 2008 by Lippincott Williams & Wilkins. Reprinted with permission.

Holistic Assessment: Integrating What We Know to Ensure Quality Care

Over the past 15 years, cancer survivorship has been increasingly recognized as an important area of clinical care and research. Yet, clinical consensus guidelines and research evidence on the management of cancer survivors in general are still limited, and even less evidence is available about older adult survivors (Earle, 2007; Rowland & Bellizzi, 2008). To ensure high-quality care for older adult survivors, ambulatory care oncology nurses must keep informed of the most recent research evidence and clinical care recommendations. In addition, approaching survivors' care from a holistic nursing perspective—a perspective that recognizes the complex nature of caring for older adults—and using the SCP as the basis for care planning will facilitate high-quality care.

Ambulatory care oncology nurses should consider framing their holistic assessment in the context of the demographic trends previously described and current knowledge from research findings. Using these data as a framework, oncology nurses should then ask each cancer survivor about his or her personal situation and experiences, ensuring that individuals' needs are identified and care planning is tailored appropriately. Ambulatory care oncology nurses should then fully assess survivors' individual situations and personal preferences. Minority populations are increasing and aging. Little survivorship research has focused on older adult minority survivors, so unfortunately oncology nurses have limited information in this area. Findings from a study with a sample of 693 Hispanics (mean age 63) suggested that acculturation influences life satisfaction (Stephens, Stein, & Landrine, 2010). Specifically, and perhaps surprisingly, less acculturated Hispanic survivors had higher life satisfaction. Low acculturated Hispanics reported higher levels of spirituality and perceived social support, both of which improved their satisfaction with life during survivorship. Therefore, understanding how such concepts as acculturation, spirituality, and social support affect minority survivors' coping and adaptation will influence survivorship care.

Survivorship research findings are generally inconclusive, and studies have limitations. For example, study samples frequently include wide age ranges, so findings specific to survivors 65 years and older cannot be readily determined. In addition, study designs are frequently cross-sectional, providing data on the survivorship experience at one point in time, rather than longitudinal, which describe the survivorship experience over time. However, knowledge of research findings to date in areas such as health promotion activities, coping and adjustment, health-related QOL, and symptom experience can assist ambulatory care oncology nurses as they approach their holistic assessment of older adult survivors.

The importance of health promotion in survivorship is emphasized in the SCP core elements. In addition, a cancer diagnosis is considered an opportunity to address lifestyle practices and health promotion (Denmark-Wahnefried,

Aziz, Rowland, & Pinto, 2005; Horning, 2008; Rowland, 2008b). Research evidence on the extent to which survivors are pursuing positive lifestyle changes is mixed. Some studies suggest that significant numbers of cancer survivors are pursuing appropriate changes (Aziz, 2007; Rowland, 2008b). Other studies suggest that survivors participate in positive health behavior practices at about the same rate as the general population, which unfortunately is poor (Fairley, Hawk, & Pierre, 2010; Park & Gaffey, 2007). A health promotion approach to managing survivors' care will potentially decrease recurrence, improve comorbid conditions, and improve QOL (Aziz, 2007; Haylock et al., 2007). With knowledge that not all survivors are adopting positive health habits after their cancer diagnosis, ambulatory care oncology nurses caring for older adult survivors have the opportunity to assess individuals' health habits and intervene, educate, and provide appropriate support and resources needed to modify behaviors.

Research findings suggest that cancer survivors generally are resilient and that for some people, cancer may lead to post-traumatic growth with increased sense of mastery and self-esteem, reestablishment of priorities, and increased appreciation for life (Jim & Jacobsen, 2008; Rowland, 2008b). Other survivors, however, may experience prolonged symptoms of distress, including intrusive thoughts, avoidance, mood disturbances, and hypervigilance (Alfano & Rowland, 2006; Earle, Neville, & Fletcher, 2007; Jim & Jacobsen, 2008). Study findings indicate that positive adaptation and post-traumatic growth are facilitated by (a) access to state-of-the-art care, (b) participation in one's care by being physically, emotionally, and cognitively engaged in the care process, (c) perceived social support, (d) a sense of purpose and meaning in one's life, and (e) stress management (Alfano & Rowland, 2006; Jim & Jacobsen, 2008; Rowland, 2008b). Ambulatory care oncology nurses must understand that survivors' responses to their cancer experience will vary, and knowledge of factors that potentially hinder (see Figure 6-3) and facilitate adaptation (see Figure 6-4) will assist nurses in assessing survivors and planning appropriate care.

Cancer survivors' subjective experience continues to be a research area of great interest. Research to date has focused on the areas of QOL and health-related QOL (HRQOL) and symptom experience and burden. Although discussion of this research is beyond the scope of this chapter, it is important to note some of the recent findings on HRQOL and symptom burden described in the literature. Specifically, HRQOL and symptom burden measure different concepts (Burkett & Cleeland, 2007). HRQOL is a multidimensional construct that typically measures four dimensions: physical function, psychological function, social role function, and disease- and treatment-related symptoms (Burkett & Cleeland, 2007). Symptom burden, on the other hand, is "a summative indicator of the severity of the symptoms that are most associated with a disease or treatment and a summary of the patient's perceptions of the impact of these symptoms on daily living" (Cleeland & Reyes-Gibby, 2002, p. 65). Numerous studies have documented that survivors report high levels of HRQOL and at the same time report high levels of symptoms (Burkett & Cleeland, 2007). Therefore, information on survivors' HRQOL may provide inadequate information on survivors' symptom burden. Hence, it is essential that ambulatory care oncology nurses fully assess symptoms in order to appropriately track late and long-term disease and treatment effects (Burkett & Cleeland, 2007).

Figure 6-3. Risk Factors for Poor Adaptation to Cancer

Medical
- More advanced disease
- More intense or aggressive treatment(s)
- Other/multiple comorbid medical conditions
- Fewer rehabilitative options
- Poorer patient/doctor relationship

Psychological
- Prior psychiatric history
- Past trauma history
- Rigid or inflexible coping style
- Helpless/hopeless outlook
- Low income/education
- Multiple social stressors
- Younger age
- Poor marital/interpersonal relationship

Social
- Lack of social support
- Limited access to service resources
- Cultural biases
- Social stigma

Note. Based on information from Weisman & Worden, 1976–1977.

From "What Are Cancer Survivors Telling Us?" by J. Rowland, 2008, *The Cancer Journal, 14,* p. 365. doi:10.1097/PPO.0b013e31818ec48e. Copyright 2008 by Lippincott Williams & Wilkins. Reprinted with permission.

Figure 6-4. Factors Associated With Good Adaptation and Potentially Improved Survival

- Accessing state-of-the-art care
- Being an active participant (engaged) in the treatment and healing process, including both mental and physical
- Having and—as needed—using social support
- Having a sense of meaning or purpose in life

Note. From "What Are Cancer Survivors Telling Us?" by J. Rowland, 2008, *The Cancer Journal, 14,* p. 365. doi:10.1097/PPO.0b013e31818ec48e. Copyright 2008 by Lippincott Williams & Wilkins. Reprinted with permission.

Nursing assessment and care planning for older adult cancer survivors must consider the complex medical and psychosocial needs of this population. Ambulatory care oncology nurses are encouraged to use a holistic perspective that incorporates knowledge of demographic trends and SCPs that emphasize health promotion. Oncology nurses are encouraged to remain informed of the research evidence based on older adult cancer survivors, particularly related to areas such as health promotion, coping and adjustment, HRQOL, and symptom experience. A holistic approach to assessment, care planning, and communication will contribute to the goal of high-quality survivorship care for the older adult.

Conclusion

In 2006, the Institute of Medicine's seminal report *From Cancer Patient to Cancer Survivor: Lost in Transition* focused attention on the state of survivorship care in the United States (Hewitt et al., 2006). Cancer organizations and institutions, clinicians, and researchers have embraced many of the IOM recommendations in an effort to address the needs of cancer survivors and improve the quality of health care for this population. Ambulatory care oncology nurses have a unique opportunity to assess patients and plan for individualized post-treatment survivorship care.

This chapter has identified several areas essential to ensuring high-quality survivorship care for older adults—survivorship issues, SCPs, long-term and late effects of cancer and cancer treatment, and recommendations for a holistic approach to assessing older adult cancer survivors. Ambulatory care oncology nurses are encouraged to (a) understand demographic trends and their potential impact on their older adult cancer survivors, (b) facilitate the use of individualized survivorship care plans to ensure well-coordinated and clearly communicated care, and (c) seek out the most current research and clinical evidence on older adult survivorship. Synthesizing these three areas will facilitate ambulatory care oncology nurses' ability to holistically assess and plan high-quality care designed to meet the complex needs of older adult cancer survivors.

References

Administration on Aging. (2009). *A profile of older Americans: 2009.* Retrieved from http://www.aoa.gov/AoARoot/Aging_Statistics/Profile/2009/docs/2009profile_508.pdf

Alfano, C., & Rowland, J. (2006). Recovery issues in cancer survivorship: A new challenge for supportive care. *Cancer Journal, 12,* 432–443. doi:10.1097/00130404-200609000-00012

American Cancer Society. (2010). *Cancer facts and figures 2010.* Retrieved from http://www.cancer.org/acs/groups/content/@epidemiologysurveillance/documents/document/acspc-026238.pdf

American Society of Clinical Oncology. (2010a, October 14). About survivorship. Retrieved from http://www.cancer.net/patient/Survivorship/About+Survivorship

American Society of Clinical Oncology. (2010b, October 14). Late effects. Retrieved from http://www.cancer.net/patient/Survivorship/Late+Effects

Aziz, N. (2007). Cancer survivorship research: State of knowledge, challenges and opportunities. *Acta Oncologica, 46,* 417–432. doi:10.1080/02841860701367878.

Aziz, N., & Rowland, J. (2003). Trends and advances in cancer survivorship research: Challenge and opportunity. *Seminars in Radiation Oncology, 13,* 248–266. doi:10.1016/S1053-4296(03)00024-9

Baravelli, C., Krishnasamy, M., Pezaro, C., Schofield, P., Lotfi-Jan, K., Rogers, M., ... Jefford, M. (2009). The views of bowel cancer survivors and health care professionals regarding survivorship care plans and post treatment follow-up. *Journal of Cancer Survivorship, 3,* 99–108. doi:10.1007/s11764-009-0086-1

Burkett, V., & Cleeland, C. (2007). Symptom burden in cancer survivorship. *Journal of Cancer Survivorship, 1,* 167–175. doi:10.1007/s11764-007-0017-y

Cheung, W., Neville, B., Cameron, C., Cook, E., & Earle, C. (2009). Comparisons of patient and physician expectations for cancer survivorship care. *Journal of Clinical Oncology, 27,* 2489–2495. doi:10.1200/JCO.2008.20.3232

Cleeland, C., & Reyes-Gibby, C. (2002). When is it justified to treat symptoms? Measuring symptom burden. *Oncology, 16*(9, Suppl. 10), 64–70.

Denmark-Wahnefried, W., Aziz, N., Rowland, J., & Pinto, B. (2005). Riding the crest of the teachable moment: Promoting long-term health after the diagnosis of cancer. *Journal of Clinical Oncology, 23,* 5814–5830. doi:10.1200/JCO.2005.01.230

Earle, G. (2006). Failing to plan is planning to fail: Improving the quality of care with survivorship care plans. *Journal of Clinical Oncology, 24,* 5112–5116. doi:10.1200/JCO.2006.06.5284

Earle, G. (2007). Cancer survivorship research and guidelines: Maybe the cart should be beside the horse. *Journal of Clinical Oncology, 25,* 3800–3801. doi:10.1200/JCO.2007.12.2325

Earle, C., Neville, B., & Fletcher, R. (2007). Mental health service utilization among long-term cancer survivors. *Journal of Cancer Survivorship, 1,* 156–160. doi:10.1007/s11764-007-0013-2

Fairley, T., Hawk, H., & Pierre, S. (2010). Health behaviors and quality of life of cancer survivors in Massachusetts, 2006: Data use for comprehensive cancer control. *Preventing Chronic Disease, 7*(1). Retrieved from http://www.cdc.gov/pcd/issues/2010/jan/09_0062.htm

Ganz, P., Casillas, J., & Hahn, E. (2008). Ensuring quality care for cancer survivors: Implementing the survivorship care plan. *Seminars in Oncology Nursing, 24,* 208–217. doi:10.1016/j.soncn.2008.05.009

Grunfeld, E. (2009). Optimizing follow-up after breast cancer treatment. *Current Opinion in Obstetrics and Gynecology, 21,* 92–96. doi:10.1097/GCO.0b013e328321e437

Haylock, P., Mitchell, S., Cox, T., Temple, S., & Curtiss, C. (2007). The cancer survivor's prescription for living. *American Journal Nursing, 107*(4), 58–70.

Hewitt, M., Greenfield, S., & Stovall, E. (Eds.). (2006). *From cancer patient to cancer survivor: Lost in transition.* Retrieved from http://www.nap.edu/catalog.php?record_id=11468

Hewitt, M., Rowland, J., & Yancik, R. (2003). Cancer survivors in the United States: Age, health and disability. *Journals of Gerontology Series A: Biological Sciences and Medical Sciences, 58,* 82–91.

Hill-Kayser, C., Vachani, C., Hampshire, M., Jacobs, L., & Metz, J. (2009). An Internet tool for creation of cancer survivorship care plans for survivors and health care providers: Design, implementation, use and user satisfaction. *Journal of Medical Internet Research, 11*(3), e39. doi:10.2196/jmir.1223

Hoffman, B., & Stovall, E. (2006). Survivorship perspectives and advocacy. *Journal of Clinical Oncology, 24,* 5154–5159. doi:10.1200/JCO 2006.06.5300.

Holland, J., & Weiss, T. (2008). The new standard of quality cancer care: Integrating the psychosocial aspects in routine cancer from diagnosis through survivorship. *Cancer Journal, 14,* 425–428. doi:10.1097/PPO.0b013e31818d8934

Horning, S. (2008). Follow-up of adult cancer survivors: New paradigms for survivorship care planning. *Hematology/Oncology Clinics of North America, 22,* 201–210. doi:10.1016/j.hoc.2008.01.005

Houldin, A., Curtiss, C.P., & Haylock, P.J. (2006). Executive summary: The state of the science on nursing approaches to managing late and long-term sequelae of cancer and cancer treatment. *Cancer Nursing, 29,* 6–11. doi:10.1097/00002820-200603002-00003

Jacobs, L., Palmer, S., Schwartz, L., DeMichele, A., Mao, J., Carver, J., ... Meadows, A. (2009). Adult cancer survivorship: Evolution, research, and planning care. *CA: A Cancer Journal for Clinicians, 59,* 391–410. doi:10.3322/caac.20040

Jacobsen, P. (2009). Clinical practice guidelines for the psychosocial care of cancer survivors: Current status and future prospects. *Cancer, 115*(Suppl. 18), 4419–4429. doi:10.1002/cncr.24589

Jim, H., & Jacobsen, P.B. (2008). Posttraumatic stress and posttraumatic growth in cancer survivorship: A review. *Cancer Journal, 14,* 414–419. doi:10.1097/PPO.0b013e31818d8963

Lewis, L. (2006). Discussion and recommendations: Addressing barriers in the management of cancer survivors. *Cancer Nursing, 29,* 91–95. doi:10.1097/00002820-200603002-00032

Mellon, S. (2002). Comparisons between cancer survivors and family members on meaning of the illness and family quality of life. *Oncology Nursing Forum, 29,* 1117–1125. doi:10.1188/02.ONF.1117-1125

Meneses, K., & Benz, R. (2010). Quality of life in cancer survivorship: 20 years later. *Seminars in Oncology Nursing, 26,* 36–46. doi:10.1016/j.soncn.2009.11.006

Miller, R. (2008). Implementing a survivorship care plan for patients with breast cancer. *Clinical Journal of Oncology Nursing, 12,* 479–487. doi:10.1188/08.CJON.479-487

Miller, K., & Triano, L. (2008). Medical issues in cancer survivors—A review. *Cancer Journal, 14,* 375–384. doi:10.1097/PPO.0b013e31818ee3dc

Morgan, M. (2009). Cancer survivorship: History, quality-of-life issues, and the evolving multidisciplinary approach to implementation of cancer survivorship care plans. *Oncology Nursing Forum, 36,* 429–436. doi:10.1188/09.ONF.429-436

Park, C., & Gaffey, A. (2007). Relationships between psychosocial factors and health behavior change in cancer survivors: An integrative review. *Annals of Behavioral Medicine, 34,* 115–134. doi:10.1007/BF02872667

Reuben, S. (2004). *Living beyond cancer: Finding a new balance* [Annual report]. Retrieved from http://deainfo.nci.nih.gov/advisory/pcp/annualReports/pcp03-04rpt/Survivorship.pdf

Rose, J., O'Toole, E., Koroukian, S., & Berger, N. (2009). Geriatric oncology and primary care: Promoting partnerships in practice and research. *Journal of the American Geriatrics Society, 57*(Suppl. 2), S235–S238. doi:10.1111/j.1532-5415.2009.02500.x

Rowland, J. (2008a). Cancer survivorship: Rethinking the cancer control continuum. *Seminars in Oncology Nursing, 24,* 145–152. doi:10.1016/j.soncn.2008.05.002

Rowland, J. (2008b). What are cancer survivors telling us? *Cancer Journal, 24,* 361–368. doi:10.1097/PPO.0b013e31818ec48e

Rowland, J., & Bellizzi, K. (2008). Cancer survivors and survivorship research: A reflection on today's successes and tomorrow's challenges. *Hematology/Oncology Clinics of North America, 22,* 181–200. doi:10.1016/j.hoc.2008.01.008

Rowland, J., & Yancik, R. (2006). Cancer survivorship: The interface of aging, comorbidity, and quality care. *Journal of National Cancer Institute, 98,* 504–505. doi:10.1093/jnci/djj154

Shulman, L.N., Jacobs, L.A., Greenfield, S., Jones, B., McCabe, M.S., Syrjala, K., ... Ganz, P.A. (2009). Cancer care and cancer survivorship care in the United States: Will we be able to care for these patients in the future? *Journal of Oncology Practice, 5,* 119–123. doi:10.1200/JOP.0932001

Smith, B.D., Smith, G.L., Hurria, A., Hortobagyi, G.N., & Buchholz, T.A. (2009). Future of cancer incidence in the United States: Burdens upon an aging, changing nation. *Journal of Clinical Oncology, 27,* 2758–2765. doi:10.1200/JCO.2008.20.8983

Stephens, C., Stein, K., & Landrine, H. (2010). The role of acculturation in life satisfaction among Hispanic cancer survivors: Results of the American Cancer Society's study of cancer survivors. *Psycho-Oncology, 19,* 376–383. doi:10.1002/pon.1566

Thorne, S., Hislop, G., Armstrong, E., & Oglov, V. (2007). Cancer care communication: The power to harm and the power to heal? *Patient Education and Counseling, 71,* 34–40. doi:10.1016/j.pec.2007.11.010

Uijtdehaage, S., Hauer, K., Stuber, M., Go, V., Rajagopalan, S., & Wilkerson, L. (2009). Preparedness for caring of cancer survivors: A multi-institutional study of medical students and oncology fellows. *Journal of Cancer Education, 24,* 28–32. doi:10.1080/08858190802665260

Weisman, A., & Worden, J. (1976–1977). The existential plight in cancer: Significance of the first 100 days. *International Journal Psychiatry in Medicine, 7,* 1–15. doi:10.2190/UQ2G-UGV1-3PPC-6387

Wolff, S.N., Nichols, C., Ulman, D., Miller, A., Kho, S., Lofye, D., ... Armstrong, L. (2005). Survivorship: An unmet need of the patient with cancer—Implications of a survey of the Lance Armstrong Foundation (LAF). *Journal of Clinical Oncology, 23*(Suppl. 16), Abstract 6032.

Wonghongkul, T., Moore, S.M., Musil, C., Schneider, S., & Deimling, G. (2000). The influence of uncertainty in illness, stress appraisal, and hope in coping on survivors of breast cancer. *Cancer Nursing, 23,* 422–429. doi:10.1097/00002820-200012000-00004

Yabroff, K., Lawrence, W.F., Clauser, S., Davis, W., & Brown, M. (2004). Burden of illness in cancer survivors: Findings from a population-based national sample. *Journal of the National Cancer Institute, 96,* 1322–1330. doi:10.1093/jnci/djh255

CHAPTER 7

Psychosocial Issues

Mary Pat Lynch, MSN, CRNP, AOCN®, and Dana Marcone DeDonato, MSW, LSW

Introduction

Psychosocial care plays a critical role in the oncologic management of older adults with cancer. Psychosocial issues in cancer can be overwhelming for patients and families, often affecting every aspect of their medical care. Untreated psychosocial issues can have negative effects on a patient's well-being and treatment adherence. For older adults with cancer, psychosocial issues may present barriers that prevent them from accessing quality care. It is important for nurses to understand these issues and identify them in their patient populations to assist older adults in overcoming these barriers and promote psychosocial health. This chapter will cover assessment tools, the role of social work, and sources of support, both financial and emotional. It will also discuss advance care planning and provide resources for patients.

Psychosocial Care

Psychosocial care has many definitions. The National Council for Hospice and Specialist Palliative Care Services (2000, p. 1) defines *psychosocial care* as "concerned with the psychological and emotional well-being of the patient and their family, including issues of self-esteem, insight into an adaptation to the illness and its consequences, communication, social functioning, and relationships." The Institute of Medicine defines psychosocial health services as "psychological and social services and interventions that enable patients, their families, and healthcare providers to optimize biomedical health care and to manage the psychological/behavioral and social aspects of illness and its consequences as to promote better health" (Adler & Page, 2008, p. 9). These definitions highlight the nonmedical component of care. Psychosocial care encompasses a number of different issues, from anxiety and depression to transportation and financial issues, all of which, if left untreated, can negatively affect a patient's medical care (Hendrick & Cobos, 2010).

Psychosocial Assessment

Assessment Tools

The older patient population is characterized by physical and psychosocial conditions that can influence how they are treated. They differ in their abilities to perform activities of daily living (ADLs). A significant percentage (9.5%) of older Americans may suffer from moderate to severe cognitive impairment (Balducci, 2003). The National Comprehensive Cancer Network (NCCN) recommends that all patients aged 70 and older undergo some form of geriatric assessment (Winn & McClure, 2003). A comprehensive geriatric assessment (CGA) has not been standardized, but there is a consensus that the elements of a CGA should include assessment of functional status, comorbidities, socioeconomic issues, nutritional status, polypharmacy, and geriatric syndromes (Balducci, 2003; Extermann & Hurria, 2007).

Psychosocial distress is common and occurs at all stages of cancer care. Screening, assessment, and management of psychosocial distress in patients with cancer have improved in recent years. Psychosocial care is considered an essential component of quality cancer care since the 2008 Institute of Medicine report *Cancer Care for the Whole Patient: Meeting Psychosocial Health Needs* (Adler & Page, 2008) requiring integration of psychosocial care into the routine care of patients with cancer (NCCN, 2010; Holland & Alici, 2010). NCCN chose the term *distress* to minimize the stigma attached to terms such as *psychiatric*, *psychological*, or *emotional*.

Distress in patients with cancer is defined as "a multifactorial unpleasant emotional experience of a psychological (cognitive, behavioral, emotional), social, and/or spiritual nature that may interfere with the ability to cope effectively with cancer, its physical symptoms and its treatment" (NCCN, 2011, p. MS-5). Rather than a single symptom, distress can have multiple causes. It may represent physical, social, and emotional components and can occur at any time from initial diagnosis to after completion of treatment (Vitek, Rosenzweig, & Stollings, 2007). Up to 43% of patients with cancer report measurable levels of psychosocial distress; this number is likely underestimated (Abrahamson, 2010). Psychosocial distress can influence treatment decisions, compliance, quality of life, and disease progression. Ambulatory care oncology nurses can improve the recognition and management of cancer-related distress, as they are on the front lines of cancer care. Nurses can utilize assessment tools and interviewing techniques when meeting with patients and families to elicit symptoms of distress and can provide referrals to other professionals, such as social workers, psychologists, and physicians for management of those symptoms.

The Distress Thermometer (DT) (NCCN, 2010) is one useful tool in identifying distress (Figure 7-1). This tool consists of a thermometer-like diagram on which patients are asked to rate their level of distress on a 0–10 scale. The tool also contains a 35-item problem list that prompts patients to identify their

Figure 7-1. NCCN Guidelines: Distress Management

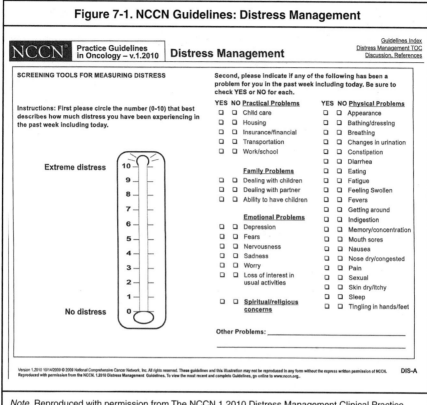

Note. Reproduced with permission from The NCCN 1.2010 Distress Management Clinical Practice Guidelines in Oncology. National Comprehensive Cancer Network, 2009. Available at: http://www.nccn.org. Accessed September 27, 2010. To view the most recent and complete version of the guideline, go online to www.nccn.org.

problems in five categories: practical, family, emotional, spiritual/religious, and physical (NCCN, 2010). Scores of 4 or higher suggest a level of distress that has clinical significance. Mild distress (a DT score of 4 or lower) is usually managed by the primary cancer care team. If the patient's score is moderate or severe (a DT score of 4 or more), referral to a social worker, spiritual counselor, or mental health professional may be indicated.

Role of the Social Worker

Oncology social workers play an important role in the care of the older adult with cancer. They can assist with performing a comprehensive psychosocial assessment or use brief screening tools to help identify high-risk patients (Kennedy, 1996). Table 7-1 illustrates a psychosocial assessment specifically tailored to the needs of older adults, developed by one geriatric oncology

Table 7-1. Psychosocial Assessment: Living Well Program for Older Adults With Cancer

Measure	Questions	Action
In home need • Functional status		
– ADLs/IADLs[1,2]	Are you independent with daily care, household tasks, etc?	Evaluate for home care, private pay help, or referral to local area Agency on Aging.
– Mobility[3]	Do you get around OK? Observe use of wheelchair, walker. Do you have stairs? Can you climb them?	Evaluate need for PT referral. Evaluate need for durable medical equipment.
– Medication management[4]	Do you take your medications on time/correctly? Do you ever forget or miss doses?	Administer Folstein MMSE[5]. Refer to psychology for cognitive assessment. Inform MD/CRNP.
– Household size	Do you live alone? Are you the primary caregiver for another member of your household?	Evaluate need for additional support. Refer to local Agency on Aging.
– Meals	Are you able to food shop? Cook meals?	Evaluate for home-delivered meal programs.
Transportation	How do you get back and forth to your medical appointments?	Evaluate for use of public transportation services or other transportation resources (e.g., American Cancer Society).
Insurance	Do you have coverage (health and prescription)? Questions about coverage? Have you received bills? Questions about paying for treatment?	Insurance counseling referral to state insurance counseling hotline or assistance applying for medical assistance. Information about prescription coverage programs.
Finances	What does your income consist of (social security, retirement, etc.)? Do you have any financial concerns?	Financial assistance referrals (i.e., supportive care grant). Co-pay assistance if related to medical bills.
Support system	Who supports you? Family close by? Church? Community? Is caregiver present? Caregiver coping style?	Evaluate for support groups. Evaluate for caregiver strain[6]. Evaluate need for psychology referral for caregiver.

(Continued on next page)

Table 7-1. Psychosocial Assessment: Living Well Program for Older Adults With Cancer (Continued)

Measure	Questions	Action
Coping	How are you coping with your diagnosis/treatment? During the last month, how often have you been bothered by 1) feeling down, depressed, or hopeless, 2) little interest or pleasure in doing things?[7]	Administer Geriatric Depression Scale.[8] Supportive counseling. Evaluate need for psychology referral.

[1]Mahoney, F.I., & Barthel, D. (1965). Functional evaluation: The Barthel Index. *Maryland State Medical Journal, 14,* 56–61.

[2]Lawton, M.P., & Brody, E.M. (1969). The Instrumental Activities of Daily Living Scale. *Gerontologist, 9,* 179–186.

[3]Get Up and Go Test. (2008). Retrieved from http://www.gericareonline.net/tools/eng/falls/attachments/Falls_Tool_2_Get_Up_and_Go_Test.pdf

[4]Svarstand, B.L., Chewning, B.A., Sleath, B.L., & Claesson, C. (1999). The Brief Medication Questionnaire: A tool for screening patient adherence and barriers to adherence. *Patient Education and Counseling, 37,* 113–124.

[5]Folstein, M.F., Folstein, S.E., & McHugh, P.R. (1975). Mini-Mental State. A practical method of grading the cognitive state of patients for the clinician. *Journal of Psychiatric Research, 12,* 189–198.

[6]Robinson, B. (1983). Validation of a caregiver strain index. *Journal of Gerontology, 38,* 344–348.

[7]Depression Screen. (2008). Retrieved October 31, 2008, from http://www.gericareonline.net/tools/eng/depression/attachments/Dep_01_DepressionScreen.pdf

[8]Yesavage, J.A., Brink, T.L., Rose, T.L., Lum, O., Huang, V., Adey, M., & Leirer, V.O. (1983). Development and validation of a geriatric depression screening scale: A preliminary report. *Journal of Psychiatric Research, 17,* 37–49.

Note. Table courtesy of Joan Karnell Cancer Center at Pennsylvania Hospital. Used with permission.

program. Social workers can help to create a psychosocial care plan based on needs identified during assessment and knowledge of available resources. After needs identification, oncology social workers can collaborate with other members of the multidisciplinary team to help mobilize resources and address identified needs.

Social workers can assist older adults in accessing community resources to address issues related to home care, transportation, and finances. Older adults with limited support or comorbidities may require intensive home- and community-based resources to support them through treatment. Other patients may need additional emotional support to cope with feelings arising from existential and end-of-life concerns, decreasing functional reserves, and diminishing social support networks. To assist with emotional issues, oncology social workers can use a broad range of treatment modalities. They can work with patients and caregivers individually or provide supportive counseling to the family unit. Figure 7-2 illustrates reasons for ambulatory care oncology nurses to recommend a referral to social work.

Figure 7-2. Social Work Referral Guidelines

Needs Assessment
- Episodic counseling
- Crisis intervention
- Caregiver distress

Assistance With
- Transportation
- Finances
- Medication costs
- Health insurance
- Wigs
- Home health services

Information About
- Support groups
- Educational programs

Patient Demographics
- Older than age 80
- Lives alone
- Diminished functional status

Finding Support

In-home services: Older adults have access to a variety of support services aimed at maintaining health and independence in the home and community setting. Home care may be useful for some older adults who have difficulty accessing medical care because of a lack of financial or social support. Homecare agencies provide access to medical equipment and visits by registered nurses, physical therapists, and social workers. They can assist with meal preparation, personal hygiene, and medication delivery. Medicare provides some reimbursement for these services, and the local health department keeps a registry of licensed homecare agencies.

For older adults requiring additional care at home, the Older Americans Act of 1965 established authority for grants to states for community planning, social services, and personnel training in the field of aging. The services are administered by the Administration on Aging and provide care to seniors including personal care, meal delivery, transportation, escorts, and shopping services. See Table 7-2 for information on how older adults can access these services.

Transportation: Older adults may face challenges in accessing medical care because of a lack of adequate transportation. Transportation should always be assessed with older adults and should be reassessed for those patients who are frequently late or miss medical appointments. Table 7-2 highlights resources to assist patients with transportation-related concerns.

Housing: Older adults without access to adequate housing may have higher levels of psychosocial distress. Programs exist to help older adults find affordable housing or improve functioning and safety in their own home by making appropriate home modifications. See Table 7-2 for more information.

Financial Resources

As the cost of cancer care continues to rise, patients and families may experience an increase in their out-of-pocket costs. Concerns about the cost of care and the financial impact for patients and families can lead to negative outcomes and increased psychological distress (Meropol et al., 2009). To date, no universal tool has been established for identifying patients in financial need; however, some research exists about this problem and its impact on patient care. Mathews and Park (2009) reported that patients may not be open about

Table 7-2. Resources for Older Adults With Cancer

Identified Need	Agency/Contact Information	Mission
In-home support; transportation	Eldercare Locator 800-677-1116 www.eldercare.gov	Connects older adults and their caregivers to community agencies
Transportation	National Center on Senior Transportation 866-528-NCST http://seniortransportation.easterseals.com	Connects older adults to transportation resources and provides information for older adults who do not drive
Home modification	Homemods.org www.homemods.org	Provides a national directory of home modification and repair resources
Housing	U.S. Department of Housing and Urban Development 800-FED-INFO www.hud.gov	Provides resoures to help people find shelter or stay in their homes
Long-term care planning	National Clearinghouse for Long-Term Care Information www.longtermcare.gov	Provides information and resources to help patients/families plan for long-term care needs
Insurance counseling	State Health Insurance Counseling and Assistance Programs (SHIPs) www.medicare.gov/contacts	Connects consumers to their local SHIP
Financial assistance	American Cancer Society 800-ACS-2345 www.cancer.org/Treatment/Findingand PayingforTreatment/index	Assists patients in obtaining assistance to pay for treatment
Financial assistance	CancerCare 800-813-HOPE www.cancercare.org/pdf/fact_sheets/fs_ financial_en.pdf	Provides some financial assistance to patients and connects them with financial resources

their financial concerns, and these concerns may change over time as treatments and insurance reimbursements change. Furthermore, some older adults may elect not to receive various cancer treatments because of cost (Meropol et al., 2009). It is important for nurses to understand the financial issues facing these patients and possess an understanding of available resources to help older adults navigate the complex healthcare system.

Patients are paying more for their cancer care as insurance reimbursements decrease and cost-sharing obligations increase. In the Kaiser Family Foundation national survey of families affected by cancer, 25% said they used all or most of their savings on cancer-related costs, and 1 in 10 reported being unable to pay for daily living expenses such as food, heat, and housing (USA Today, Kaiser Family Foundation, & Harvard School of Public Health, 2006). Rising medical bills are due, in part, to increasing out-of-pocket costs associated with care. Increased cost sharing for patients is achieved through the use of co-payments, co-insurances, deductibles, and lifetime maximums (see Figure 7-3).

Resources exist to assist patients in financial need. Private philanthropic organizations have been established to help patients reduce cost-sharing obligations related to chemotherapy. Medical and financial criteria must be met in order to qualify for these programs. Table 7-3 highlights a list of national organizations and the diseases they support.

Figure 7-3. Insurance Definitions

Deductible: The amount of money a person must pay before insurance will pay anything toward the cost of the person's medical expenses
Co-payment: The fixed amount a person must pay for each medical service (e.g., doctor visit, emergency department visit)
Co-insurance: The cost-sharing percentage a person must pay for medical services (e.g., 20% chemotherapy co-insurance)
Maximum benefit: The amount after which the insurance will no longer pay for any medical services (may be yearly or lifetime)

Older adults may have questions about insurance coverage related to Medicare. The State Health Insurance Counseling and Assistance Programs (SHIPs) aid the elderly as they choose a healthcare plan, decide between original Medicare and Medicare Advantage Plans, and understand their health plan choices. Older adults should contact their SHIP office for further assistance in finding coverage that meets their needs (see Table 7-2).

Emotional Coping Resources

People with cancer and their families face many challenges, and most, if not all, will have emotional and psychological reactions to the diagnosis. Nurses and other healthcare professionals can provide psychosocial interventions to help patients and families meet these challenges. Psychosocial interventions can be educational and therapeutic approaches that are designed to strengthen the patient's adaptation to having cancer and its effect on one's life (Massie, Holland, & Straker, 1990). Three primary psychosocial interventions are emotional support, education, and psychotherapy. All three can be accessed one-on-one or in a group setting. Emotional support is a common component

---

Table 7-3. Co-Pay Relief and Prescription Assistance Programs for People With Cancer

Organization/ Contact Information	Program Information*
Cancer*Care* Co-Payment Assistance Foundation 866-55-COPAY www.cancercarecopay.org	Provides co-payment assistance for pharmaceutical products to insured individuals who are covered by private insurance or employer-sponsored health plans or have Medicare Part D or Medicare Advantage. Household income must be at or within 400% of U.S. federal poverty guidelines for people residing and receiving treatment in the U.S. or its territories. Must be U.S. citizen or valid resident alien. Conditions covered include • Breast cancer • Lung cancer • Colorectal cancer • Pancreatic cancer • Gastric cancer • Glioblastoma • Head and neck cancer • Prostate cancer • Renal cell cancer.
Chronic Disease Fund 877-968-7233 www.cdfund.org	Co-payment assistance for pharmaceutical products for patients with private insurance or Medicare Part D. Patients who utilize a participating pharmacy can have their out-of-pocket expenses remitted by the fund directly to the pharmacy. Patients using nonparticipating pharmacies can submit receipts for reimbursement. The conditions covered are • Breast cancer • Colorectal cancer • Multiple myeloma • Non-small cell lung cancer • Thyroid cancer • Liver cancer • Prostate cancer • Pancreatic cancer.

(Continued on next page)

Table 7-3. Co-Pay Relief and Prescription Assistance Programs for People With Cancer *(Continued)*

Organization/ Contact Information	Program Information*
HealthWell Foundation 800-675-8416 www.healthwellfoundation.org	Addresses the needs of individuals who cannot afford their insurance co-payments, premiums, co-insurance, or other out-of-pocket healthcare costs. Offers assistance for the following specific conditions: • Breast cancer • Bone metastases • Carcinoid tumors and related symptoms • Chronic myeloid leukemia • Chemotherapy-induced anemia/neutropenia • Colorectal cancer • Cutaneous T-cell lymphoma • Head and neck cancer • Metastatic melanoma • Non-Hodgkin lymphoma • Non-small cell lung cancer • Wilms tumor.
The Leukemia and Lymphoma Society's Co-Pay Assistance Program 877-557-2672 www.LLS.org/copay	The program helps patients meet their health insurance or Medicare Plan B or D premiums or co-payment obligations. Household income must be at or within 500% above the U.S. federal poverty guidelines for people residing in the U.S. and Puerto Rico. Offered assistance for the following conditions: • Chronic lymphocytic leukemia • Lymphoma • Multiple myeloma • Myelodysplastic syndrome • Waldenström macroglobulinemia
National Organization for Rare Disorders 800-999-6673 (voicemail only) 203-744-0100 www.rarediseases.org	Assists uninsured or underinsured individuals in securing life-saving or life-sustaining medications including Trisenox®, TheraCys®, and Matulane®. Offers co-payment assistance for • Advanced renal cell carcinoma • Hodgkin lymphoma • Paroxysmal nocturnal hemoglobinuria • Peripheral T-cell lymphoma.
Partnership for Prescription Assistance 888-477-2669 www.pparx.org	Offers a single point of access to more than 150 programs offered by pharmaceutical companies. Includes assistance for the uninsured.

(Continued on next page)

Table 7-3. Co-Pay Relief and Prescription Assistance Programs for People With Cancer *(Continued)*

Organization/ Contact Information	Program Information*
Patient Access Network Foundation 866-316-7263 www.panfoundation.org	Assists patients who cannot access the treatments they need because of out-of-pocket healthcare costs, including deductibles, co-payments, and co-insurance. Offers assistance for the following: • Breast cancer • Chronic lymphocytic leukemia • Colorectal cancer • Cutaneous T-cell lymphoma • Multiple myeloma • Myelodysplastic syndrome • Non-Hodgkin lymphoma • Non-small cell lung cancer • Pancreatic cancer • Prostate cancer • Renal cell carcinoma • Thyroid cancer.
Patient Advocate Foundation's Co-Pay Relief Program 866-512-3861 www.copays.org	Provides direct co-payment assistance for pharmaceutical products to insured patients (including Medicare Part D beneficiaries) who financially and medically qualify. Offers assistance for the following: • Bladder cancer • Breast cancer • Colon cancer • Lung cancer • Lymphoma • Kidney cancer • Malignant brain tumors • Multiple myeloma • Myelodysplastic syndrome • Prostate cancer • Sarcoma.
Patient Services, Inc. 800-366-7741 www.patientservicesinc.org	Assists patients in locating health insurance policies. Provides health insurance premium assistance (including COBRA) and co-payment assistance (including helping satisfy Medicare Part D true-out-of-pocket). Offers assistance with the following conditions: • Bone metastases • Chronic myeloid leukemia • Cutaneous T-cell lymphoma • Gastrointestinal stromal tumors.

*Funding may change; contact agency for up-to-date information.

of nursing care that can include providing the patient with an opportunity to talk about the illness and its impact on his or her life, as well as recognition and expressions of feelings and beliefs. Education about the disease and its treatment can help the patient manage some of the stress of the diagnosis, allowing the person to gain a sense of control over the frightening unknowns of living with cancer. Nurses can utilize patient education as a psychosocial intervention at any point in the cancer trajectory.

When emotional support and education do not relieve the patient's psychosocial distress, psychotherapy should be considered. Psychotherapy with patients with cancer differs from psychotherapy with psychiatric patients, as patients with cancer may primarily need help adjusting to their diagnosis and its affect on their lives, relationships, and mood. Psychotherapy can decrease existing symptoms or behavior patterns and promote positive growth and development. It can help patients identify and live with the "new normal" in their lives as cancer survivors and help them process the experience of living with and through cancer.

Psychosocial Support Programs

Patients with cancer and their families may seek programs or services that can help them understand their disease and its treatment, cope with their diagnosis, meet others who are living with cancer, and help them actively participate in their health care. A psychosocial support program is defined as two or more individuals with a common need who meet one or more times (Johnson & Johnson, 1998). The program can be led by a professional or peer leader or may have team leadership. The purpose for a psychosocial support group is to provide accurate information, enhance coping skills, advance problem solving skills, and foster mutual support. With the increase in early diagnosis and survival in the past two decades, the number of support programs has also increased. Psychosocial support programs can include peer-to-peer support, facilitator-led support groups, peer-led support groups, telephone support, online support, and individual counseling.

Psychoeducational programs are usually structured and time limited with clear goals. Support groups bring together individuals with similar diagnoses or problems for peer support and education. One-to-one peer support involves a cancer survivor willing to share their experience and coping strategies with a more newly diagnosed patient. Older adults with cancer can benefit from any type of support program but may find that peer-to-peer support is helpful when transportation to groups is an issue. Alternatively, a group of older adults with cancer can provide an opportunity to socialize and promote discussion of shared experiences and a sense of usefulness.

Table 7-4 lists organizations that provide general and specific cancer support through a variety of programs. Table 7-5 lists specific programs offered by the American Cancer Society.

Table 7-4. General and Specific Cancer Information/Support

Organization/Contact Information	Description
General Cancer Information	
American Cancer Society www.cancer.org 800-227-2345	Provides programs and services to help people with cancer understand cancer, manage their lives through treatment and recovery, and find emotional support
Cancer*Care* www.cancercare.org 800-813-HOPE	Oldest, largest national nonprofit agency offering support and practical information
The Cancer Journey www.thecancerjourney.org 866-257-4667	Oncology Nursing Society's patient Web site provides information on treatment, side effects, survivorship, and other cancer topics
Cancer.Net www.cancer.net 703-299-0150	American Society of Clinical Oncology's patient Web site, designed to help patients make informed healthcare decisions
Fertile Hope www.fertilehope.org 888-994-HOPE	Provides reproductive information, support, and hope to patients with cancer whose medical treatments present the risk of infertility
Gilda's Club Worldwide www.gildasclub.org 888-445-3248	Free support community for people living with cancer
Lance Armstrong Foundation www.laf.org 512-236-8820	Survivor resources and support, survivorship programs, national advocacy initiatives, and scientific and clinical research grants
National Cancer Institute www.cancer.gov 800-4-CANCER	Information on cancer types, treatments, support, and research
National Coalition for Cancer Survivorship www.canceradvocacy.org 877-NCCS-YES	National network of organizations and individuals serving people with cancer
National Family Caregivers Association www.nfcacares.org 800-896-3650	Support for family caregivers
The Wellness Community www.thewellnesscommunity.org 888-793-WELL	Provides free psychological and emotional support to patients and families, support groups on stress reduction, educational workshops, and social events

(Continued on next page)

Table 7-4. General and Specific Cancer Information/Support *(Continued)*

Organization/Contact Information	Description
Brain Cancer	
American Brain Tumor Association www.abta.org 800-866-2282	Information about brain tumors, treatment options, clinical trials, and living with a brain tumor
National Brain Tumor Foundation www.braintumor.org 800-934-CURE	Provides patient resources, information, education, and funds research
Breast Cancer	
Breastcancer.org www.breastcancer.org	Dedicated to providing the most reliable, complete, and up-to-date information about breast cancer
Living Beyond Breast Cancer www.lbbc.org 888-753-LBBC	Provides educational conferences, newsletter, outreach to medically underserved women, and a help line
Sisters Network www.sistersnetwork.org 866-781-1808	National African American breast cancer survivors support organization
Susan G. Komen for the Cure www.komen.org 877-GO-KOMEN	Eradicating breast cancer by advancing research, education, screening, and treatment
Y-ME National Breast Cancer Organization www.y-me.org 800-221-2141 (English) 800-986-9505 (Spanish)	Provides information and support through its 24/7 hotline with interpreters in 150 languages
Colorectal Cancer	
Colon Cancer Alliance www.ccalliance.org 877-422-2030	Provides support and information for those battling colorectal cancer
National Colorectal Cancer Research Alliance www.eifoundation.org 818-760-7722	Dedicated to providing education about colon cancer prevention
Gynecologic Cancer	
Gynecologic Cancer Foundation www.thegcf.org 800-444-4441	Ensures public awareness of gynecologic cancer prevention, early diagnosis, and proper treatment and supports research and training related to gynecologic cancers

(Continued on next page)

Table 7-4. General and Specific Cancer Information/Support *(Continued)*

Organization/Contact Information	Description
National Cervical Cancer Coalition www.nccc-online.org 800-685-5531	Dedicated to serving women with, or at risk for, cervical cancer and human papillomavirus disease
Hospice	
National Hospice and Palliative Care Organization www.nhpco.org 800-658-8898	Association of programs that provide hospice and palliative care
Leukemia and Lymphoma	
Leukemia and Lymphoma Society www.leukemia-lymphoma.org 800-995-4LSA	Fights leukemia, lymphoma, multiple myeloma, and Hodgkin disease through research, education, patient services, and advocacy
Lung Cancer	
Alliance for Lung Cancer Advocacy, Support and Education www.alcase.org 800-298-2436	Offers programs to improve quality of life of people with lung cancer, education, psychosocial support, and advocacy
American Lung Association www.lungusa.org 800-LUNG-USA	Offers information, programs, press releases, legislative advocacy, and referrals
Lung Cancer Alliance www.lungcanceralliance.org 800-298-2436	Helps individuals with lung cancer improve their quality of life
Lymphedema	
National Lymphedema Network www.lymphnet.org 800-541-3259	Works to standardize quality treatment for patients with lymphedema
Multiple Myeloma	
Institute for Myeloma and Bone Cancer Research www.imbcr.org 310-623-1210	Working to find improved treatment and a cure for multiple myeloma
International Myeloma Foundation www.myeloma.org 800-452-CURE	Supports education, treatment, and research for multiple myeloma; assistance provided in many languages

(Continued on next page)

Table 7-4. General and Specific Cancer Information/Support *(Continued)*

Organization/Contact Information	Description
Oral and Head and Neck Cancer	
Support for People with Oral and Head and Neck Cancer www.sponhc.org www.800-377-0928	Survivor to survivor network providing information, support and encouragement
Ovarian Cancer	
CancerConsultants.com www.cancerconsultants.com	Provides comprehensive information on prevention and treatment of ovarian cancer and clinical trials listings
National Ovarian Cancer Coalition www.ovarian.org 888-OVARIAN	Promotes awareness and provides education and referrals for people affected by ovarian cancer
Pancreatic Cancer	
Pancreatic Cancer Action Network www.pancan.org 877-272-6226	Provides public and professional education on research, effective treatments, prevention programs, and early detection methods
Prostate Cancer	
National Prostate Cancer Coalition www.pcacoalition.org 888-245-9455	Provides information, counseling, and educational meetings to help men with prostate cancer make decisions about their treatment and support
Sarcoma	
The National Leiomyosarcoma Foundation www.nlmsf.org	Supporting research and improving treatment outcomes and awareness
The Sarcoma Alliance www.sarcomaalliance.org 415-381-7236	Strives to extend and improve the lives of patients with sarcoma through accurate diagnosis, improved access to care, guidance, education, and support

Table 7-5. American Cancer Society* Support Programs and Services	
Program	**Description**
Cancer Survivors Network	Online community by and for people with cancer and their families
Road to Recovery	Rides to cancer treatment
Hope Lodge	Lodging for patients with cancer and families
TLC	Catalog and magazine for women, featuring hair loss and mastectomy products
Reach to Recovery	Breast cancer support provided by matching patients with other trained breast cancer survivors
Man to Man	Prostate cancer support
I Can Cope	Cancer education classes
I Can Cope Online	Online cancer education classes
Look Good … Feel Better	Trained volunteer cosmetologists teach women how to cope with skin changes and hair loss
Look Good … Feel Better for Teens	Helps patients aged 13–17 to cope with how cancer treatment and side effects can change the way they look
Circle of Sharing	Personalizes cancer information, and offers information and resources for coping
Tell Your Story	Allows patients to share a story and give hope to someone else facing cancer
*More information is available at www.cancer.org or by calling 800-227-2345.	

Advance Care Planning

Advance care directives are specific instructions, prepared in advance, that are intended to direct a person's medical care if he or she becomes unable to do so in the future. They are legal documents that clearly state the individual's wishes about medical decisions. Some types of advance directives include the following.

- A durable power of attorney for health care (also called a *medical power of attorney* or *healthcare proxy*) is a written legal document in which someone is named to make medical decisions for the patient if the patient is unable to communicate his or her wishes. This document provides for power to make medical decisions only, not legal or financial decisions.

- A living will gives directions about the use of certain medical treatments at the very end of life. This document ensures that the patient's wishes are followed if he or she becomes too ill to make decisions.
- Organ donation can still be an option for patients with cancer and should be included in the advance directive document.
- A do-not-resuscitate order (often referred to as a DNR order) states that cardiopulmonary resuscitation is not to be performed should the patient stop breathing or should his or her heart stop. The doctor can write this order after discussions with the patient and family.

Oncology nurses should encourage communication with patients and families about advance care planning. Early discussions about goals of care can normalize these difficult topics so that patients and family members become more comfortable with end-of-life discussions before they reach that point. Nurses can help to explain medical terminology and promote discussions among patients, families, and medical providers. Table 7-6 lists organizations that can initiate discussions around advance care planning and provide resources to help patients to develop appropriate documents.

Table 7-6. Resources to Assist With Advanced Care Planning	
Name/Contact Info	Purpose
Caring Connections 800-658-8898 www.caringinfo.org	Provides information and resources for "planning ahead." Provides free downloadable advance directive form by state.
Aging With Dignity–5 Wishes 888-5WISHES (594-7437) www.agingwithdignity.org	Easy-to-use packet for patients/families that enhances the conversation around advance care planning. Packets can be purchased for a cost.

Conclusion

Psychosocial care is a vital component of all cancer care for older adults. Psychosocial needs encompass both the practical and emotional. Issues surrounding transportation, housing, finances, advance care planning, and coping with distress should all be included in a psychosocial assessment. Psychosocial issues may prevent older adults from accessing quality cancer care, so it is important for ambulatory care oncology nurses to be aware of these issues and to provide education and support.

Resources and organizations exist to help older adults cope with the psychosocial issues they may face during their cancer care. Oncology nurses can collaborate with oncology social workers to address psychosocial needs and mobilize community resources. Adequate management of psychosocial needs can help older adults throughout their cancer treatment by improving adherence and promoting well-being. Oncology nurses and social workers can provide a caring, empathetic resource for managing psychosocial distress in older adults with cancer.

References

Abrahamson, K. (2010). Dealing with cancer-related distress. *American Journal of Nursing, 110,* 67–69. doi:10.1097/01.NAJ.0000370162.07674.f6

Adler, N.E., & Page, A.E.K. (Eds.). (2008). *Cancer care for the whole patient: Meeting psychosocial health needs.* Washington, DC: National Academies Press.

Balducci, L. (2003). New paradigms for treating elderly patients with cancer: The comprehensive geriatric assessment and guidelines for supportive care. *Journal of Supportive Oncology, 1*(4, Suppl. 2), 30–37.

Extermann, M., & Hurria, A. (2007). Comprehensive geriatric assessment for older adults with cancer. *Journal of Clinical Oncology, 25,* 1824–1831. doi:10.1200/JCO.2007.10.6559

Hendrick, S.S., & Cobos, E. (2010). Practical model for psychosocial care. *Journal of Oncology Practice, 6,* 34–36. doi:10.1200/JOP.091066

Holland, J.C., & Alici, Y. (2010). Management of distress in cancer patients. *Journal of Supportive Oncology, 8,* 4–12.

Johnson, J., & Johnson, M.B. (1998). Programmatic approaches to psychosocial support. In R.M. Carroll-Johnson, L.M. Gorman, & N.J. Bush (Eds.), *Psychosocial nursing care along the cancer continuum* (pp. 315–327). Pittsburgh, PA: Oncology Nursing Society.

Kennedy, V.N. (1996). Supportive care of the patient with pancreatic cancer: The role of the oncology social worker. *Oncology, 10*(Suppl. 9), 35–37.

Massie, M.J., Holland, J., & Straker, N. (1990). Psychotherapeutic interventions. In J. Holland & J.H. Rowland (Eds.), *Handbook of psychooncology: Psychological care of the patient with cancer* (pp. 455–518). New York: Oxford University Press.

Mathews, M., & Park, A.D. (2009). Identifying patients in financial need: Cancer care providers' perceptions of barriers. *Clinical Journal of Oncology Nursing, 13,* 501–505. doi:10.1188/09.CJON.501-505

Meropol, N.J., Schrag, D., Smith, T.J., Mulvey, T.M., Langdon, R.M., Blum, D., … Schnipper, L.E. (2009). American Society of Clinical Oncology guidance statement: The cost of cancer care. *Journal of Clinical Oncology, 27,* 3868–3874. doi:10.1200/JCO.2009.23.1183

National Comprehensive Cancer Network. (2010). *NCCN Clinical Practice Guidelines in Oncology: Distress management* [v.1.2011]. Retrieved from http://www.nccn.org/professionals/physician_gls/PDF/distress.pdf

National Council for Hospice and Specialist Palliative Care Services. (2000). What do we mean by 'psychosocial'? *Briefing Bulletin, 4,* 1–2.

USA Today, Kaiser Family Foundation, & Harvard School of Public Health. (2006, November). National survey of households affected by cancer. Retrieved from http://www.kff.org/kaiserpolls/upload/7591.pdf

Vitek, L., Rosenzweig, M.Q., & Stollings, S. (2007). Distress in patients with cancer: Definition, assessment, and suggested interventions. *Clinical Journal of Oncology Nursing, 11,* 413–418. doi:10.1188/07.CJON.413-418

Winn, R.J., & McClure, J. (2003). The NCCN Clinical Practice Guidelines in Oncology: A primer for users. *Journal of the National Comprehensive Cancer Network, 1,* 5–13. Retrieved from http://www.jnccn.org/content/1/1/5.long

CHAPTER 8

Considering the Future of Nursing

Sarah H. Kagan, PhD, RN

Introduction

Care for older adults in the ambulatory setting is the future of cancer care delivery in America (Decker, Schappert, & Sisk, 2009). The demographics of our aging society combined with cancer epidemiology and trends in cancer therapeutics have resulted in an increase in ambulatory cancer care services delivery and consequent changes in oncology nursing (Beverly, Burger, Maas, & Specht, 2010; Erikson, Salsberg, Forte, Bruinooge, & Goldstein, 2007; Griffith, Lyman, & Blackhall, 2010). Older adults account for more than 65% of current cancer diagnoses, consume the bulk of cancer care provided, and represent the majority of cancer survivors (Adler & Page, 2008). Approximately 96% of Americans older than 65 live independently in owned or rented dwellings and seek health care within their communities (Fendrich & Hoffmann, 2007; U.S. Census Bureau, 2010). Cancer accounts for more deaths than heart disease in people younger than 85 (Siegel, Ward, Brawley, & Jemal, 2011). Increasingly, the majority of cancer diagnoses result in patterns of chronic treatment and long-term survivorship, even among older adults (Avis & Deimling, 2008; Malek & Silliman, 2007). Importantly, cancer may produce significant morbidity during treatment and throughout survivorship, resulting in extensive use of ambulatory cancer and other healthcare services (Avis & Deimling, 2008; Kurtz, Kurtz, Given, & Given, 2006; Malek & Silliman, 2007).

This chapter will project future aspects of ambulatory cancer care and explore issues relevant to several domains of nursing practice in this setting. Changes in demographics and epidemiology as they affect the future of ambulatory oncology nursing practice will be discussed. Strategies to meet expanding and changing needs of older patients and their families will be considered in light of changes in demographics and consequent shifts in volume of care, service projections, and resource use. Matters of cost, reimbursement, and reform, as well as how they may shape the provision of cancer care in ambulatory and other settings, are connected to effectiveness, utility, and matters of ageism. Finally, the chapter will conclude with the synthesis of necessary leadership in nursing practice, education, research, and policy to transform the future of ambulatory cancer care for older adults and their families.

Ambulatory Oncology Care

Ambulatory settings progressively offer complex, single- and multimodality cancer therapeutics. Medical therapeutics, including chemotherapy, biotherapy, and targeted agents, are almost exclusively delivered in infusion centers and other outpatient settings (Extermann, Crane, & Boulware, 2010; Malek & Silliman, 2007). Radiation therapy, usually administered on an outpatient basis, is often a primary treatment modality for older adults with solid tumors and is commonly offered as palliative care for frail older adults (Malek & Silliman, 2007). Surgical treatment is increasingly relying on minimally invasive techniques that reduce functional sequelae and employ day hospitalization and outpatient follow-up care, quickly returning older patients to presurgical patterns of daily living (McGory et al., 2009). The nursing care that older adults in ambulatory settings require increasingly spans all therapeutic modalities. Thus, the future of ambulatory oncology nursing practice will mandate a direct focus on older adults, specialized clinical skills, and coordination of care.

Future Influences on Ambulatory Oncology Nursing Practice

Epidemiology

Nurses caring for patients in ambulatory settings should expect increases in the number of older patients and even the number of very old adults seeking active oncologic treatment (Fendrich & Hoffmann, 2007). Cancer incidence affects older adults of all ages, including nonagenarians (Avis & Deimling, 2008; Smith, Smith, Hurria, Hortobagyi, & Buchholz, 2009). Young-old (65–75 years old) and old (75–85 years) adults commonly face first cancer diagnoses and active treatment in the context of comorbid, age-related diseases such as hypertension, coronary artery disease, and arthritis (Malek & Silliman, 2007; Rowe & Kahn, 1997). Old-old (older than 85 years) adults are more likely to have advanced cancers on diagnosis as well as higher rates of second cancers and a greater prevalence of functional debility (Extermann et al., 2010; Kanapuru, Posani, Muller, & Ershler, 2008; Min et al., 2009; Robine, Michel, & Herrmann, 2007; Rowe & Kahn, 1997). In the coming years, the number of older patients treated in ambulatory oncology centers is projected to grow dramatically (Beverly et al., 2010; Levit, Smith, Benz, & Ferrell, 2010). Their complex, unique oncologic and nononcologic clinical needs will heighten the demand for specialized knowledge, care, and services from nurses and interdisciplinary oncology teams (Beverly et al., 2010; Erikson et al., 2007; Levit et al., 2010).

Geriatric Generalist/Oncology Specialist

Oncology nurses practicing in ambulatory care settings of the future must fundamentally be geriatric generalists and oncologic specialists (Beverly et al., 2010; Erikson et al., 2007). Optimal oncologic care for older adults receiving diagnostic evaluation, oncologic therapy, and survivorship services relies on three essential components. The first is assessment that balances aging and function, age-related disease, and cancer (Extermann et al., 2005; Overcash, Beckstead, Moody, Extermann, & Cobb, 2006). The second is intervention that considers oncologic and nononcologic health and social care needs in the context of aging to promote and support patient wishes and adherence to cancer treatment (Bomba & Vermilyea, 2006; Griffith et al., 2010). The third is careful coordination of services and oncologic and geriatric resources with facilitation of transitions in care (Chumbler et al., 2007; Kizer & Dudley, 2009). Translating components of assessment, intervention, and coordination into ambulatory care for the future will necessitate the use of available evidence and best practices while incorporating emerging evidence as it becomes available. Many models in research and practice outline integration of assessment, intervention, and coordination for older adults who have cancer and their families.

Geriatric assessment, both focal and comprehensive, is among the best established aspects of ambulatory cancer care for older adults. Geriatric assessment has long offered the means to identify and monitor comorbid conditions in frail older adults (Boyd et al., 2007; Extermann et al., 2005; Karampeazis & Extermann, 2009). Overcash and colleagues (2006) lead in generating evidence that adapts and supports the utility of comprehensive geriatric assessment (CGA) in outpatient oncology settings (Brunello, Sandri, & Extermann, 2009; Extermann et al., 2005; Overcash et al., 2006). Their work establishes the use of CGA to identify individual needs and set goals for assistance (Extermann et al., 2005; Karampeazis & Extermann, 2009; Overcash et al., 2006). Many publications outline strategies to facilitate CGA; however, these are not well implemented in practice (Karampeazis & Extermann, 2009; Klepin, Mohile, & Hurria, 2009; Overcash et al., 2006). Future improvements in practice must integrate mechanisms for CGA in all ambulatory cancer care settings.

Recent research suggests reframing paradigms of care to include early initiation of advance care planning, palliative care, and physician orders for life-sustaining treatment (POLST) with older adults diagnosed with cancer (Bomba & Vermilyea, 2006; Griffith et al., 2010; Temel et al., 2010). Better use of advance directives, palliative care, and POLST and effective communication with patients and their families present opportunities to improve satisfaction with care, functional outcomes, and healthcare costs (Bach, 2007; Decker et al., 2009; Extermann et al., 2005; Kelley & Meier, 2010; Meropol & Schulman, 2007; Temel et al., 2010). Patient and family education promotes treatment adherence and concordance between older patients and their clinicians (Jansen, van Weert, van Dulmen, Heeren, & Bensing, 2007). Further, such education may enhance and improve decision making to support older patients' wishes through cancer survivorship (Min et al., 2009).

Built on assessment data, effective decision making in future ambulatory cancer care focuses on the wishes and concerns of older adults and their families while accounting for the clinical realities of cancer, comorbid conditions, and frailty (Bayliss, Edwards, Steiner, & Main, 2008; Bomba & Vermilyea, 2006; Gosney, 2009; Klepin et al., 2009; Min et al., 2009). Effective and knowledgeable assessment and communication in the absence of ageist assumptions will support this balance (Sifer-Rivière, Girre, Gisselbrecht, & Saint-Jean, 2010). Advance care planning may facilitate better decision making and realization of necessary shifts in aims and care settings (Bomba & Vermilyea, 2006; Kelley & Meier, 2010; Lorenz et al., 2008). Integration of home care and community services supports ambulatory care by avoiding preventable decline and easing transitions in and out of institutional care (Bayliss et al., 2008; Chumbler et al., 2007; Wolff, Roter, Given, & Gitlin, 2009). Finally, refined approaches to end-of-life decision making that supports older adult and family desires may improve function and survival and compensate for ineffective and costly healthcare expenditures in the last year of life (Bomba & Vermilyea, 2006; Lorenz et al., 2008; Temel et al., 2010; Yabroff, Davis, et al., 2007; Yabroff et al., 2008; Yabroff, Warren, & Brown, 2007).

Advances in Oncology Care

Rapid proliferation of oncologic therapeutics and minimally invasive systems and settings for daily delivery of those therapies transform the setting and practice of oncology nursing (Beverly et al., 2010; Ma & Adjei, 2009). While trends in all oncologic treatment modalities move toward ambulatory settings, analyses project significant increases in patient volume and a decrease in the supply of oncologists (Beverly et al., 2010; Erikson et al., 2007; Ma & Adjei, 2009; Smith et al., 2009). These trends suggest that oncology nurses must realign practice patterns, structures, and systems to become competent in the care of older patients, thereby meeting future needs (Beverly et al., 2010; Committee on the Future Health Care Workforce for Older Americans, 2008; Mezey, Stierle, Huba, & Esterson, 2007). Current ambulatory cancer care generally lacks geriatric competence among nurses and other staff. Future education of nurses and others in care of older adults is necessary to create new "geriatric friendly" standards of care (Mezey, Mitty, Burger, & McCallion, 2008; Mezey et al., 2007). Nurses can achieve geriatric competence, in part, by enhancing knowledge and skills within the categories of assessment, intervention, and care coordination specific to patient and family education, monitoring and surveillance, and symptom and distress management.

Innovations in therapeutics mandate advances in assessment, intervention, and coordination. Patient and family education must clearly reflect therapeutic advances, and nursing and interdisciplinary assessment and intervention must similarly keep pace. Concomitant changes in decision making, supportive care, care coordination, and communication emerge through therapeutic innovation. Adherence to oral antineoplastic regimens illustrates the extent to which these changes represent the future of ambulatory practice (Banna et al., 2010; Kav et al., 2008; Moore, 2007). New interventions to ensure adherence encompass a range of educational and technologic strategies (George, Elliott, & Stewart, 2008). Comparative effectiveness research evaluates comparable interventions and, as such, offers important direction for future practice (Beverly et al., 2010; Ma & Adjei, 2009). Advances in assessment and in surveillance and monitoring similarly require integral use of electronic data collection, management, and analysis within electronic medical records; Web-based applications for patient and clinician communication; and telehealth initiatives (Blayney et al., 2009; Galligioni et al., 2009; Reidel, Tamblyn, Patel, & Huang, 2008).

Care Coordination

Monitoring and surveillance links patient and family education and decision making to care coordination. These processes augment patient and family education and self-care by creating a partnership between nurses and their patients (Bayliss et al., 2008). This partnership can aid in early identification of side effects and complications, initiation of timely symptom management that addresses risks of necessary polypharmacy, and detection of disease progression with advancing symptoms (Bayliss et al., 2008; Gosney, 2009; Sokol, Knudsen, & Li, 2007). Given the implications of cancer and comorbid disease accompanied by complex coexisting treatment regimens, comprehensive symptom and distress management and early introduction of palliative care are critical components of care (Chumbler et al., 2007; Holland & Weiss, 2008; Hurria et al., 2009; Temel et al., 2010). Similarly, care coordination involving primary and other specialty care providers as well as psychological, social, and spiritual services must advance to integrate home- and community-based resources to facilitate self-care and family caregiving (Bayliss et al., 2008; Chumbler et al., 2007; Kizer & Dudley, 2009; Taplin & Rodgers, 2010). Research in transitional care suggests that enormous opportunity exists to improve care coordination and to prevent older adults from "slipping through the cracks" (Bodenheimer, 2008; Boyd et al., 2007; Coleman, 2003). Nonetheless, as with geriatric assessment, transitions in care and coordination have received little attention in ambulatory oncology settings. Future ambulatory cancer care nursing practice must embrace care coordination and the tenets of transitional care to achieve the best outcomes for older adults (Coleman, 2003).

Healthcare Reform and Effectiveness of Cancer Care

The potential for national reform of the U.S. healthcare system has become reality with initial legislation passed in 2010 (Iglehart, 2009; Oberlander, 2010). Current costs of cancer care for older adults show greatest expenditures in the first year after diagnosis and in the last year of life, with stable costs in intervening years but great variability according to diagnosis (Yabroff, Davis, et al., 2007; Yabroff et al., 2008; Yabroff, Warren, et al., 2007). Considerable human costs as well as financial inequities exist for older adults who are treated for cancer within the current system (Meropol & Schulman, 2007; Yabroff, Davis, et al., 2007). These costs are compounded by absent evidence and suboptimal practices often magnified by ageism (Kagan, 2008). The present legislation offers little specific planning to address projected increases in the volume and complexity of cancer care for our aging society. Nonetheless, oncology nurses possess both perspective and capability to influence reform of ambulatory cancer care for older adults at local, regional, and national levels.

Leveraging existing evidence and resources, while fostering scientific innovations and comparative effectiveness research, potentiates future improvements to systems of ambulatory cancer care. Variation in cancer care and deviation from evidence and best practices limits the determination of effective care and evaluation of outcomes (Desch et al., 2008; Extermann et al., 2010). Implementing standard treatment and supportive care creates a platform from which to gauge effectiveness and outcomes. Integrated electronic communication and recordkeeping within and across care settings supports such programmatic implementation (Boyd et al., 2007). Further, these systems offer enhanced opportunities for care coordination, bundled education and intervention, and opportunities for improved evaluation (Chumbler et al., 2007). However, implementation of practices without processes to judge options is insufficient for an environment marked by limited resources and growing demands for services. Comparative effectiveness research, as a leading scientific perspective, develops evidence necessary to achieve effective care and just use of scarce commodities while avoiding wasteful or ineffective care and resource use (Murray & McElwee, 2010).

Ageism

Ageism in cancer practice and research persists as a lingering and often still socially acceptable form of discrimination (Kagan, 2008). Older adults are dramatically underrepresented in cancer clinical trials. Many of those trials tend to represent samples of artificially healthy participants because they are designed to avoid the complicating factors of comorbid disease and previous cancer and cancer treatment (Kagan, 2008). Analysis of cancer care shows some variations attributable to misperceptions of chronologic age and absent application of extant evidence (Lapid et al., 2007; Leonard et al., 2010; Thompson & Chochinov, 2009). Ageism in research and practice limits applicable evidence, thus jeopardizing current and future best practices. Although ageism remains accepted in healthcare culture, measures to identify and correct current misinformation should anticipate more widely cast efforts to transform those cultural precepts. Furthermore, as they age, the Baby Boomers and Generation X may add pressures with different expectations and tolerance for discriminatory judgments hinged on age. Nonetheless, altered attitudes and specific knowledge are long overdue. Modernizing attitudes in care is the foundation from which shifting expectations of care, implementing age-sensitive research paradigms, and ensuring intolerance for current ageism are possible.

Geriatric Competence

Geriatric competence provides the fundamental knowledge, attitudes, and practices necessary to deliver adequate health care for an aging society (Mezey et al., 2008). Achieving widespread geriatric competence requires continuing education of practicing clinicians, teaching students differently, and rethinking models of care (Committee on the Future Health Care Workforce for Older Americans, 2008; Leipzig et al., 2009). Nurses who frequently work with older adults must be competent to care for them even though they are not geriatric specialists (Beverly et al., 2010; Diachun, Van Bussel, Hansen, Charise, & Rieder, 2010; Leipzig et al., 2009). However, some older adults and their families have complex needs requiring geriatric specialty care. In the absence of geriatric specialists, interdisciplinary teams that include mental health specialists, social workers, and physical and occupational therapists offer a potential bridge to meeting these more complex needs (Kagan, 2010).

Leadership for the Future

Future ambulatory geriatric oncology nursing practice requires educating for general geriatric competence, developing gero-oncology nursing experts, and implementing geriatric assessment, intervention, and care coordination. More specifically, ambulatory oncology nursing care of the future must integrate sophisticated knowledge, advanced skills, and positive attitudes in advance care planning, care coordination and transitional care, patient and family education, and sophisticated monitoring and surveillance. Definitive assessment and intervention that considers the unique needs of older adults and their families limits iatrogenesis and controls or manages treatment complications (Bodenheimer, 2008; Boyd et al., 2007). Together, such actions on the part of oncology nursing leaders acknowledge that older adults are the primary focus of adult ambulatory oncology care. Recognizing that older adults are the majority among oncology patients fosters development of education for nurses and programs for older adults and their families that enhance patient care and optimize outcomes (Bayliss et al., 2008; Kizer & Dudley, 2009; Klepin et al., 2009).

Nursing Education

Movement toward ambulatory cancer care as the main care delivery setting in an aging society mandates transformation of curricula and teaching materials from undergraduate through advanced practice and continuing education (Mezey et al., 2008). Reframing cancer care as nursing practice with older adults suggests a variety of shifts in content. Future-oriented curricula will examine the needs of community-dwelling older adults and their families; outpatient treatment administration, monitoring, and supportive services; and geriatric competence as well as interdisciplinary assessment and intervention. Such content is easily shaped to address the needs of nursing students who will benefit from didactic education and clinical placements in ambulatory cancer care settings. Self-assessment and targeted learning goals potentiate integration of geriatric approaches and content in graduate and continuing education. The phenomenon of "I see/take care of older people every day" heightens concerns that both practicing nurses and students alike understand that older people are the majority of patients in cancer care and that they may require different assessment or intervention (Diachun et al., 2010; Kagan, 2009). While acknowledging how often older patients are treated in a clinical setting is important, it may lead to a false sense of familiarity and a failure to see limits of geriatric knowledge (Diachun et al., 2010; Kagan, 2009). Thus, activities to enhance awareness may promote active engagement in learning about the knowledge, skills, and attitudes necessary to improve care for older adults (Kagan, 2009).

Research

Research, coupled with effective plans for dissemination and implementation of evidence, ultimately contributes to paradigm shifts and practice improvement. By defining phenomena in care of older people in ambulatory cancer care settings for investigation, future research offers the promise of evidence to support improved practice. Moreover, research guided by this frame of ambulatory geriatric oncology can ascertain outcomes of implementing already available assessment and intervention strategies, care coordination systems, and oncology and geriatric services and resources for older adults and their families. Future research should take full advantage of a variety of ambulatory settings. Older participant groups are important. However, further benefit emerges from consideration of comparative participant groups that represent older as well as younger adults to distinguish needs related to age and generation. Mixing methodologies that capture older adult perspectives as well as outcomes with augment future comparative effectiveness research to codify best practices (Murray & McElwee, 2010).

Advocacy

Advocacy and policy making support future changes in nursing practice, education, and research to meet requisite growth in ambulatory cancer care for older adults (Erikson et al., 2007). Practice, research, and education change only with necessary impetus, resources, and leadership. Much of oncology nursing remains centered on the care of young and midlife adults and focuses on inpatient settings as the axis of care delivery. Undergraduate and graduate curricula in nursing currently limit cancer care content and fail to represent oncology nursing adequately in demographic and epidemiologic terms (Ferrell & Winn, 2006). Research in emerging treatment effects, survivorship, utility, and effectiveness lags behind investigation into more familiar phenomena such as symptom management or stress and coping with generally younger participants. Active leadership must transform these omissions and commissions into education, research, advocacy, and policy to create the future of cancer care: ambulatory cancer care for older adults.

Conclusion

The ambulatory setting is rapidly becoming the central location for oncology care delivery to older adults. Oncology nursing practice must adapt to the needs of the older adult population and to advances in oncology treatment by becoming geriatric generalists and oncology specialists. Cultivating competence in the care of older adults requires continuing education to ensure that nurses assess, refer, and intervene in ways targeted to improve patient experiences and outcomes. Care coordination is critical to ensure that older adults receive necessary services to promote function and avoid adverse outcomes. Leadership for the future of ambulatory geriatric oncology nursing practice then requires redesigned entry-level and continuing education, expanded programs of research, and forward-thinking advocacy for policy improvements.

References

Adler, N.E., & Page, A.E.K. (Eds.). (2008). *Cancer care for the whole patient: Meeting psychosocial health needs.* Washington, DC: Institute of Medicine.

Avis, N.E., & Deimling, G.T. (2008). Cancer survivorship and aging. *Cancer, 113*(Suppl. 12), 3519–3529. doi:10.1002/cncr.23941

Bach, P.B. (2007). Costs of cancer care: A view from the Centers for Medicare and Medicaid Services. *Journal of Clinical Oncology, 25,* 187–190. doi:10.1200/JCO.2006.08.6116

Banna, G.L., Collovà, E., Gebbia, V., Lipari, H., Giuffrida, P., Cavallaro, S., ... Ferraù, F. (2010). Anticancer oral therapy: Emerging related issues. *Cancer Treatment Reviews, 36,* 595–605. doi:10.1016/j.ctrv.2010.04.005

Bayliss, E.A., Edwards, A.E., Steiner, J.F., & Main, D.S. (2008). Processes of care desired by elderly patients with multimorbidities. *Family Practice, 25,* 287–293. doi:10.1093/fampra/cmn040

Beverly, C., Burger, S.G., Maas, M.L., & Specht, J.K.P. (2010). Aging issues: Nursing imperatives for healthcare reform. *Nursing Administration Quarterly, 34,* 95–109. doi:110.1097/NAQ.1090b1013e3181d91718

Blayney, D.W., McNiff, K., Hanauer, D., Miela, G., Markstrom, D., & Neuss, M. (2009). Implementation of the quality oncology practice initiative at a University Comprehensive Cancer Center. *Journal of Clinical Oncology, 27,* 3802–3807. doi:10.1200/JCO.2008.21.6770

Bodenheimer, T. (2008). Coordinating care—A perilous journey through the health care system. *New England Journal of Medicine, 358,* 1064–1071. doi:10.1056/NEJMhpr0706165

Bomba, P.A., & Vermilyea, D. (2006). Integrating POLST into palliative care guidelines: A paradigm shift in advance care planning in oncology. *Journal of the National Comprehensive Cancer Network, 1,* 819–829.

Boyd, C.M., Boult, C., Shadmi, E., Leff, B., Brager, R., Dunbar, L., ... Wegener, S. (2007). Guided care for multimorbid older adults. *Gerontologist, 47,* 697–704. doi:10.1093/geront/47.5.697

Brunello, A., Sandri, R., & Extermann, M. (2009). Multidimensional geriatric evaluation for older cancer patients as a clinical and research tool. *Cancer Treatment Reviews, 35,* 487–492. doi:10.1016/j.ctrv.2009.04.005

Chumbler, N.R., Kobb, R., Harris, L., Richardson, L.C., Darkins, A., Sberna, M., ... Kreps, G.L. (2007). Healthcare utilization among veterans undergoing chemotherapy: The impact of a cancer care coordination/home-telehealth program. *Journal of Ambulatory Care Management, 30,* 308–317. doi:10.1097/01.JAC.0000290399.43543.2e

Coleman, E.A. (2003). Falling through the cracks: Challenges and opportunities for improving transitional care for persons with continuous complex care needs. *Journal of the American Geriatrics Society, 51,* 549–555. doi:10.1046/j.1532-5415.2003.51185.x

Committee on the Future Health Care Workforce for Older Americans. (2008). *Retooling for an aging America: Building the health care workforce.* Washington, DC: National Academies Press.

Decker, S.L., Schappert, S.M., & Sisk, J.E. (2009). Use of medical care for chronic conditions. *Health Affairs, 28,* 26–35. doi:10.1377/hlthaff.28.1.26

Desch, C.E., McNiff, K.K., Schneider, E.C., Schrag, D., McClure, J., Lepisto, E., ... Edge, S.B. (2008). American Society of Clinical Oncology/National Comprehensive Cancer Network quality measures. *Journal of Clinical Oncology, 26,* 3631–3637. doi:10.1200/JCO.2008.16.5068

Diachun, L., Van Bussel, L., Hansen, K.T., Charise, A., & Rieder, M.J. (2010). "But I see old people everywhere": Dispelling the myth that eldercare is learned in nongeriatric clerkships. *Academic Medicine, 85,* 1221–1228. doi:1210.1097/ACM.1220b1013e3181e0054f

Erikson, C., Salsberg, E., Forte, G., Bruinooge, S., & Goldstein, M. (2007). Future supply and demand for oncologists: Challenges to assuring access to oncology services. *Journal of Oncology Practice, 3,* 79–86. doi:10.1200/JOP.0723601

Extermann, M., Aapro, M., Bernabei, R., Cohen, H.J., Droz, J.P., Lichtman, S., ... Topinkova, E. (2005). Use of comprehensive geriatric assessment in older cancer patients: Recommendations from the task force on CGA of the International Society of Geriatric Oncology (SIOG). *Critical Reviews in Oncology/Hematology, 55,* 241–252. doi:10.1016/j.critrevonc.2005.06.003

Extermann, M., Crane, E.J., & Boulware, D. (2010). Cancer in nonagenarians: Profile, treatments and outcomes. *Journal of Geriatric Oncology, 1,* 27–31. doi:10.1016/j.jgo.2010.03.003

Fendrich, K., & Hoffmann, W. (2007). More than just aging societies: The demographic change has an impact on actual numbers of patients. *Journal of Public Health, 15,* 345–351. doi:10.1007/s10389-007-0142-0

Ferrell, B.R., & Winn, R. (2006). Medical and nursing education and training opportunities to improve survivorship care. *Journal of Clinical Oncology, 24,* 5142–5148. doi:10.1200/JCO.2006.06.0970

Galligioni, E., Berloffa, F., Caffo, O., Tonazzolli, G., Ambrosini, G., Valduga, F., ... Forti, S. (2009). Development and daily use of an electronic oncological patient record for the total management of cancer patients: 7 years' experience. *Annals of Oncology, 20,* 349–352.

George, J., Elliott, R.A., & Stewart, D.C. (2008). A systematic review of interventions to improve medication taking in elderly patients prescribed multiple medications. *Drugs and Aging, 25,* 307. doi:10.2165/00002512-200825040-00004

Gosney, M. (2009). General care of the older cancer patient. *Clinical Oncology, 21,* 86–91. doi:10.1016/j.clon.2008.11.005

Griffith, J., Lyman, J., & Blackhall, L. (2010). Providing palliative care in the ambulatory care setting. *Clinical Journal of Oncology Nursing, 14,* 171–175. doi:10.1188/10.CJON.171-175

Holland, J., & Weiss, T. (2008). The new standard of quality cancer care: Integrating the psychosocial aspects in routine cancer from diagnosis through survivorship. *Cancer Journal, 14,* 425–428. doi:10.1097/PPO.1090b1013e31818d38934

Hurria, A., Li, D., Hansen, K., Patil, S., Gupta, R., Nelson, C., ... Kelly, E. (2009). Distress in older patients with cancer. *Journal of Clinical Oncology, 27,* 4346–4351. doi:10.1200/JCO.2008.19.9463

Iglehart, J.K. (2009). The struggle for reform—Challenges and hopes for comprehensive health care legislation. *New England Journal of Medicine, 360,* 1693–1695. doi:10.1056/NEJMp0902651

Jansen, J., van Weert, J., van Dulmen, S., Heeren, T., & Bensing, J. (2007). Patient education treatment in cancer care: An overview of the literature on older patients' needs. *Cancer Nursing, 30,* 251–260. doi:10.1097/1001.NCC.0000281735.0000225609.af

Kagan, S.H. (2008). Ageism in cancer care. *Seminars in Oncology Nursing, 24,* 246–253. doi:10.1016/j.soncn.2008.08.004

Kagan, S.H. (2009). The plateau of recognition in specialty acute care. *Geriatric Nursing, 30,* 130–131. doi:10.1016/j.gerinurse.2009.01.005

Kagan, S.H. (2010). Revisiting interdisciplinary teamwork in geriatric acute care. *Geriatric Nursing, 31,* 133–136. doi:10.1016/j.gerinurse.2010.02.007

Kanapuru, B., Posani, K., Muller, D., & Ershler, W.B. (2008). Decreased cancer prevalence in the nursing home. *Journal of the American Geriatrics Society, 56,* 2165–2166. doi:10.1111/j.1532-5415.2008.01864.x

Karampeazis, A., & Extermann, M. (2009). Assessment and impact of comorbidity in older adults with cancer. In A. Hurria & L. Balducci (Eds.), *Geriatric oncology: Treatment, assessment and management* (pp. 95–111). New York, NY: Springer.

Kav, S., Johnson, J., Rittenberg, C., Fernadez-Ortega, P., Suominen, T., Olsen, P., ... Clark-Snow, R. (2008). Role of the nurse in patient education and follow-up of people receiving oral chemotherapy treatment: An international survey. *Supportive Care in Cancer, 16,* 1075–1083. doi:10.1007/s00520-007-0377-x

Kelley, A.S., & Meier, D.E. (2010). Palliative care—A shifting paradigm. *New England Journal of Medicine, 363,* 781–782. doi:10.1056/NEJMe1004139

Kizer, K.W., & Dudley, R.A. (2009). Extreme makeover: Transformation of the veterans health care system. *Annual Review of Public Health, 30,* 313–339. doi:10.1146/annurev.publhealth.29.020907.090940

Klepin, H., Mohile, S., & Hurria, A. (2009). Geriatric assessment in older patients with breast cancer. *Journal of the National Comprehensive Cancer Network, 7,* 226–236.

Kurtz, M., Kurtz, J., Given, C., & Given, B. (2006). Predictors of use of health care services among elderly lung cancer patients: the first year after diagnosis. *Supportive Care in Cancer, 14,* 243–250. doi:10.1007/s00520-005-0877-5

Lapid, M.I., Rumanns, T.A., Brown, P.D., Frost, M.H., Johnson, M.E., Huschka, M.M., ... Clark, M.M. (2007). Improving the quality of life of geriatric cancer patients with a structured multidisciplinary intervention: A randomized controlled trial. *Palliative and Supportive Care, 5,* 107–114. doi:10.1017/S1478951507070174

Leipzig, R.M., Granville, L., Simpson, D., Anderson, M.B., Sauvigné, K., & Soriano, R.P. (2009). Keeping Granny safe on July 1: A consensus on minimum geriatrics competencies for graduating medical students. *Academic Medicine, 84,* 604–610. doi:10.1097/ACM.0b013e31819fab70

Leonard, R.C., Barrett-Lee, P.J., Gosney, M.A., Willett, A.M., Reed, M.W., & Hammond, P.J. (2010). Effect of patient age on management decisions in breast cancer: Consensus from a national consultation. *Oncologist, 15,* 657–664. doi:10.1634/theoncologist.2009-0284

Levit, L., Smith, A.P., Benz, E.J., & Ferrell, B. (2010). Ensuring quality care through the oncology workforce. *Journal of Oncology Practice, 6,* 7–11. doi:10.1200/JOP.091067

Lorenz, K.A., Lynn, J., Dy, S.M., Shugarman, L.R., Wilkinson, A., Mularski, R.A., ... Shekelle, P.G. (2008). Evidence for improving palliative care at the end of life: A systematic review. *Annals of Internal Medicine, 148,* 147–159.

Ma, W.W., & Adjei, A.A. (2009). Novel agents on the horizon for cancer therapy. *CA: A Cancer Journal for Clinicians, 59,* 111–137. doi:10.3322/caac.20003

Malek, K., & Silliman, R. (2007). Cancer survivorship issues in older adults. In P.A. Ganz (Ed.), *Cancer survivorship* (pp. 215–224). New York, NY: Springer.

McGory, M.L., Kao, K.K., Shekelle, P.G., Rubenstein, L.Z., Leonardi, M.J., Parikh, J.A., ... Ko, C.Y. (2009). Developing quality indicators for elderly surgical patients. *Annals of Surgery, 250,* 338–347. doi:10.1097/SLA.0b013e3181ae575a

Meropol, N.J., & Schulman, K.A. (2007). Cost of cancer care: Issues and implications. *Journal of Clinical Oncology, 25,* 180–186. doi:10.1200/JCO.2006.09.6081

Mezey, M., Mitty, E., Burger, S.G., & McCallion, P. (2008). Healthcare professional training: A comparison of geriatric competencies. *Journal of the American Geriatrics Society, 56,* 1724–1729. doi:10.1111/j.1532-5415.2008.01857.x

Mezey, M., Stierle, L.J., Huba, G.J., & Esterson, J. (2007). Ensuring competence of specialty nurses in care of older adults. *Geriatric Nursing, 28*(6), 9–14. doi:10.1016/j.gerinurse.2007.10.013

Min, L., Yoon, W., Mariano, J., Wenger, N.S., Elliott, M.N., Kamberg, C., & Saliba, D. (2009). The Vulnerable Elders-13 survey predicts 5-year functional decline and mortality outcomes in older ambulatory care patients. *Journal of the American Geriatrics Society, 57,* 2070–2076. doi:10.1111/j.1532-5415.2009.02497.x

Moore, S. (2007). Facilitating oral chemotherapy treatment and compliance through patient/family-focused education. *Cancer Nursing, 30,* 112–122. doi:10.1097/01.NCC.0000265009.33053.2d

Murray, R.K., & McElwee, N.E. (2010). Comparative effectiveness research: Critically intertwined with health care reform and the future of biomedical innovation. *Archive of Internal Medicine, 170,* 596–599. doi:10.1001/archinternmed.2010.50

Oberlander, J. (2010). A vote for health care reform. *New England Journal of Medicine, 362,* e44. doi:10.1056/NEJMp1002878

Overcash, J.A., Beckstead, J., Moody, L., Extermann, M., & Cobb, S. (2006). The abbreviated comprehensive geriatric assessment (aCGA) for use in the older cancer patient as a prescreen: Scoring and interpretation. *Critical Reviews in Oncology/Hematology, 59,* 205–210. doi:10.1016/j.critrevonc.2006.04.003

Reidel, K., Tamblyn, R., Patel, V., & Huang, A. (2008). Pilot study of an interactive voice response system to improve medication refill compliance. *BMC Medical Informatics and Decision Making, 8,* 46. doi:10.1186/1472-6947-8-46

Robine, J.M., Michel, J.P., & Herrmann, F.R. (2007). Who will care for the oldest people in our ageing society? *BMJ, 334,* 570–571. doi:10.1136/bmj.39129.397373.BE

Rowe, J.W., & Kahn, R.L. (1997). Successful aging. *Gerontologist, 37,* 433–440. doi:10.1093/geront/37.4.433

Siegel, R., Ward, E., Brawley, O., & Jemal, A. (2011). Cancer statistics, 2011: The impact of eliminating socioeconomic and racial disparities on premature cancer deaths [Online version]. *CA: A Cancer Journal for Clinicians.* doi:10.3322/caac.20121

Sifer-Rivière, L., Girre, V., Gisselbrecht, M., & Saint-Jean, O. (2010). Physicians' perceptions of cancer care for elderly patients: A qualitative sociological study based on a pilot geriatric oncology program. *Critical Reviews in Oncology/Hematology, 75,* 58–69. doi:10.1016/j.critrevonc.2010.04.001

Smith, B.D., Smith, G.L., Hurria, A., Hortobagyi, G.N., & Buchholz, T.A. (2009). Future of cancer incidence in the United States: Burdens upon an aging, changing nation. *Journal of Clinical Oncology, 27,* 2758–2765. doi:10.1200/JCO.2008.20.8983

Sokol, K.C., Knudsen, J.F., & Li, M.M. (2007). Polypharmacy in older oncology patients and the need for an interdisciplinary approach to side-effect management. *Journal of Clinical Pharmacy and Therapeutics, 32,* 169–175. doi:10.1111/j.1365-2710.2007.00815.x

Taplin, S.H., & Rodgers, A.B. (2010). Toward improving the quality of cancer care: Addressing the interfaces of primary and oncology-related subspecialty care. *Journal of the National Cancer Institute Monographs, 2010*(40), 3–10. doi:10.1093/jncimonographs/lgq006

Temel, J.S., Greer, J.A., Muzikansky, A., Gallagher, E.R., Admane, S., Jackson, V.A., ... Lynch, T.J. (2010). Early palliative care for patients with metastatic non–small-cell lung cancer. *New England Journal of Medicine, 363,* 733–742. doi:10.1056/NEJMoa1000678

Thompson, G.N., & Chochinov, H.M. (2009). Palliative care: Special considerations for older adults with cancer. In A. Hurria & L. Balducci (Eds.), *Geriatric oncology: Treatment assessment and management* (pp. 293–324). New York, NY: Springer.

U.S. Census Bureau. (2010, May). Older Americans month: May 2010. Retrieved from http://www.census.gov/newsroom/releases/archives/facts_for_features_special_editions/cb10-ff06.html

Wolff, J.L., Roter, D.L., Given, B., & Gitlin, L.N. (2009). Optimizing patient and family involvement in geriatric home care. *Journal for Healthcare Quality, 31,* 24–33. doi:10.1111/j.1945-1474.2009.00016.x

Yabroff, K.R., Davis, W.W., Lamont, E.B., Fahey, A., Topor, M., Brown, M.L., & Warren, J.L. (2007). Patient time costs associated with cancer care. *Journal of the National Cancer Institute, 99,* 14–23.

Yabroff, K.R., Lamont, E.B., Mariotto, A., Warren, J.L., Topor, M., Meekins, A., & Brown, M.L. (2008). Cost of care for elderly cancer patients in the United States. *Journal of the National Cancer Institute, 100,* 630–641. doi:10.1093/jnci/djn103

Yabroff, K.R., Warren, J.L., & Brown, M.L. (2007). Costs of cancer care in the USA: A descriptive review. *Nature Clinical Practice in Oncology, 4,* 643–656. doi:10.1038/ncponc0978

Resources

Gerontology Centers

American Nurses Association GeroNurseOnline: www.geronurseonline.org
Web site for Nurse Competence in Aging Initiative providing best practice information on care of older adults.

Concept Healthcare: www.cohealth.org
Educational material and training in the use of psychological concepts for professionals interacting with patients and their families to increase the quality and efficiency of care delivery with older adults.

ConsultGeriRN.org: www.consultgerirn.org
Geriatric clinical nursing Web site of the Hartford Institute for Geriatric Nursing offering evidence-based content on elder patient care.

Hartford Institute for Geriatric Nursing: www.hartfordign.org
Web site promoting excellence in geriatric nursing practice, education, research, and policy to improve the quality of care provided to older adults.

Associations and Societies

AARP (formerly American Association of Retired Persons): www.aarp.org
Nonprofit membership organization for individuals age 50 and older that focuses on promoting quality of life and positive social change through information, advocacy, and service to members.

Alliance for Aging Research: www.agingresearch.org
Nonprofit organization supporting research and educational endeavors to improve the quality of life and health of aging individuals. Educational in-

formation is available for patients and caregivers on a broad range of topics pertinent for older adults.

American Geriatrics Society: www.americangeriatrics.org
Nonprofit membership organization of healthcare professionals dedicated to improving the quality of life of all older individuals by implementing and advocating for programs in patient care, research, professional and public education, and healthcare policy.

American Society on Aging: www.asaging.org
The largest organization of multidisciplinary professionals in the field of aging. Resources, publications, and educational opportunities are provided to improve the knowledge and skills for individuals caring for older adults and their families.

Gerontological Society of America: www.geron.org
Nonprofit multidisciplinary professional organization dedicated to the promotion of scientific study of aging and the promotion of quality of life for older adults.

National Council on Aging: www.ncoa.org
Nonprofit organization with a national network of more than 14,000 organizations providing programs to support and facilitate healthy, independent living for older adults.

Statistics and Government Sites

Administration on Aging: www.aoa.gov
Comprehensive information about home and community services, news, benefits, and government programs for elderly individuals to assist in health maintenance and independent community living.

Aging Stats: www.agingstats.gov
The Federal Interagency Forum on Aging-Related Statistics coordinates the development and use of statistical databases among the following federal agencies: National Institute on Aging, National Center for Health Statistics and Census Bureau, Administration on Aging, Agency for Healthcare Research and Quality, Bureau of Labor Statistics, Centers for Medicare and Medicaid Services, Department of Veterans Affairs, Employee Benefits Security Administration, Environmental Protection Agency, Office of Management and Budget, Office of the Assistant Secretary for Planning and Evaluation in Health and Human Services, Social Security Administration, and the Substance Abuse and Mental Health Services Administration.

Centers for Disease Control and Prevention: www.cdc.gov
- **FastStats:** www.cdc.gov/nchs/fastats
  Public health statistics organized alphabetically for quick access.
- **National Center for Health Statistics:** www.cdc.gov/nchs
  United States public health statistics, including diseases, pregnancies, births, aging, and mortality.

National Institute on Aging: www.nia.nih.gov
  Information and publications for older adults on health promotion activities and diseases. Information on National Institute on Aging research programs, including studies on mechanisms on aging, the processes of aging, aging and the nervous system, and aging in relation to health and disease.

Index

The letter f after a page number indicates that relevant content appears in a figure; the letter t, in a table.

A

AARP, 191
Abbreviated Comprehensive Geriatric Assessment (aCGA), 48
absorption, of medications, 29*t*, 104*t*
acinar cells, 21, 90
activities of daily living (ADLs), 9, 57, 160*t*
Activities of Daily Living scale, 44, 45*f*, 48
adjuvant analgesics, 105
Administration on Aging (AoA), 143, 192
advance care planning, 129, 131, 169–174, 174*t*, 179
advocacy, 185
ageism, 182–183
ageusia, 18, 59
aging
　normal progression of, 12–13
　physiologic changes of, 14–28
　theories of, 10, 11*t*–12*t*
　trajectories of, 12–13
Aging Stats, 192
Aging With Dignity—5 Wishes, 174*t*
aid in dying, 133
Alliance for Aging Research, 191–192
Alliance for Lung Cancer Advocacy, Support and Education, 171*t*
allodynia, 104
Alzheimer disease (AD), 16, 63
ambulatory oncology care, 4, 5*f*, 178
　assessment in, 38–48. *See also* comprehensive geriatric assessment
　future influences on, 178–181

nursing role in, 4–5, 127, 130–131
American Brain Tumor Association, 170*t*
American Cancer Society, 143, 163*t*, 169*t*, 173*t*
American Geriatrics Society, 192
American Lung Association, 171*t*
American Nurses Association
　on end-of-life care, 133
　GeroNurseOnline, 191
American Society of Clinical Oncology, 146*f*
American Society on Aging, 192
Americans with Disabilities Act, 147
amyloid deposits, 15–16
anemia, 22, 27
anorexia, 58–59
　assessment of, 60–61
　etiology of, 59–60, 60*f*
　management of, 61–62
"anorexia of aging," 22, 59
anticholinergics, for dyspnea management, 95
antidepressants
　for fatigue management, 99
　for pain management, 105
antidiuretic hormone (ADH), 23, 28
antiemetics, constipation from, 78–79
antipsychotics, 74
anxiety, dyspnea with, 95
appetite changes, 22, 59, 135
appetite stimulants, 61–62
arteriosclerotic changes, 19, 23
ascites, 134
aspiration pneumonia, 83, 92

assessment. *See also* comprehensive geriatric assessment
  of anorexia/weight loss, 60–61
  of caregiver strain, 42*f*, 44
  case study of, 48–50
  of cognitive impairment, 45*f*, 46, 66–69, 70*f*–72*f*
  of constipation, 79–81, 80*f*
  of depression, 38, 45*f*, 45–46
  of fatigue, 41–42, 42*f*
  of functional status, 44–45, 45*f*
  holistic, 150–153, 152*f*
  of pain, 42*f*, 42–43
  by phone, 48
  self-administration of, 47–48
  of sexual dysfunction, 42*f*, 43
  of sleep problems, 42*f*, 43
atherosclerotic changes, 19, 65

B

baroreceptors, 19
behavioral modifications, for constipation management, 82
benign prostatic hypertrophy, 24
benzodiazepines, for dyspnea management, 95
bereavement, 136–137
beta agonists, for dyspnea management, 95
bile changes, 23
biotherapy, cognitive impairment from, 66
bisacodyl, for constipation, 83*t*
bladder function, 23–24
bladder prolapse, 24
blood pressure, 19, 88
blood urea nitrogen (BUN), 88
body mass, 29
body mass index (BMI), 60–61
bone formation, 26
bone loss, 25–26
bone marrow reserves, 26–27
bone-resorbing cytokines, 26
bone resorption, 26
brain cancer, 66, 170*t*
brain weight, 15
breakthrough pain, 101
breast cancer
  depression with, 45
  incidence rates, 3
  resources on, 170*t*

Breastcancer.org, 170*t*
Brief Fatigue Inventory, 98
Brief Male Sexual Function Inventory, 42*f*, 43
Brief Pain Inventory (BPI), 42, 42*f*, 102
bulk-forming laxatives, 83*t*, 84
bupropion, for fatigue management, 99
burnout, 137–138

C

cachexia, 22, 59
Cancer*Care*, 163*t*, 165*t*, 169*t*
CancerConsultants.com, 172*t*
Cancer Dyspnea Scale, 94
Cancer Journey, 169*t*
Cancer.net, 148, 169*t*
cancer-related fatigue (CRF). *See* fatigue
cancer survivorship. *See* survivorship
cardiac changes, 19
cardiovascular changes, 18–19, 149*f*
care coordination, 181
caregiver stress
  assessment of, 42*f*, 44
  dementia and, 74
  at end of life, 130
  and sexual function, 108
CARES program, 138
Caring Connections, 174*t*
cartilage changes, 26
cascara, for constipation, 83*t*
Centers for Disease Control and Prevention (CDC), 193
cerebral blood flow (CBF), 15, 65
cerebrovascular resistance, 15, 65
chemobrain, 66
chemotherapy
  cognitive impairment from, 66
  constipation from, 78–79
  long-term/late effects from, 149
Cheyne-Stokes respirations, 135
chlorpromazine, for cognitive impairment, 75*t*
cholinesterase inhibitors (ChEIs), for cognitive impairment, 73
chondrocytes, 26
Chronic Disease Fund, 165*t*
chronological age, 10–12
Clock Drawing Test (CDT), 46–47, 69
cognitive impairment, 16, 62–64
  from aging, 65
  assessment of, 45*f*, 46, 66–69, 70*f*–72*f*

from cancer/treatment, 66, 67*t*
drugs causing, 67*t*
management of, 72–76, 75*t*–76*t*
prevalence of, 64–65
Colon Cancer Alliance, 170*t*
colorectal cancer, 170*t*–171*t*
Common Terminology Criteria for Adverse Events (CTCAE) grading
of constipation, 79, 80*f*
of weight loss, 60
communication, in end-of-life care, 131–132
comorbid conditions, 41, 57, 60*f*, 86, 129, 147–148
compassion fatigue, 137–138
comprehensive geriatric assessment (CGA), 37, 39*f*–40*f*, 158, 179
case study application of, 48–50
components of, 38–41
definition/development of, 38–47
rapid assessments in, 47–48
Concept Healthcare, 191
confusion, 15, 63, 76, 136. *See also* cognitive impairment
constipation, 76–77
from aging, 78
assessment of, 79–81, 80*f*
from cancer/treatment, 78–79, 79*f*
management of, 81–84, 83*t*
medications causing, 77–78, 79*f*, 84–85, 105
prevalence of, 77–78
risk factors for, 77*f*
Constipation Assessment Scale, 79
ConsultGeriRN.org, 191
co-pay assistance, 165*t*–167*t*
coping strategies/resources, 73, 138, 161, 164–168
corticosteroids
for anorexia management, 61–62
for fatigue management, 99–100
for pain management, 105
cortisol, 28
creatinine clearance, 23, 29*t*
cross link theory of aging, 11*t*
cystocele, 24
cytochrome P450 (CYP450), 30

D

"death rattle," 135
dehydration, 85

from aging, 85–86
assessment of, 87*f*, 87–88
from cancer/treatment, 86–87, 87*f*
at end of life, 135
management of, 89
prevalence of, 85
signs/symptoms of, 87*f*
delirium, 46, 63–65, 64*f*, 136
management of, 73–74, 75*t*, 75–76, 76*t*
dementia, 15–16, 47, 62–63
assessment of, 38, 46
prevalence of, 64–65
dementia with Lewy bodies, 62, 73
demographics, of aging population, 1–2, 2*f*, 6, 143–145
dentition, 21, 92
depression
assessment of, 38, 45*f*, 45–46
case study of, 48–50
risk factors for, 45
dermal papillae, 25
dexamethasone, for anorexia management, 61–62
diarrhea
chemotherapeutic agents causing, 87*f*
dehydration from, 87, 89
diastolic BP, 19
dietary counseling, 61
dietary fiber intake, 81–82, 83*t*
diffuse cerebral atrophy, 66
disposable soma theory of aging, 11*t*
distress, 158
Distress Thermometer (DT), 158–159, 159*f*
distribution, of medications, 29*t*, 104*t*
dizziness, 15
docusate, for constipation, 83*t*, 84
donepezil, for cognitive impairment, 73
do-not-resuscitate (DNR) order, 174
drusen, 16
dry mouth, 21, 90–92
durable power of attorney for health care, 169–173
dysesthesia, 104
dysgeusia, 18, 59
dysphagia, 83, 89–90
from aging, 89–90
assessment of, 91, 91*f*
management of, 91–93
prevalence of, 90
signs/symptoms of, 91*f*
dyspnea, 20, 93–95, 94*f*–95*f*, 136
Dyspnea-12 scale, 94

E

early satiety, 22, 59
Eastern Cooperative Oncology Group performance status, 68, 135
education, nursing, 184
Eldercare Locator, 163*t*
endocrine changes, 27–28, 149*f*
end of life, 131–132, 174. *See also* hospice care
 ethical issues during, 132–133
 physiologic changes at, 135–136
 prognostication during, 134–135
 symptom management and, 133
enteral feeding, 92, 133–134
error theory of aging, 11*t*
established incontinence, 24
estrogen, 24, 26
estrogen replacement, 26
ethical issues, at end of life, 132–133
euthanasia, 133
excretion, of medications, 29*t*, 104*t*
exercise
 and cognitive function, 73
 for constipation management, 82
 for fatigue management, 99
expiratory flow rate, 20, 21*t*
exquisite empathy, 137–138

F

Faces Pain Scale, 42, 42*f*
falls, 15
 risk assessment for, 38, 45*f*, 46–47, 49–50
family meetings, 132
FastStats, 193
fatigue, 41, 96
 from aging, 96–97
 assessment of, 41–42, 42*f*, 97–98
 from cancer/treatment, 97, 97*f*
 at end of life, 135
 management of, 98–100
 outcomes from, 97*f*
 prevalence of, 96
Female Sexual Functional Index, 42*f*, 43
Fertile Hope, 169*t*
fiber intake, 81–82, 83*t*
financial concerns/resources, 160*t*, 162–164, 163*t*, 164*f*, 165*t*–167*t*
5-Item Geriatric Depression Scale, 45*f*, 46–47

fluid intake
 constipation and, 78, 81–82
 dehydration and, 85, 87, 89
 at end of life, 135
follow-up care, after assessment, 50
free-radical theory of aging, 11*t*
Functional Activities Questionnaire (FAQ), 68
Functional Assessment of Anorexia/Cachexia Therapy (FAACT), 60
Functional Assessment of Cancer Therapy–Fatigue (FACT-F), 98
Functional Assessment of Cancer Therapy–General (FACT-G), 98
functional reserve capacity, 13–14, 14*f*
functional status, 9
 assessment of, 44–45, 45*f*, 135, 160*t*

G

gag reflex, 91, 136
galantamine, for cognitive impairment, 73
gallstones, 23
gastrointestinal changes, 20–22, 59, 149*f*
genitourinary changes, 23–24
geriatric competence, 183
Geriatric Depression Scale (GDS), 45*f*, 45–46, 48
geriatric generalists, 179
geriatric syndromes, 47
Gerontological Society of America, 192
gerontology centers, 191
GeroNurseOnline, 191
Gilda's Club Worldwide, 169*t*
glomerular filtration rate, 23
glucocorticoids, 28
glycerin suppositories, for constipation, 83*t*
grief, 136–137
grip strength measurement, 47
growth hormone, 28
Gynecologic Cancer Foundation, 171*t*

H

haloperidol
 for cognitive impairment, 75*t*
 at end of life, 136
Hartford Institute for Geriatric Nursing, 43–44, 46, 191

healthcare proxy, 169–173
healthcare reform, 182–183
health insurance, 147, 160*t*, 163*t*, 164, 164*f*
health-related QOL (HRQOL), 151–152
HealthWell Foundation, 166*t*
hearing changes, 17, 76*t*
heart size, 19
hematopoiesis, changes in, 26–27
hepatic changes, 22–23
hepatocytes, 23
holistic assessment, 150–153, 152*f*
Homemods.org, 163*t*
homeostenosis, 13–14, 14*f*
hormonal changes, 27–28
hospice care
    ethical issues in, 132–133
    vs. palliative care, 125–128, 128*f*
    symptom management in, 133
    transition to, 130–132
hospice care, 130, 125–128, 128*f*
housing needs, 162, 163*t*
hyperalgesia, 104
hypoalgesia, 104
hypogeusia, 18, 59
hyponatremia, 86
hypotension/hypertension, 19
hypothermia, 25

I

immune function, 26–27, 82
immunity theory of aging, 12*t*
immunosenescence, 26–27
incidence rates, of cancer in aging, 2–4, 3*f*, 6
insomnia. *See also* sleep problems
    assessment of, 43
    fatigue from, 99
Insomnia Severity Index, 43
Institute for Myeloma and Bone Cancer Research, 172*t*
Institute of Medicine (IOM)
    on cancer survivorship, 145, 153
    on psychosocial distress, 157–158
instrumental activities of daily living, 9, 68, 160*t*
Instrumental Activities of Daily Living Scale, 44, 45*f*, 48
insulin, 27–28
integumentary changes, 24–25

International Myeloma Foundation, 172*t*
Internet resources
    on aging, 191–193
    on cancer, 163*t*, 169*t*–172*t*
    for survivorship care plans, 146*f*
Iowa Sleep Disturbance Scale, 42*f*, 43
ischemia, 15, 23

J

joints, changes in, 26
Journey Forward, 146*f*

K

Karnofsky Performance Status, 68, 135
kidney function, changes in, 23, 29*t*, 86

L

lactulose, for constipation, 83*t*
Lance Armstrong Foundation, 169*t*
last reflex breathing, 135
late effects, of cancer, 147–149, 149*f*
laxatives, for constipation management, 82, 83*t*, 84
Leukemia and Lymphoma Society, 171*t*
    Co-Pay Assistance Program, 166*t*
leukoencephalopathy, 66
Lewy body disease, 63, 73
life expectancy, 144
lipid-soluble drugs, 29
liver function, 22–23, 28–29, 29*t*
LIVESTRONG, 146*f*
Living Beyond Breast Cancer, 170*t*
living will, 173
long-term effects, of cancer, 147–149, 149*f*
lorazepam
    for cognitive impairment, 75*t*
    at end of life, 136
loss, 136–137
lubricants, for constipation, 83*t*
lung cancer
    dyspnea with, 93
    resources on, 171*t*
Lung Cancer Alliance, 171*t*
lung changes, 19–20, 21*t*
lymphedema, 171*t*
lymphocytes, 27

M

macular degeneration, 16
magnesium citrate/magnesium hydroxide, for constipation, 83t
malnutrition, 22, 58, 61
medical power of attorney, 169–173
Medicare, 164
  hospice benefit, 127–128, 130
medications. See also pharmacokinetics
  affecting cognition, 67t
  causing constipation, 77–78
  causing dehydration, 86
  for cognitive impairment, 73–74, 75t
megestrol acetate, 62
memantine, for cognitive impairment, 73
memory, 16, 62
menopause, 24, 26
  sleep problems during, 43
metabolic syndrome, 65
metabolism, of medications, 29t, 104t
methylcellulose, for constipation, 81, 83t
methylnaltrexone, for constipation, 83t, 84
methylprednisolone, for anorexia management, 61–62
metoclopramide, for constipation, 83t
middle-old adults, 1
mild cognitive impairment (MCI), 62, 72–73
mineral oil, for constipation, 83, 83t
Mini-Cog, 45f, 46, 69
Mini-Mental State Exam (MMSE), 46, 48, 68–69
minority populations, 150
mixed pain syndrome, 101
Modified Caregiver Strain Index, 42f, 43
mortality rates
  from cancer, 4, 143
  from falls, 46
mu antagonists, for constipation, 83t
mucociliary escalator, 20
mucositis, 91
Multidimensional Fatigue Symptom Inventory–Short Form (MFSI-SF), 98
multiple myeloma, 172t
muscle mass, loss of, 20, 25, 86, 97
musculoskeletal changes, 25–26, 149f
mutation accumulation theory of aging, 11t

N

naloxone, for constipation, 83t, 84
National Ambulatory Medical Care Survey, 4, 5f
National Brain Tumor Foundation, 170t
National Cancer Institute, 169t
National Center for Health Statistics, 193
National Center on Senior Transportation, 163t
National Cervical Cancer Coalition, 171t
National Clearinghouse for Long-Term Care Information, 163t
National Coalition for Cancer Survivorship, 170t
National Colorectal Cancer Research Alliance, 171t
National Comprehensive Cancer Network (NCCN)
  on geriatric assessment, 38. See also comprehensive geriatric assessment
  on palliative care, 126–127
  on survivorship care plans, 146f
National Council for Hospice and Specialist Palliative Care Services, 157
National Council on Aging, 192
National Family Caregivers Association, 170t
National Hospice and Palliative Care Organization, 130, 171t
National Institute on Aging, 193
National Leiomyosarcoma Foundation, 172t
National Lymphedema Network, 171t
National Organization for Rare Disorders, 166t
National Ovarian Cancer Coalition, 172t
National Prostate Cancer Coalition, 172t
National Social Life, Health, and Aging Project, 109
neuroendocrine theory of aging, 12t
neuroleptic malignant syndrome, 74
neuroleptics, 74
neurologic changes, 15–16, 136, 149f
neuropathic pain, 101, 102f, 103–105
Neuropsychiatric Inventory Questionnaire (NPI-Q), 69, 70f–72f
neurotransmitters, changes in, 15, 65
nociception, 101
nociceptive pain, 101, 103

nonopioids, for pain management, 105
nonsteroidal anti-inflammatory drugs
    (NSAIDs), 105, 106*f*
normal aging, 12–13
numeric rating
    of fatigue, 41–42
    of pain, 42, 42*f*, 102
nursing advocacy, 185
nursing education, 184
nursing research, 184
nursing role, in ambulatory oncology
    care, 4–5, 127, 130–131
nutrition counseling, 61

O

olanzapine, for cognitive impairment,
    74, 75*t*
oldest-old adults, 1, 63, 178
olfactory changes, 17–18, 59
oncology social worker, role of, 159–161,
    160*t*–161*t*, 162*f*
oncology specialists, 179
online resources
    on aging, 191–193
    on cancer, 163*t*, 169*t*–172*t*
    for survivorship care plans, 146*f*
opioid antagonists, for constipation, 83*t*
opioid rotation, 84
opioids
    constipation from, 77, 84–85, 105
    for dyspnea management, 95
    for pain management, 105–107, 106*f*
    side effects from, 105
oral hygiene, 92
organ donation, 173
osmotic laxatives, 82, 83*t*
osteoporosis, 22, 25–26
ovarian cancer, 172*t*
overactive bladder, 24
oxidative stress theory of aging, 11*t*
oxygen therapy, for dyspnea, 95

P

pain, 100
    assessment of, 42*f*, 42–43, 102–104,
        103*t*
    at end of life, 133, 136
    etiology of, 101, 102*f*
    incidence/prevalence of, 100

    management of, 76*t*, 104*t*, 104–107,
        106*f*
    outcomes of, 100
Pain Assessment in Advanced Dementia
    (PAINAD) scale, 102, 103*t*
palliative care, 128–130, 179
    goal transitions in, 130–132
    vs. hospice care, 125–128, 128*f*
    symptom management in, 133
Palliative Performance Scale, 135
Pancreatic Cancer Action Network,
    172*t*
parathyroid hormone, 28
parenteral feeding, 135
Parkinson disease, 63
paroxetine, for fatigue management, 99
Partnership for Prescription Assistance,
    166*t*
Patient Access Network Foundation,
    167*t*
Patient Advocate Foundation, 167*t*
patient-controlled analgesia, 106
Patient-Generated Subjective Global As-
    sessment (PG-SGA), 60
Patient Self-Determination Act, 133
Patient Services, Inc., 167*t*
pelvic floor dysfunction, 77, 82
percutaneous endoscopic gastrostomy
    (PEG) tubes, 92, 133–134
peripheral vision, 16
persistent effects, of cancer, 147–149, 149*f*
pharmacokinetics, 28–30, 29*t*, 104*t*
phenothiazines, for dyspnea manage-
    ment, 95
phonation, 136
phone assessments, 48
photoaging, 25
physical activities of daily living, 9
physical activity
    and cognitive function, 73
    for constipation management, 82
    for fatigue management, 99
physical functioning, 9
physician-assisted suicide, 133
physician orders for life-sustaining treat-
    ment (POLST), 179–180
physiologic age, 10–12
physiologic changes, of aging, 14–28
physiologic reserve capacity, 13–14, 14*f*
physiologic stress, altered response to,
    13–14, 14*f*, 28
Pittsburgh Sleep Quality Index (PSQI),
    42*f*, 43, 49

plaques, 15–16
platinums, constipation from, 79
pleural effusion, 134
PLISSIT model, for sexual assessment/
intervention, 109–110
polyethylene glycol (PEG), for constipation, 83*t*
polypharmacy, dehydration from, 86
post-traumatic growth, 151, 152*f*
postural maneuvers, for dysphagia, 92–93
prednisolone, for anorexia management,
61–62
pre-renal azotemia, 23
presbycusis, 17
presbyopia, 16
Prescription for Living Care Plan, 146*f*
pressure ulcers, 135
primary care providers (PCPs), 49
programmed aging, 11*t*
progressively lowered stress threshold
(PLST) model, 74–76
prokinetics, for constipation, 83*t*
prolactin, 28
prostate cancer
incidence rates, 3
resources on, 172*t*
psychosocial assessment, 158–168, 159*f*,
160*t*–161*t*, 162*f*
tools for, 158–159, 159*f*
psychosocial care, 157, 168, 169*t*–173*t*
psychosocial distress, 158
psychostimulants, for fatigue management, 99
psyllium, for constipation, 81, 83*t*
pulmonary changes, 19–20, 21*t*, 149*f*

Q

quality of life (QOL), 37–38, 48–50, 57,
147, 151–152

R

radiation necrosis, 66
radiation therapy
cognitive impairment from, 66
diarrhea from, 87
long-term/late effects of, 149
palliative, 134
rapid assessment technique, 47–48
rate of living, 12*t*

rating scale
for fatigue, 41–42
for pain, 42, 42*f*, 102
reaction time, 15
renal function, 23, 29, 29*t*, 149*f*
renin-angiotensin system, 23
research, nursing, 184
reserve capacities, 13–14, 14*f*, 30
residual lung volume, 20, 21*t*
resources
on aging, 191–193
on cancer, 163*t*, 169*t*–172*t*
on survivorship care plans, 146*f*
Respiratory Distress Observation Scale,
94
respiratory functioning, 19–20, 21*t*
risperidone, for cognitive impairment,
74, 75*t*
rivastigmine, for cognitive impairment,
73

S

saline laxatives, 83*t*
salivary gland dysfunction, 21, 90
sarcoma, 172*t*
sarcopenia, 20, 25, 86, 97
satiety, 22, 59
Saunders, Dame Cecily, 129
self-care, for healthcare workers, 138
senescence, 9
senile emphysema, 20
senna, for constipation, 83*t*, 84
sensory changes, 16–18, 149*f*
sensory overload, 76*t*
serum creatinine, 88
sexual dysfunction, 107–108
assessment of, 42*f*, 43, 109–110
from cancer/treatment, 109–110
comorbidities and, 109
management of, 110, 110*f*
prevalence of, 108–109
shortness of breath. *See* dyspnea
Simplified Nutritional Appetite Questionnaire (SNAQ), 60
Sisters Network, 170*t*
skeletal changes, 25–26
skin changes, 24–25
skin turgor, 88
sleep problems, 18, 65, 99
assessment of, 42*f*, 43
case study of, 48–50

with delirium, 76*t*
smell identification, 17–18, 59
smoking history, 93, 95
social support, 73, 160*t*
social worker, role of, 159–161, 160*t*–
161*t*, 162*f*
somatic mutation theory of aging, 11*t*
somatic pain, 101
State Health Insurance Counseling and
Assistance Programs (SHIPs),
163*t*, 164
stimulant laxatives, 82, 83*t*, 84
stomatitis, 91–92
stool softeners, 83*t*, 84
stroke, 63
successful aging, 13
sun exposure, cumulative effects of, 25
Support for People with Oral and Head
and Neck Cancer, 172*t*
survivorship, 143, 151–153
health promotion in, 150–151
transitioning to, 145
survivorship care plan (SCP), 146*f*, 146–
147, 150
Susan G. Komen for the Cure, 170*t*
swallowing difficulties, 21–22, 136. *See*
also dysphagia
swallowing exercises, 91–93
symptom burden, 151–152
syncope, 15
systolic BP, 19, 88

T

tacrine, for cognitive impairment, 73
taste changes, 18, 59
teeth, 21, 92
telomere senescence theory of aging, 11*t*
temozolomide, constipation from, 79
testosterone, 26
thalidomide, constipation from, 79
theories of aging, 10, 11*t*–12*t*
thermoregulation, 25
thirst, 86. *See also* dehydration
3-item recall test, 46, 69
thyroid hormones, 28
thyroid-stimulating hormone, 28
tidal volume, 20, 21*t*
Timed Up and Go assessment, 47
tissue fibrosis, 91
tongue-hold exercise, 92
total body fluid, 85–86

total lung capacity, 20, 21*t*
total pain, 129
trajectories
of advanced cancer/death, 129–131
of aging, 12–13
transient incontinence, 24
transient ischemic attacks, 15
transitions, in healthcare goals, 130–132
transportation needs, 162, 163*t*
assessment of, 38, 44, 160*t*
treatment plans, 49–50. *See also* assessment
tube feeding, 92, 133–134

U

urethral prolapse, 24
urinary frequency/urgency, 24, 49
urinary incontinence, 23–24, 49
Urinary Incontinence Assessment in Older Adults, 49
urine studies, for dehydration assessment, 88
U.S. Department of Housing and Urban
Development, 163*t*
usual aging, 13

V

vascular dementia (VaD), 15, 62
vestibulo-ocular reflex, 15
vinca alkaloids, constipation from, 79
visceral pain, 101, 103
vision, changes in, 16–17, 76*t*
visual analog scale
for dyspnea, 94
for fatigue, 41, 42*f*, 98
for pain, 42
vital capacity, 20, 21*t*
vitreous detachment, 16–17
volume of distribution (Vd), 29

W

water-soluble drugs, 29
weight loss, 58–59
assessment of, 60–61
etiology of, 59–60, 60*f*
management of, 61–62
Wellness Community, 170*t*

whole brain radiation therapy, 66
World Health Organization (WHO)
    pain ladder, 104–105
    on palliative care, 126

X

xerostomia, 21, 90–92

Y

Y-ME National Breast Cancer Organization, 170*t*
young-old adults, 1